THE ENCYCLOPEDIA OF

ALZHEIMER'S DISEASE

THE ENCYCLOPEDIA OF

ALZHEIMER'S DISEASE

Carol Turkington

Foreword by
James E. Galvin, M.D., M.Sc.

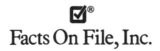

Facts On File, Inc.

The Encyclopedia of Alzheimer's Disease

Facts On File, Inc.
132 West 31st Street
New York NY 10001

Library of Congress Cataloging-in-Publication Data

Turkington, Carol.
The encyclopedia of Alzheimer's disease / Carol Turkington ; foreword by James E. Galvin.
p. cm.
Includes bibliographical references and index.
ISBN 0-8160-4818-5 (HC)
1. Alzheimer's disease—Encyclopedias. I. Title.
[DNLM: 1. Alzheimer Disease—Encyclopedias. WT 13
T939e 2002]
RC523.T87 2003
616.8'31'003—dc21
2002011981

Facts On File books are available at special discounts when purchased in bulk quantities for businesses, associations, institutions, or sales promotions. Please call our Special Sales Department in New York at (212) 967-8800 or (800) 322-8755.

You can find Facts On File on the World Wide Web at http://www.factsonfile.com

Text and cover design by Cathy Rincon

Printed in the United States of America

VB Hermitage 10 9 8 7 6 5 4 3 2 1

This book is printed on acid-free paper.

To my wife, Doris, and my sons, Chris, Jake, and Conor.
They are my source of inspiration and strength.

—J.E.G.

CONTENTS

FOREWORD

Dementia is a major public health problem, crossing gender, socioeconomic, and ethnic lines. It is not a single disease but, rather, a symptom of many conditions causing brain dysfunction. It is associated with a wide range of symptoms, modes of onset, clinical courses, and therapeutic responses. This diverse and rich background of clinical symptoms provides researchers with valuable "testing grounds" for developing theories and insights into the basic inner workings of the brain and of the mind.

From a layperson's perspective, however, dementia is a "thief" that steals away a person's knowledge, memory, and awareness. The affected individuals become, in effect, something other than who they were. The basic human attributes that distinguish each of us—personality, language, behavior, judgment, abstract reasoning, and social skills—are stripped away, leaving behind a victim who is uncommunicative, uncomprehending, and unresponsive. I use the term *victim* deliberately, because anyone who has seen a loved one changed by the progression of these relentless disorders knows this image is apt.

I often look upon my patients with sorrow because I am all too aware of what changes to expect. I am in awe of the inner strength and resolve of so many caregivers who strive to provide their loved ones with the care they deserve and look for answers—and for hope.

These are not uncommon problems. There is a good chance that everyone who opens this book will know someone with dementia. The prevalence of Alzheimer's disease (AD), the most common

dementing disorder, increases with age for every decade after 65. It is currently estimated that there are more than 4.5 million Americans with AD, up to half of whom may be undiagnosed.

About one in 10 individuals over the age of 65 and half of everyone over age 85 will develop dementia. In addition to AD, other common causes of dementia are cerebrovascular disease and Parkinson's disease. The annual cost of caring for patients with dementia is greater than *$100 billion*.

In addition to individuals with overt clinical dementia, terms such as *mild cognitive impairment* and *age-associated memory impairment* have been proposed to characterize older individuals who have cognitive deficits (particularly in memory) with relative preservation of other cognitive abilities and function in daily life. It has been difficult to reach consensus, however, on how and when these entities should be diagnosed. Moreover, because the prevalence of dementia increases with age, and because there is wide variation in test performance among normal older adults, the boundaries between age-related cognitive decline and very early dementia are sometimes uncertain, both to the patients and to the physicians who treat them.

In the early part of the 20th century, Dr. Alois Alzheimer described his first patient (Auguste D) with the disorder that would come to bear his name. A psychiatrist, Dr. Alzheimer examined Auguste D in an institutionalized setting after she was admitted for delusions of extreme jealousy and spousal infidelity. She lived but four and a half years after admission to the sanitarium. Dr. Alzheimer performed an autopsy and described the classic "senile" degenerative changes that have come to be synonymous with AD. For three-quarters of a century after that, the diagnosis of AD was largely relegated to individuals confined to nursing homes and psychiatric institutions, bedridden and incontinent, unaware of their surroundings. People living at home who had memory problems were often told they were just getting old or a "little senile." Memory problems were misdiagnosed as "hardening of the arteries" or "part of the normal aging process." In general, there was little effort to search for either the cause of the disease or for treatments.

Two factors dramatically changed these perceptions. The first was the creation of the National Institute on Aging (NIA) within the National Institutes of Health. From this point onward, significant focus was placed on the public policy implications of the aging American population, a significant proportion experiencing some form of memory impairment. One of the first actions was to create centers of excellence for clinical and basic science research investigating AD and other forms of dementia. There are now 32 such centers operating in the United States. Other branches of NIH have followed the lead of NIA and have established centers to investigate other diseases of the elderly such as cancer and Parkinson's disease.

The second important discovery was the chemical analysis of the proteins found in the brain lesions of AD: amyloid beta-protein in the senile plaques, and tau protein in the neurofibrillary tangles. With targets of scientific inquiry and funding available for scientists to pursue these new avenues of research, the chase was on. Neuroscience research is now one of the largest areas of scientific growth, along with cancer and cardiovascular disease.

This interest from the federal government and academia also has a noticeable effect on the pharmaceutical industry. With advances in the molecular understanding of AD, the first medication for the treatment of AD (tacrine, Cognex) was approved in 1992. In 1996 donepezil (Aricept) was approved. Donepezil was followed by rivastigmine (Exelon) in 2000 and galantamine (Reminyl) in 2001. There are now more than 100 new compounds undergoing clinical trial for the treatment of dementia.

The future of the care of dementia patients looks much brighter. With the advent of advances in molecular biology, genetics, pharmacology, and biochemistry, we have learned so much about the disease process that mechanistic approaches to both diagnosis and treatment now seem possible. The search for biomarkers of the disease has greatly advanced. In the next few years it will be possible to take a blood test to make a diagnosis of AD. We will soon be able to image the pathology of AD in a living person's brain, enabling the clinicians to accurately diagnose an individual at the earliest possible stage of dementia.

Treatment options will also greatly expanded. In addition to the symptomatic treatment from the cholinesterase inhibitors, mechanism-based approaches will enable clinicians to prevent the production of the amyloid protein and enhance its removal from the brain.

There is still so much more to do, however. It is estimated that within one generation (the year 2050) there will be more than 14 million Americans with dementia. AD patients currently make up half of all nursing home populations, and AD is the fourth leading cause of death in individuals over age 65. Part of the problem still lies in the underrecognition of the disorder. Fewer than half of the individuals with dementia are correctly diagnosed, and more important, even in the face of diagnosis, less than half of all persons with dementia are treated with the only medications currently approved to treat the disease. This is not the case with other diseases of the elderly, such as hypertension, diabetes, or heart disease. If the field is to advance further, families and clinicians must be more aware of the problem so that as new treatments become available, eligible patients are prescribed them. Knowledge is power!

I first became interested in dementia observing my grandfather's battle with Parkinson's disease and dementia. He was diagnosed during my junior year in high school. Over the next 15 years I watched a vital, strong-willed individual decline both physically and mentally until he was essentially immobile, mute, and unaware of his surroundings. Ultimately, the only response my grandfather was able to consistently make was to his visual hallucinations, causing him eventually to fall and fracture his hip. Although the surgeon succeeded in repairing his facture, my grandfather never recovered, passing away in his sleep at the rehabilitation hospital. This experience combined with my interest in science led to the pursuit of a career in neurology, focusing on geriatric disorders.

Sadly, back then I was not able to provide my grandmother with information that might have prevented Grandfather's death, or at the very least made both their lives a little bit easier. Hopefully, we have succeeded in providing such useful information with this volume.

When I was first approached to assist in this project, I questioned the value of producing an encyclopedia about Alzheimer's disease (AD). I wondered about the individuals who would read it, and more important, why they would want to read it? In today's world most medical information is readily available on the Internet or at university libraries. The information is also available from most family physicians.

I have dedicated my professional career to helping individuals with dementia and their families, and I provide a substantial amount of (what I con-

sider) useful information to each family from the time of the first office visit through the terminal portion of the patient's life. Should I really take the time to put all of this information down in one place so that it is readily available to someone searching for answers?

Of course, that is when I came to understand the true value of this project. The real question is not *should* I help put together this volume, but rather *why I had not done it before?*

Volumes such as the *Facts On File* series provide families and patients with Alzheimer's disease and other forms of dementia the information and resources they need and provide it in an easy-to-understand and easy-to-read format.

—James E. Galvin, M.D.
   Assistant Professor, Neurology
   Director, Memory Diagnostic Center
   Director, Laboratories for Dementia Research
   Alzheimer's Disease Research Center
   Washington University School of Medicine

ACKNOWLEDGMENTS

The creation of a detailed encyclopedia involves the help and guidance of a wide range of experts, without whom this book could not have been possible.

Thanks to the staffs of the National Institute on Aging, the National Institute of Neurological Disorders and Stroke, the National Institute of Mental Health, and the National Institute of Nursing Research.

Thanks also to the Alzheimer's Association, the American Association for Retired Persons, the American Medical Association, American Society on Aging, National Association of Area Agencies on Aging, National Council on the Aging, the Alzheimer's Disease Education and Referral Center, the Alzheimer's Foundation, and the John Douglas French Alzheimer's Foundation.

Thanks also to the librarians at the Hershey Medical Center medical library, the National Library of Medicine, the Reading Public Library, and the Pennsylvania State Library.

Finally, thanks to my agent, Gene Brissie of James Peter Associates, my editor at Facts On File, James Chambers, and Sarah Fogarty, also at Facts On File.

—Carol Turkington

I would like to acknowledge the sources of my research support, including the National Institute on Aging, the National Institutes of Health, the American Federation for Aging Research, the Missouri Alzheimer Disease and Related Disorders Program, the Longer Life Foundation, and the generous support of Alan A. and Edith L. Wolff. Most of all, I wish to thank all my patients, their families, and caregivers, who have taught me so much but constantly show me that I have so much more yet to learn.

—James E. Galvin, M.D.

INTRODUCTION

Scientists have produced an extraordinary amount of research into Alzheimer's disease in the past 25 years. Many of these results have explored the genetic and biological changes that underlie the disease, and offer possible targets for treatment.

Researchers have studied a number of medications that may potentially counteract the structural changes that occur in Alzheimer's; so far, four have received the approval of the U.S. Food and Drug Administration (FDA). None of the four will cure the disease, and only some of the mildly to moderately affected patients respond to any of the drugs at all. Another 17 drugs are in the research pipeline and are currently being developed.

With ongoing genetic breakthroughs, scientists are making strides in identifying genes linked with the condition, which enable doctors to determine who is at higher risk for developing Alzheimer's. As studies continue, scientists hope that someday they will be able to understand the earliest pathological and clinical signs of Alzheimer's, perhaps 10 or 20 years before an actual clinical diagnosis can be made.

At the same time, a variety of approaches have been introduced to improve how we provide care for Alzheimer's patients, easing the burden with which caregivers struggle, and lessening the need for institutionalization.

Meanwhile, the search for understanding in Alzheimer's has also helped define the characteristics of normal aging. Research is beginning to shed light on how healthy adults learn and remember, and ways in which it may be possible to minimize normal, age-related cognitive decline.

The National Institutes of Health (NIH) has launched two new initiatives that build on current activities and give a new focus to future work. The first, called the NIH Alzheimer's Disease Prevention Initiative, is designed to speed up the progress of finding effective medications, and other approaches to delaying or preventing the onset of Alzheimer's disease. Scientists are taking new approaches to basic biologic and epidemiologic research, increasing the focus on drug discovery and development, improving methods to identify early those people who are at increased risk, getting possible new treatments into the clinic sooner for testing in clinical trials, and actively pursuing research into drug and nondrug strategies for treating behavioral disturbances in Alzheimer's patients.

Scientists have identified a number of potential candidates that might help prevent Alzheimer's. These include estrogen-like compounds, anti-inflammatory agents, and antioxidants, as well as drugs that target cell death, the buildup of abnormal lesions such as plaques and tangles, and other harmful processes involved in Alzheimer's. The evidence on which these interventions are based was largely unknown only a few years ago, and the pace of discovery is increasing each year.

The first NIH clinical trial aimed at preventing or delaying the onset of clinically diagnosed Alzheimer's disease in people at risk (called the Memory Impairment Study) was launched in March 1999, and a major prevention trial of two anti-inflammatory drugs has been started. Other trials will be added to already ongoing studies that are investigating treatments or prevention strategies for other conditions.

The second initiative, called the President's Initiative on Alzheimer's Disease, was announced by President Clinton on July 16, 2000. In this effort, the NIH set aside $50 million through 2005 to support new research on Alzheimer's disease, which will include basic research as a part of preclinical studies, and clinical interventions to treat or prevent Alzheimer's by targeting areas such as amyloid plaques and neurofibrillary tangles. A major component of the President's Initiative will be efforts to address promising immunological strategies to prevent amyloid deposition.

Research is not limited simply to finding out how to prevent the disease. Experts also are focusing on issues related to supporting patients and family members, friends, and providers who care for patients.

Today scientists in both public and private sectors are working together to understand more about the disease. The major supporters of Alzheimer's research—the National Institute on Aging, the National Institute of Neurological Disorders and Stroke, the National Institute of Mental Health, and the National Institute of Nursing Research—make up the NIH Alzheimer's Disease Working Group.

This book has been designed as a guide and reference to a wide range of subjects important to the understanding of Alzheimer's disease. It includes a wide variety of contact information for organizations and governmental agencies affiliated with the condition, including current website addresses and phone numbers. However, the book is not designed as a substitute for prompt assessment and treatment by experts trained in the diagnosis and support of Alzheimer's disease.

In this encyclopedia we have tried to present the latest information in the field, based on the newest research and current FDA approvals of new treatments. Readers will find the most up-to-date information on the suspected causes (and controversies), risks, diagnoses, prevention, and treatments.

Although information in this book comes from the most up-to-date medical journals and research sources, readers should keep in mind that changes occur very quickly in neurology. A bibliography has been included for those who seek additional sources of information.

—Carol Turkington
Cumru, Pennsylvania

ENTRIES A–Z

abstract language Slang, figures of speech, proverbs, sarcasm, innuendo, idioms, jokes, and homonyms are all difficult for most patients even in the early stages of Alzheimer's disease to understand. Patients may have trouble following long, detailed conversations. They may have trouble understanding that "his" book refers to "Peter" and they may need much longer to formulate a response to questions.

abuse Abuse of a patient with Alzheimer's disease may be physical, psychological, financial, material, or any combination of these. Because patients with Alzheimer's are demented, they are vulnerable to a wide range of abuse by others—either caregivers, family, friends, or strangers. In an institution, a patient may be abused not only by a staff member, but by another patient, an intruder, or a visitor.

Physical abuse is usually easy to spot, but other types of abuse may be more insidious. Emotional abuse includes verbal assaults, threats of abuse, harassment, and intimidation. Neglect is usually the responsibility of a caregiver who fails to provide food, clothing, shelter, or medical care. Financial abuse involves misusing or withholding the patient's money.

Sometimes, sexual abuse may be a problem; this could involve anything from inappropriate touching or fondling to any sexual activity when the patient is unable to understand, unwilling to consent, or physically forced to participate.

Family members who don't live with the patient can guard against abuse by routinely asking questions directly related to abuse or neglect. If the patient confirms abuse, family members should examine the patient thoroughly and document findings, including the person's statements, behavior, and appearance. Family members should maintain well-documented medical records and photographs that can provide concrete evidence and may be crucial in any legal case.

Many states require physicians to report suspected elder abuse and neglect to a designated state agency. A doctor's duty to report suspected abuse supersedes doctor-patient confidentiality issues; failure to report the problem can make doctors liable.

acetylcholine A chemical messenger that brain cells use to communicate with each other, especially in parts of the brain important for thought, memory and judgment. Acetylcholine is a critical neurotransmitter in the process of forming memories, and it is the neurotransmitter commonly used by nerve cells in the HIPPOCAMPUS and CEREBRAL CORTEX—regions devastated by Alzheimer's disease. Normally, acetylcholine is produced by these brain cells, released to carry signals, and then broken down for reuse by enzymes. When brain cells are damaged by Alzheimer's disease, they produce less acetylcholine, which disrupts communication in the brain.

Since low acetylcholine levels were first discovered in patients with Alzheimer's disease, the chemical has been the subject of hundreds of studies. Scientists have found that acetylcholine levels can be as much as 90 percent lower in people with Alzheimer's. They have also discovered that low levels are linked to memory problems.

Other neurotransmitters have also been implicated in Alzheimer's disease. For example, serotonin, somatostatin, and noradrenaline levels are reduced by at least 50 percent in some Alzheimer's patients, which may contribute to sensory disturbances, aggressive behavior, and brain cell death. Most neurotransmitter research, however, continues to focus on acetylcholine because of its steep decline in Alzheimer's disease and its close ties to memory formation and reasoning.

However, scientists aren't sure if the drop in acetylcholine and other neurotransmitters is the cause of the disease, or whether the low levels occur as a result of the disease process. Scientists do know that drugs that boost acetylcholine levels in the brain can improve memory. These drugs include DONEPEZIL, RIVASTIGMINE, GALANTAMINE, and others.

acetylcholinesterase　An enzyme that breaks down ACETYLCHOLINE, a neurotransmitter that helps to conduct messages throughout the brain. As Alzheimer's disease gets worse, the level of acetylcholine found in the brain drops significantly.

acetylcholinesterase inhibitors　See DRUG TREATMENTS.

active lifestyle　People who are physically and mentally active in midlife may have a better chance of avoiding Alzheimer's disease later in life. According to experts, recreational activities such as physical exercise, playing a musical instrument, or using board games play a key role in preventing Alzheimer's. In fact, people who are involved in only minimal physical activity are at least three times more likely to suffer from Alzheimer's disease.

One recent study investigated how much activity Alzheimer's disease patients participate in five years before symptoms appeared. Subjects answered questions about mental activity (such as reading and painting), physical activity such as sports and gardening, and passive activity like social interaction and going to church. The study was composed of 193 people with Alzheimer's disease and 358 without. The participants without Alzheimer's disease had been more active between the ages of 40 and 60 than were those with Alzheimer's, no matter the age, GENDER, economic status, or education of the subjects.

While earlier research had linked Alzheimer's disease to less active individuals with low educational and occupational status, the more recent findings show that it is activity alone, not job and educational factors, that affects the risk of getting the disease.

activities　Patients with Alzheimer's disease benefit from activities that boost their sense of involvement, accomplishment, and well-being. As long as the activities are not too confusing or overstimulating, it is usually helpful for patients with Alzheimer's to maintain their sense of self-esteem in the face of constant deterioration. Anything from going to a restaurant to taking a trip to a museum may be suitable, depending on the patient's level of function and the stage of the disease. However, while many patients who are more active seem to maintain better physical and mental function, others can't tolerate anything other than a very simple activity. Elaborate trips—such as a visit to a theme park—even for a mildly demented patient may cause serious confusion with devastating results.

This is why it's important that a patient's tolerance to activity must be determined on an individual basis. Regular activities in familiar locations should be encouraged, but trips that require staying overnight in a strange environment should be considered carefully.

The types of activities that a patient may benefit from will almost certainly change as the disease progresses. In general, patients with Alzheimer's tend to have problems concentrating and following directions, which can turn even the simplest activities into a challenge. Many patients may simply sit or stand in one place, or pace the room for long periods of time; unless directed, it is quite common for patients not to initiate an activity on their own; even when they do, they may have trouble carrying out the activity.

A daily routine can help patients feel good about themselves as they maintain more of their normal day-to-day life.

When planning an activity schedule for patients, caregivers should consider how to adapt the person's past interests and hobbies to the current situation. It may be possible to adapt a hobby, such as ham radio or model trains, in ways that would still be manageable by someone with even significant limits.

Structure and schedules will give most patients a sense of security, so caregivers should think about providing the same activities in the same way at the same time each day. Caregivers should expect to offer constant guidance and supervision, helping the patient through the activity with simple, step-by-step directions.

Daily activities as basic as dusting or running the vacuum may please a patient with Alzheimer's. If someone used to love to read the paper while having a cup of morning coffee, this may still be enjoyable even if the person can no longer make sense of the daily news. The fact that it is a familiar activity will often make it enjoyable.

It is also important that caregivers be able to understand the implications of the disease. If a patient suddenly insists she doesn't want to do something, it may be that the person can't do it or is afraid.

Just because a patient "always" was a fabulous cook in the past does not mean she can still function at the same level—but she may still enjoy part of the process of baking a cake, for example. If the person has lost the ability to follow a complicated recipe, caregivers can help by separating the tasks involved in baking a cake, taking over the steps that are too much for the patient. Caregivers might count the eggs and break them into a bowl, and then hand the bowl to the patient to stir.

Involving patients in activities that are important in keeping the household running is a good way to help the person maintain self-esteem. This might include activities such as sweeping, gardening, taking out the trash, or raking leaves. Working alongside the patient setting the table, drying the dishes, or emptying the wastebaskets, can boost the person's feeling of being useful and sociable. Patients may also enjoy helping prepare for family picnics or birthdays, although caregivers should be careful to prevent the patient from feeling overwhelmed. Activities before and during the event should be simple and well organized.

While it's important for patients to stay busy, they don't need to be involved in a 24-hour whirlwind of activities. A mixture of rest and brief, simple activities is a good way to take advantage of the patient's limited ability to concentrate. Patients would probably not be able to spend five hours helping to reorganize the kitchen cabinets, but 20 minutes of helping to wipe down shelves would be helpful.

Most patients benefit from activities that tie in with former jobs and responsibilities, because they are reassuring and familiar. For example, a patient who used to work in a business office might enjoy putting stamps or address labels on envelopes, or putting papers in a file. A former florist might enjoy puttering in the yard, setting out tomato plants, or planting seeds.

While patients may not be able to perform complicated procedures, self-expression is still important. Many patients still enjoy drawing and painting, working in clay, dancing and singing, or playing a musical instrument. People with Alzheimer's respond very well to familiar songs and music from their past, so playing, singing, or performing songs and hymns can be important.

Exercise is also important for patients, who may enjoy playing Ping-Pong, taking regular walks around a mall (during quiet times, not peak shopping hours), playing catch with a soft ball, or playing badminton in the backyard.

Even as the disease continues, patients may enjoy looking at magazines, photo albums, or books. Many patients enjoy being read to from the newspaper or a magazine, or listening to poetry or favorite stories.

Tasks involving separating and organizing may interest patients, who may be able to sort nuts and bolts, buttons, or coins. Other patients may enjoy working with cloth, folding laundry, or sewing together different types of material, such as denim and corduroy.

Many patients benefit from getting in touch with past experiences and memories, so old TV shows or movies from earlier decades are often a good choice. Some patients may enjoy going to a sports event, such as a tennis match or golf tournament, riding in the car, or taking a trip to the zoo or an art museum.

activities of daily living The collective term for personal care activities necessary for everyday living, such as eating, bathing, grooming, dressing, and toileting. People with Alzheimer's disease may not be able to perform these functions without help. Geriatric professionals often assess a person's activities of daily living as a way of determining what type of care is needed.

acupuncture New research with Alzheimer's disease suggests that acupuncture may increase a patient's verbal and motor skills and improve mood and cognitive function, according to two separate studies, one at the Wellesley College Center for Research on Women and the other at the University of Hong Kong. The studies suggest that acupuncture may significantly reduce DEPRESSION and anxiety in patients with DEMENTIA. Experts hope that acupuncture might improve the life of Alzheimer's patients by altering their mood, behavioral symptoms, and overall sense of well-being.

Acupuncture is most often practiced by inserting needles into specified points in the patient's body, which is believed to unblock the flow of energy through the body. Acupuncture is also believed to increase blood flow to the brain and lessen inflammation, which is a problem associated with Alzheimer's.

Acupuncture has been recognized as a potentially effective therapy by the World Health Organization and by the National Institutes of Health's Center for Complementary and Alternative Medicine.

AD7C test A controversial test that measures levels of neural thread protein (NTP) found in spinal fluid or urine. High levels of NTP have been found in people with Alzheimer's disease, as well as in those who suffer from brain tumors, strokes, and other neurological disorders. Because patients with other neurological problems besides Alzheimer's disease can test positive on this assessment, a result showing higher-than-average levels of NTP in spinal fluid or urine can't by itself indicate or rule out Alzheimer's disease.

For this reason, many experts (including the ALZHEIMER'S ASSOCIATION) don't recommend using the AD7C as a test for diagnosing or ruling out Alzheimer's disease.

At this time, there is no consensus among Alzheimer experts that this test is useful; many experts believe that the use of AD7C for the diagnosis of Alzheimer's disease should remain experimental.

ADAPT (Alzheimer's Disease Anti-inflammatory Prevention Trial) A clinical research study testing a possible link between certain ANTI-INFLAMMATORY DRUGS and the prevention of Alzheimer's disease. Researchers have noted that people who regularly take anti-inflammatory medicines seem less likely to develop Alzheimer's disease.

The study began on January 30, 2001, at four study centers across the country. Sponsored by the NATIONAL INSTITUTE ON AGING, ADAPT is following 2,625 healthy participants with a family history of Alzheimer's disease for up to seven years. Participants will take Aleve (naproxen sodium), a nonprescription NONSTEROIDAL ANTI-INFLAMMATORY DRUG (NSAID), Celebrex (CELECOXIB), a prescription NSAID, or a placebo. Each subject will undergo cognitive and physical tests three times in the first year of the study and twice a year after that, and will participate in a telephone interview twice a year.

The study is being conducted by the Johns Hopkins Medical Institutions, the University of Rochester Medical Center, Boston University School of Medicine, and Sun Health Research Institute in Arizona.

adult day services Programs that provide clients with opportunities to interact with others in a community-based center or facility. Adult day services are designed to meet the needs of patients with Alzheimer's disease through an individual plan of care. These structured, comprehensive programs provide a variety of health, social, and other related support services in a protective setting during any part of a day. Typically, an adult day center operates programs during normal business hours five days a week. Some programs offer services in the evenings and on weekends. At a typical center, clients can participate in various activities such as music programs and support groups. Transportation is often provided.

Adult day centers are designed to serve adults with physical problems or mental confusion, and who may require supervision, more social opportunities, and help with personal care or other daily living activities. The average age of a client is 76; two-thirds of all participants are women. One survey found that about half of all clients of these centers had some cognitive impairment, and a third required nursing services at least weekly.

In the 1940s, adult day care began in psychiatric day hospitals such as the Yale Psychiatric Clinic, primarily to assist patients following release from mental institutions. During the 1960s, the day care concept shifted from a single psychiatric focus to other health maintenance. Centers began in Arizona, Pennsylvania, and Minnesota. In 1978, the government published a directory of nearly 300 adult day care centers. Today, there are more than 4,000 adult day centers operating in every state of the United States, most of which are nonprofit or public. Many are affiliated with larger organizations such as skilled nursing facilities, medical centers, or multipurpose senior organizations.

The typical adult day center offers a wide range of services which may include transportation, social services, meals, nursing and personal care, counseling, therapeutic activities, and rehabilitation.

Regulations regarding adult day service differ from state to state. The Standards and Guidelines for Adult Day Care developed by the NATIONAL ADULT DAY SERVICES ASSOCIATION (NADSA, formerly the National Institute on Adult Daycare) of THE NATIONAL COUNCIL ON THE AGING provide important guidelines for states that have chosen to regulate adult day services. Funding sources also define the range of services for which they will pay while an eligible participant is at an adult day center. Besides the voluntary NADSA standards, there are no uniform national standards governing either the operation of centers or the qualifications of staff members.

NADSA offers a certification process for program assistants and is developing the same for administrators and directors.

Daily fees for adult day services vary depending on location and the type of available services, and there is quite a variable range. Funding for adult day services comes from participant fees as well as public and charitable sources. The average cost of a day at an adult day center is often much less than a visit from a home health nurse and about half the cost of skilled nursing facility care.

A high-quality adult day center will:

- assess a client's needs
- provide an active day program that meets the client's social, recreational, and rehabilitation needs
- develop an individualized treatment plan for each client and regularly monitor each person's progress
- provide referrals to other needed services in the community
- develop clear criteria for service and guidelines for termination of service, based upon the functional status of each client
- provide a full range of in-house services
- provide a safe, secure environment
- hire qualified and well-trained staff and volunteers
- follow existing state and national standards and guidelines

advance directive A written document, completed and signed when a person is legally competent, that explains what the person would or would not want if unable to make decisions about medical care. Common advance directives include:

- HEALTH CARE PROXY (or health care power of attorney) that gives another person the authority to make decisions for the patient when the patient is unable to do so
- LIVING WILL, which directs a doctor to not start or stop treatment that is keeping a dying patient alive when the patient can't make those wishes known
- NON-HOSPITAL DO NOT RESUSCITATE ORDER (DNR) that directs emergency staff not to resuscitate a person when not in a hospital or other health care facility

Advance directives are an important part of the management of the affairs for a patient with Alzheimer's disease, because an advance directive allows someone else to make treatment decisions on a patient's behalf when the person is no longer capable of making those decisions. In particular, patients with early Alzheimer's disease should ask themselves what would they want to happen if they stopped eating because of their disease.

Patients should prepare and sign advance directives that comply with state law, and give copies to family, friends, and doctors. The document should reflect the patient's wishes and appoint someone to make decisions who is willing to carry out those wishes.

Advil See NONSTEROIDAL ANTI-INFLAMMATORY DRUGS.

African Americans Recent studies suggest the risk of Alzheimer's disease may be higher for African Americans than for Caucasians. Other studies have found that first-degree relatives of African Americans with Alzheimer's have a higher cumulative risk of dementia than do those of whites with Alzheimer's.

These studies underscore the critical need for more research to find the unknown factors that are responsible for the differences in risk. In one study of more than 1,000 people in New York City who did not carry a copy of the gene for Alzheimer's, the risk of the disease was four times higher in African Americans than for Caucasians. In another study published in the *Journal of the American Medical Association,* researchers compared the risk of Alzheimer's disease among African Americans and Africans from Nigeria, and found that the risk was nearly twice as high for African Americans.

See also RACE.

age and Alzheimer's disease The single greatest risk factor for Alzheimer's disease is age. While the disease can occasionally occur in people as young as 30 or 40, the risk increases considerably after age 65. Experts estimate that half of those over age 80 will be diagnosed with Alzheimer's.

As people age, the brain undergoes a number of changes. Some brain cells in some brain regions degenerate, although most neurons important to learning remain healthy. Slowly, cells begin to shrink and stop functioning, especially in areas important to learning, memory, planning, and other complex mental activities. Neurofibrillary tangles develop in brain cells and senile plaques appear in surrounding areas in certain brain regions, such as the hippocampus.

In healthy older people, the impact of these changes may just mean that it gets a little harder to remember day-to-day details. In people who develop Alzheimer's, on the other hand, some of these changes are much more severe and have devastating consequences.

During normal metabolism, the body produces molecules called FREE RADICALS that help cells by fighting infection. However, free radicals are very reactive, and when the body produces too many, they can damage and kill cells—a major cause of the aging process. With age, the brain gets less able to cope with and eliminate free radicals. Brain cells are particularly vulnerable to attack by free radicals because they have a high metabolism and are low in natural antioxidants, the substances that destroy free radicals. Free radicals also attack DNA and RNA, brain lipids and proteins. This is why several researchers are studying whether treatment with antioxidants can slow age-related cognitive decline or development of Alzheimer's.

Because Alzheimer's often develops in older people who may already have other health problems such as heart disease or high BLOOD PRESSURE, scientists suspect that these conditions may play a role in the development of Alzheimer's. For example, Lewy bodies are the second most common cause of DEMENTIA; there is some evidence that there may be a link between Alzheimer's and strokes. High CHOLESTEROL levels that occur in old age may increase the rate of plaque formation. There are also similarities between Alzheimer's and other progressive neurodegenerative disorders that cause dementia, such as prion diseases, Parkinson's, and Huntington's disease. All of these conditions involve deposits of abnormal proteins in the brain, and new research is showing that these diseases have a number of important overlapping characteristics.

age-associated memory impairment (AAMI) A controversial idea that normal decline in memory due to aging leads to "memory lapses," such as forgetting the location of an everyday object, while retaining perfectly clear memories of personal information, such as the names of family members.

Some experts may diagnose a patient over age 50 with AAMI if all other obvious causes of memory decline have been ruled out and the person:

• has noticed a decline in memory performance
• performs below "normal" levels on a standard test of memory

A more severe memory problem may be classified as MILD COGNITIVE IMPAIRMENT (MCI), which may be an indication of the early stages of Alzheimer's disease. The memory loss associated with MCI is more severe and involves continuing problems in delayed recall of information.

Abnormal memory loss associated with Alzheimer's is characterized by even more severe problems, such as disorientation and general confusion. Research suggests that people with MCI appear to be at a higher risk of developing Alzheimer's disease when they get older. As many as 15 percent of people over the age of 65 with MCI eventually develop Alzheimer's per year, whereas only 1 percent of healthy people over age 65 develop Alzheimer's per year. Some experts believe that individuals with MCI will all develop Alzheimer's disease if followed long enough.

Agency on Aging See AREA AGENCY ON AGING.

aggression Hitting, pushing, or threatening behaviors may be exhibited by people with Alzheimer's disease, often when a caregiver tries to help with daily activities. It is important to control such behavior because aggressive patients can hurt themselves or others. Newer atypical antipsychotics, including risperidone (Risperdal), olanzapine (Zyprexa), and quetiapine (Seroquel), appear to significantly decrease symptoms of aggression while posing a very low risk for severe side effects. Carbamazepine, an antiseizure drug, may also be effective for AGITATION and DEMENTIA.

aging Aging does not necessarily cause an irreversible loss of cells in the cerebral cortex; major cell loss appears to be in the basal forebrain, in the HIPPOCAMPUS, and AMYGDALA (the sites of learning and memory). The loss of these cells, in turn, causes a drop in the production of the neurotransmitter ACETYLCHOLINE, a chemical that is vital to memory and learning. Not surprisingly, Alzheimer's disease patients have markedly low levels of this vital neurotransmitter.

Unfortunately, the hippocampus (probably one of the most important brain structures involved in memory and learning) is highly vulnerable to aging, and up to 5 percent of the nerve cells in the hippocampus break down with each decade past middle age. This could add up to a loss of up to 20 percent of total hippocampal nerve cells by the time a person enters the eighth decade of life.

Damage to this area of the brain may be caused by stress hormones such as CORTISOL. Rat studies have found that stress-induced increases in cortisol prematurely age the hippocampus. In addition, excessive amounts of FREE RADICALS (a toxic form of oxygen) can also build up as a person ages, damaging the hippocampus.

However, the aging brain can also be negatively affected by a whole host of other factors, such as malnutrition, alcohol, depression, and medications (especially the benzodiazepines used to treat anxiety). In addition, there are a range of organic problems that can occur in the brain itself. Functional brain problems may also be caused by dying neurons or decreased production of neurotransmitters (chemicals like acetylcholine that allow brain cells to communicate with each other).

In addition, there are physical changes in the aging brain; tissue actually shrinks and the cells become less efficient. In addition, hereditary problems, environmental toxins, or poor lifestyle choices such as smoking or substance abuse, can speed up the decline in brain function.

About half the elderly men and women with severe intellectual impairment have Alzheimer's disease, but another fourth suffer from vascular disorders such as strokes. The rest have a variety of problems, including brain tumors, abnormal thyroid function, infections, pernicious anemia, adverse drug reactions, and abnormalities in the cerebrospinal fluid.

The chief problem among healthy older people is a decline in their ability to perform several tasks at once, or to switch back and forth rapidly between them. While general vocabulary and knowledge about the world often stays sharp through the seventh decade of life, the ability to recognize faces and find one's car has begun to wane by the time a person enters the 20s. Memory for names begins to decline as early as the mid-30s. While long-term memory does not usually decline as a person ages, short-term and episodic memory does deteriorate with age.

Researchers believe that after age 30, most people reach an intellectual plateau which is usually maintained until about age 60; after that, there are small declines, depending on initial ability and gender.

Overall brain function, however, remains strong in most people through the 70s. In fact, many people in their 60s and 70s score significantly better in verbal skills than young people. For many people, it is not until the 80s that any sort of serious mental slowdown occurs.

Indeed, brain deterioration with age is not inevitable. Studies of nursing home populations showed that patients were able to make significant improvements in cognitive ability when given rewards and challenges. Furthermore, physical exercise and mental stimulation can even improve mental function in some people as they age. A stimulating environment strengthens the brain, while a dull environment weakens it.

Indeed, the brain often becomes less effective as a person ages because of disuse rather than disease. However, it is possible to challenge the brain to become more efficient by practicing daily mental drills, preventing intellectual breakdown and reversing a decline.

Evidence from animal research suggests that brain stimulation stops cells from shrinking and can also strengthen brain cell function. For example, studies show that rats living in an enriched environment have larger outer brain layers with healthier neurons and more cells responsible for providing food for the neurons. Rats kept in a barren cage had smaller brains than did rats with a lot of toys. Taking this into consideration, some scientists believe that humans can also improve their brain function or reverse a decline by challenging themselves with active learning or by living in an enriched environment. Scientists suggest that a person's socioeconomic status can predict mental decline because poverty often goes hand in hand with an unstimulating environment. Fewer, smaller brain cells is the price a person pays for failing to stimulate the brain.

agitation   A term used to describe many typical behaviors in patients with Alzheimer's disease, such as screaming, shouting, complaining, moaning, cursing, pacing, fidgeting, or WANDERING. As the disease progresses, many people experience agitation in addition to memory loss and other thinking problems. Abnormal behavior is considered to be agitation only if it poses risk or discomfort to a caregiver or the individual with Alzheimer's. Agitation can be a nonspecific symptom of a physical or psychological problem such as headache, pain, or depression.

Cause

Agitation may be caused by a medical problem, a drug interaction, or anything that interferes with a patient's ability to think clearly. A wide variety of situations can trigger agitation, especially changes in routine such as moving to a new home or nursing home, a different caregiver, or even altered daily routines. In addition, a patient's fuzzy thinking may lead to perceived threats, or may cause fear and exhaustion as the result of trying to make sense of a confusing world. Agitation can interfere with a patient's ability to handle ACTIVITIES OF DAILY LIVING, and it can also frighten and exhaust caregivers.

Diagnosis

A patient who experiences agitation should be thoroughly examined, especially if the problem has appeared abruptly. Agitation often may be caused by an underlying physical illness (such as infection) or medication, so a good history and physical exam are important. Proper treatment can often stabilize or even reduce symptoms.

Treatment

Agitation is usually treated first with behavioral methods; if these fail, medication can be added. Experts believe it is important to understand the cause of the behavior and change the environment or routine, which is why it is important to correctly identify what triggered agitated behavior in the first place.

Agitation may be eased by changing caregivers, living arrangements, or the environment. It is important when trying to ease agitation to avoid arguing, disagreeing, cornering, criticizing, or confronting the patient. Instead, caregivers can:

- redirect the patient's attention
- simplify routines
- limit stimulation
- reassure
- focus on pleasant events
- provide the patient with rest
- use labels as a reminder
- back off and ask permission
- turn up the lights at night
- use calm, positive statements

Medications can help manage some symptoms of agitation, but they must be used carefully and are most effective when combined with behavioral and environmental changes. Medications should target specific symptoms so that improvement can be monitored. If medication is needed to target specific symptoms, most doctors prefer to start with one drug at a low dose and carefully monitor the patient's response.

Antipsychotic medications are the most common drugs used to treat agitation, in addition to hallucinations, delusions, aggression, hostility, and uncooperativeness. These include olanzapine (Zyprexa), quetiapine (Seroquel), or risperidone (Risperdal).

Antidepressants may be used to treat low mood, depression, or irritability. Typically, a doctor will prescribe one of the newer selective serotonin reuptake inhibitors (SSRIs): citalopram (Celexa), fluoxetine (Prozac), paroxetine (Paxil), or sertraline (Zoloft).

Antianxiety drugs (anxiolytics) can treat anxiety, restlessness, verbally disruptive behavior, and resistance. Common drugs used for these symptoms include Buspar or oxazepam (Serax), which reduce anxiety.

Some doctors may prescribe an anticonvulsant/mood stabilizer such as carbamazepine (Tegretol) or divalproex (Depakote) for hostility or aggression.

Sedatives should only be used with caution because of the risk of side effects, such as incontinence, instability, or falls; they may worsen agitation.

Although the drugs haloperidol or trazodone are commonly used to treat agitation in Alzheimer's patients, the first large controlled study of behavior and drug treatments found that they are only marginally effective at best. The Alzheimer's Disease Cooperative Study (ADCS) reports that across all groups, only 34 percent of patients improved; patients getting trazodone showed the greatest improvement. Agitation worsened in 46 percent of patients, however, and did not change in 20 percent. Interestingly, 31 percent of patients receiving placebo showed improvement. This suggested that meeting regularly with a well-trained and supportive clinician may help reduce agitation.

Prevention

It is better to try to prevent agitation than to have to treat it once it appears. To head off episodes of agitated behavior, caregivers should try to create a calm, quiet, stress-free environment. Security objects, rest, and privacy may help. Caffeine should be limited, and caregivers should try to offer exercise, and soothing rituals. To some extent, agitation may be avoided by cutting down on noise, glare, and too much background distraction, such as TV.

agnosia Loss of the ability to recognize what an object is and what it is used for, despite undamaged senses of sight, smell, touch, hearing, and so on. Agnosia is one of the symptoms that may be required for a diagnosis of Alzheimer's disease.

A person with agnosia might try to use a knife instead of a spoon, a brush instead of a glass, or a ruler instead of a pen. Others with agnosia might not be able to recognize another person not because of poor memory but because the brain can't match the person's identity with information supplied by the eyes.

Alcar   The brand name for acetyl-l-carnitine hcl.

alcohol   Recent studies have found that a glass of wine may have health benefits not just for cardio-vascular function, but also for thinking ability. It appears that moderate drinking protects against dementia and the development of Alzheimer's disease, but that drinking too much leads to more cognitive problems.

In the past, various studies have identified alcohol consumption as either a risk factor for DEMENTIA or as a protection, but in a recent large Italian study, it appeared that drinking wine might help protect patients from dementia.

In that study, researchers analyzed data gathered from 15,807 patients over 65 who had taken part in a study of adverse drug reactions in hospitalized patients. Among these patients, wine was the alcoholic beverage of choice. Study authors found signs of cognitive problems in 19 percent of the participants who reported regular alcohol consumption, and in 29 percent of those who abstained from alcohol. Statistical methods ruled out other contributing factors such as age, GENDER, education, disease, or medication, but scientists did find that how much a person drank each day was an important factor.

The risk of cognitive impairment was lower among women whose daily alcohol consumption was less than 40 grams and among men who drank less than 80 grams, compared to people who did not drink at all. On the other hand, subjects who drank more than this were at increased risk of cognitive impairment when compared with both abstainers and moderate drinkers.

This study showed that among older people, moderate drinking protects against the development of cognitive impairment. However, alcohol abuse—more than one bottle of wine a day for a man, or more than a half bottle for a woman—is associated with an increased risk of cognitive dysfunction. These findings add to a body of hard scientific information developed in the last decade which suggests that alcohol confers clear health benefits on those who consume it in moderation. However, researchers caution against "prescribing" alcohol for the elderly, despite its emerging health benefits, because the risk of alcohol abuse is higher among older adults and because so many take medications that may interact with alcohol. However, people who enjoy one or two drinks a day should understand this practice is consistent with a healthy lifestyle.

Scientists aren't sure exactly why moderate drinking appears to protect patients from developing dementia in old age, but suggest that perhaps moderate alcohol consumption might protect against heart attacks and stroke, which are linked to dementia. In addition, the antioxidant components of wine might account for the specific protection against Alzheimer's disease.

Aleve   See NONSTEROIDAL ANTI-INFLAMMATORY DRUGS.

Alois Alzheimer Center   The first specialized facility dedicated to the care, treatment, and study of Alzheimer's disease in the United States. The Alois Alzheimer Center, which opened in 1987 in Cincinnati, was established because patients with Alzheimer's need special programs to enhance their quality of life. In addition, it was clear that the needs of these patients were not being met in traditional long-term care facilities. Despite the progressive nature of Alzheimer's disease and other dementias, special care programs can improve a person's independence, ability to function, and quality of life.

The specialized resident programs designed and implemented by the center include creative care techniques, methods of management that significantly decrease problem behaviors, a special physical environment, and life enrichment programs.

Because Alzheimer's disease is a progressive disease, the needs of patients will change over time.

At the Alois Alzheimer Center, the programs, environment, and approaches to care change with residents. The center encourages residents to function at their highest level, and helps clients find a sense of belonging and companionship.

The center coordinates and conducts research that will improve the care of individuals with Alzheimer's disease and dementia. Local and national research projects are continuously in process, ranging from measuring the effects of specific programs to experimental drug treatments.

For contact information, see Appendix I.

alpha-2-macroglobulin (A2M)   A gene on CHROMOSOME 12 that, when defective, may make people who inherit it more susceptible to Alzheimer's disease. The gene was discovered by researchers at Massachusetts General Hospital and the Harvard School of Public Health, who found that patients with late onset Alzheimer's were more likely to have a mutation in this gene than were siblings who had not developed the disease. Although the defective gene doesn't always cause Alzheimer's, its presence increases the risk of developing the disease.

The Alzheimer gene mutation on chromosome 12 is especially important because the protein it codes for interacts with proteins coded for by two previously identified Alzheimer genes—APOLIPOPROTEIN E (apoE) and AMYLOID PRECURSOR PROTEIN (APP). However, the exact nature of these relationships is still unclear.

The risk of developing Alzheimer's disease conferred by the A2M mutation seems to be the same as the risk conferred by the gene variant (identified above) apoE-4. However, people who carry both variants don't seem to be at higher risk. Although apoE-4 appears to affect the age at which symptoms appear, A2M doesn't affect age of onset.

The A2M gene controls the activity of enzymes that break down other proteins, and helps remove potentially toxic proteins out of the synapse (the space between neurons). Since one of the proteins A2M removes is beta amyloid, a hallmark component of the plaques and tangles that characterize Alzheimer's disease, a defective alpha-2-macroglobulin might allow beta amyloid to build up to toxic levels. Scientists believe that Alzheimer's may be caused by a failure in the process of the breakdown and removal of beta amyloid, so a flawed A2M gene may fail to help brain synapses function properly.

Scientists believe that the key event triggering Alzheimer's is the buildup of amyloid plaques made up of toxic deposits of insoluble beta amyloid protein fragments inside the brain. It could be that the A2M and apoE are involved in a sensitive, balanced system that breaks down beta amyloid and removes it from brain cells.

If A2M interfered with this system, or if a variant of apoE blocked the usual breakdown process, beta amyloid plaques could form and clog the synapses, slowing nerve signals and preventing the release of growth factors that keep cells healthy.

Three genes have been identified for the rare, early onset forms of Alzheimer's disease, which are estimated to affect between 1 and 10 percent of cases. A variant of the apoE gene is considered to be a risk factor for the more common, late onset form of the disease. ApoE comes in three forms, known as e2, e3, and e4. Every person has two of these forms, one from each parent. Many scientists believe that people with one or two e-4 forms are at higher risk for Alzheimer's.

See also HEREDITY AND ALZHEIMER'S DISEASE; CHROMOSOME 1; CHROMOSOME 10; CHROMOSOME 14; CHROMOSOME 19; CHROMOSOME 21.

alpha-tocopherol   See VITAMINS.

alprazolam   The generic name for Xanax, an antianxiety medication that is sometimes used to calm agitated patients with Alzheimer's disease. These patients may experience panic attacks and fearfulness, which may lead to demands for constant company and reassurance. Short-lived periods of ANXIETY, such as in response to a stressful event, may be helped by an antianxiety medication.

aluminum   One of the most abundant elements found in the environment, which has been from time to time suspected as one potential cause of Alzheimer's disease. Aluminum is one of 90 naturally occurring chemicals and is the third most common element found in the earth's crust. Scientists are still studying ways to clarify how aluminum affects the body and whether it is a factor in Alzheimer's disease.

Early studies in the 1960s suggested that aluminum triggered changes in an animal's brain that seemed to be similar to those in the brain of a person with Alzheimer's. However, closer analysis proved that the changes in the animals' brains were very different from the structural changes of Alzheimer's.

Human studies searching for a link between Alzheimer's and aluminum have been inconclusive and contradictory. While some researchers have found increased levels of aluminum, mercury, or other metals in the brains of patients with Alzheimer's, other scientists have not. Although some investigators still suspect that aluminum buildup may play a role in the onset of Alzheimer's disease, most believe aluminum is a result of the disorder, not its cause. Research continues in an effort to better understand this phenomenon and to determine whether the aluminum deposits are a cause or a result of the disease.

Because it is found everywhere in the earth, it's almost impossible to avoid contact with aluminum. Most people don't ingest very much because aluminum doesn't dissolve well in many of its naturally occurring forms. In fact, less than 1 percent of the aluminum a person eats or drinks is absorbed from the gastrointestinal tract. Most people ingest between 10 and 150 mg of aluminum each day from food, water, and medications, although the body eliminates most of it. The rest finds its way to the lungs, brain, kidneys, liver, and thyroid. People with poor kidney function may accumulate higher levels of aluminum in their bones.

Less than a fourth of the total intake of aluminum comes from water; the highest levels of aluminum come from food additives. For example, sodium aluminum phosphate is an emulsifier in processed cheese; potassium alum is used to whiten flour; and sodium silicoaluminate and aluminum calcium silicate are added to common table salt to help it pour freely and not cake. In the average diet, 40 to 50 mg a day may come from foods such as these. Therefore, people who eat a lot of refined foods, refined flours, baked goods,

processed cheeses, and common table salt are more likely to have higher aluminum levels in their bodies.

Some common nonprescription drugs such as antacids and buffered aspirin contain aluminum.

Although there has been some concern about whether significant levels of aluminum can leach from cookware and beverage cans, scientists have discovered that this doesn't contribute much to a person's daily intake. Aluminum beverage cans are usually coated with a polymer to minimize leaching, and the problem from aluminum cookware becomes potentially significant only when cooking highly basic or acidic foods.

Avoiding or using these products less often will reduce the ingestion of aluminum. Medicines called chelating agents also can help clear aluminum from the body more rapidly. Likewise, calcium disodium edetate (EDTA) can clear aluminum from the body when given as an intravenous treatment. Another chemical called deferoxamine can remove both iron and aluminum from the body. Some research has suggested improvement in Alzheimer's disease symptoms with deferoxamine treatment.

Although scientists can't yet prove whether aluminum is a cause or a by-product of Alzheimer's disease, experts agree it doesn't hurt to try to avoid excess levels. The best way to prevent aluminum buildup is to avoid the sources of aluminum—foods that have aluminum additives, table salt, aluminum-containing tap water, aluminum cookware, and antiperspirants containing the mineral.

Alzheimer, Alois (1864–1915) German neuropathologist who first identified the dementing disease that bears his name. Born in Markbreit, Bavaria, the young Alois excelled at science, and received his medical degree from the University of Würzburg in 1887 at the age of 23. He was then appointed clinical assistant at an asylum in Frankfurt, where he collaborated with neurologist Franz Nissl in studying the nervous system. Together they published the six-volume *Histologic and Histopathologic Studies of the Cerebral Cortex*.

In search of a post where he could combine research and clinical practice, he became research assistant to Emil Kraepelin at the Munich medical school, creating a new laboratory for brain research and publishing several papers on arteriosclerosis and Huntington's disease.

While working at the Bergholzi Clinic, a famous Swiss psychiatric institution, Dr. Alzheimer began to study "pre-senile dementia," which he thought was a different disease than dementia that occurred after age 65. He believed that pre-senile dementia occurred as the brain deteriorated, but that senile dementia was caused by vascular problems.

Using a high-resolution microscope, Alzheimer performed autopsies on patients who had been diagnosed with dementia, finding specific areas of deterioration in their brains.

One day he noticed a variety of puzzling symptoms in one of his patients, Frau August D., who experienced fits of jealousy toward her husband, together with memory loss, depression, hallucinations, and rapidly progressing dementia. She died at age 51 within five years of her first visit to Dr. Alzheimer. In his landmark 1906 paper on the case, Dr. Alzheimer discussed this "unusual case of disease in the cerebral cortex," describing the woman's unusual early symptoms and his subsequent autopsy of her brain. The autopsy revealed signs of general shrinkage and lesions, extensive distorted tissue, and cell damage in a part of the brain called the CEREBRAL CORTEX—the hallmarks of Alzheimer's disease. It was his colleague, the distinguished psychiatrist Emil Kraepelin, who named the condition after Alzheimer in a textbook in 1910.

In 1912 the University of Breslau appointed Alzheimer professor of psychiatry and director of the Psychiatric and Neurologic Institute. Alzheimer continued his research there for the next three years. In addition to his research on dementia, Alzheimer also made significant contributions to the field of histology, making important observations in epilepsy, brain tumors, Huntington's chorea, and alcoholic delirium. He was widely admired as a meticulous and dedicated researcher and a generous teacher.

On his way to Breslau in 1913 to chair the department of psychology at the Friedrich-Wilhelm University, Alzheimer caught a severe cold complicated by endocarditis, from which he never fully recovered. He died at the age of 51 and was buried next to his wife in Frankfurt am Main.

It was not until the 1960s that scientists looked at Alzheimer's work and began to diagnose Alzheimer's disease in their own patients.

Alzheimer's Association The largest national voluntary health organization committed to finding a cure for Alzheimer's and helping those affected by the disease. In 1980, a group of people committed to helping those afflicted with the disease and their families and caregivers founded the association.

Having awarded more than $100 million in research grants since then, the association ranks as the top private funding agent for research into the causes, treatments, prevention, and cure of Alzheimer's disease. The association also provides education and support for patients, their families, and caregivers, and mobilizes worldwide resources for biomedical, social, and behavioral research. It promotes, develops, and disseminates educational programs and training guidelines for health and social service professionals, and tries to increase public awareness of the disease and its impact on families and society.

The association's grants program is designed to attract more scientists to the field, and at the core of the program is a peer review system to ensure the merit of each study.

According to the National Charities Information Bureau, nonprofit organizations should spend at least 60 percent of their budget on programs, with remaining funds going to administrative and fundraising expenses. At the Alzheimer's Association, 75 percent of revenues goes to programs such as research, while the remaining money pays for management, general expenses, and program improvement.

The Alzheimer's Association's Benjamin B. Green-Field Library and Resource Center collects a wide range of materials—books, journals, audiocassettes, videos, and CD-ROMs—on Alzheimer's disease and related disorders. The center serves as a resource for family members of those with Alzheimer's, educators and students, health care professionals, social service agencies, and the general public. Library staff respond to information requests, do literature searches, lend materials, and provide referrals. Also, the library provides reading lists of books and other sources to help educate the public and others about a variety of Alzheimer's-related topics. Anyone may use materials in the library or borrow them via interlibrary loan through their public or institutional libraries or local chapters.

See also ALZHEIMER'S ASSOCIATION SAFE RETURN PROGRAM.

Alzheimer's Association Safe Return Program
A program established in 1993 by the ALZHEIMER'S ASSOCIATION, which is dedicated to finding patients who have wandered away from their home or institution. The Safe Return Program is the only nationwide program that helps identify and quickly return individuals with Alzheimer's disease and related dementias who wander and become lost.

Since its inception, the program has helped return about 6,300 people. An estimated 78,000 people are now registered with the program, which provides identification jewelry that indicates the person has a memory problem and lists a 24-hour toll-free telephone number to call if the person is found WANDERING. The association has collected data on all registered users as well as data related to both missing persons and discovery reports.

This program includes

- identification products, including wallet cards, jewelry, and clothing labels
- a national photo/information database
- a 24-hour toll-free emergency crisis line
- Alzheimer's Association local chapter support
- wandering behavior education and training for caregivers and families

Patients may register by phone with a credit card, by calling (888) 572–8566, Monday through Friday, 8 A.M. to 8 P.M. central time. The registration fee is $40, and identification jewelry costs $5. Some local Alzheimer's Association chapters offer scholarships.

If the registrant wanders and is found, the person who finds the patient can call the Safe Return toll-free number located on the wanderer's identification wallet card, jewelry, or clothing labels. The Safe Return telephone operator immediately alerts the family members or caregiver listed in the national database, so they can be reunited with the patient.

If a person is reported missing by a family member or caregiver, Safe Return can fax local law enforcement agencies the missing person's information and photograph. Local Alzheimer's Association chapters provide family support and assistance while police conduct the search and rescue.

Up to 60 percent of people with Alzheimer's disease may wander off and get lost sometime during the course of the disease, putting them at risk from traffic, the elements, and those who prey on the helpless.

Alzheimer's disease
A progressive, degenerative disease characterized by death of nerve cells in several areas of the brain. While the most obvious symptom is loss of memory, the disease also causes problems with emotional control, vision, and language.

The progressive deterioration characteristic of the disease continues for up to 20 years, although many patients die within three to five years of diagnosis. Eventually, a person with Alzheimer's disease requires 24-hour care and assistance with daily activities such as eating, grooming, and toileting. Because its impact on the affected person is so great, the condition profoundly affects family and caregivers.

Alzheimer's disease is not a normal part of aging—nor is it inevitable. It is the most common of the more than 70 forms of dementia, a condition that leads to the loss of mental and physical functions. Alzheimer's disease currently affects 4 million Americans, but experts believe that number could rise to more than 22 million by 2025 as the population ages and as people live longer. While the course of the disease varies from one person to the next, it is always progressively fatal, killing 120,000 Americans a year—the fourth cause of death among adults over 65 after heart disease, cancer, and stroke.

Alzheimer's is characterized by an accumulation of twisted protein fragments inside nerve cells in the gray matter of the brain, which appear under the microscope as a tangle of filaments called NEU-ROFIBRILLARY TANGLES. It was these tangles that were first described in 1906 by German neurologist Dr. ALOIS ALZHEIMER, who discovered them while performing an autopsy on the brain of a 55-year-old woman with dementia.

Other brain changes common in Alzheimer's disease include groups of degenerated nerve endings in the brain called plaques that disrupt electrochemical signals in the brain. The larger the number of plaques and tangles, the greater the disturbance in intellectual function and memory. Upon autopsy, the presence of plaques and tangles is the only way to definitely diagnose Alzheimer's.

History

The manifestations of Alzheimer's disease have been recognized since ancient times, when Greek and Roman writers described symptoms similar to what experts know today as Alzheimer's. In the 16th century, Shakespeare wrote about very old age as a time of "second childishness and mere oblivion," suggesting that the symptoms of Alzheimer's were known and recognized then.

Despite this long history, relatively little was known until recently about the processes in the brain that lead to Alzheimer's disease. In the past, most doctors assumed that the dementia of Alzheimer's was an inevitable part of aging, but over the past 25 years scientists have discovered much more about Alzheimer's disease—what it is, who gets it, how it develops, and what course it follows. Scientists also have made significant progress in early diagnosis and possible treatments.

Symptoms

At first, Alzheimer's disease destroys brain cells in parts of the brain that control memory, including the HIPPOCAMPUS (a structure deep in the brain that helps to encode short-term memories). As nerve cells in the hippocampus stop working properly, short-term memory fails, and a person's ability to complete familiar tasks begins to decline. Next, the disease attacks the areas responsible for language and reasoning in the CEREBRAL CORTEX, interfering with language skills, judgment, and personality. Emotional outbursts and behavior like wandering and agitation become more frequent as the disease

continues. Eventually, many other areas of the brain shrink and die, and the patient becomes bedridden, incontinent, totally helpless, and unresponsive to the outside world.

Alzheimer's vs. Normal Memory Lapses

One of the problems with the symptoms of memory loss is that many of them are quite normal, and yet many mimic the very early symptoms of Alzheimer's. Of course, not all memory complaints in later life signal Alzheimer's disease or even a mental disorder. Many memory changes are only temporary, such as those that occur during any stressful situation that makes it hard to concentrate. There are major differences between normal behavior and Alzheimer's symptoms:

- *Memory loss:* The memory loss of Alzheimer's often affects daily life and job skills. It's normal to forget occasionally a task or a person's name, but frequent forgetfulness or unexplainable confusion at home or in the workplace may signal something is wrong. It's normal for people to forget where they placed their glasses, but not that they *wear* glasses.

- *Problems with familiar tasks:* It's normal to forget a pan on the stove, but someone with Alzheimer's might forget to serve an entire meal or even that it had been made.

- *Language problems:* It's normal to forget a word sometimes, but a person with Alzheimer's disease forgets many words and also substitutes inappropriate words so that sentences become hard to understand.

- *Disorientation:* It's normal to forget momentarily what day of the week it is, but people with Alzheimer's disease not only forget the day, they get lost on their own street.

- *Poor judgment:* A person with Alzheimer's often exhibits bad judgment; for example, dressing inappropriately by wearing pajamas to the workplace or making poor financial decisions.

- *Abstract thinking problems:* Most everyone occasionally forgets a multiplication fact now and then, but people with Alzheimer's forget how to recognize numbers, and can no longer add or subtract.

- *Misplacing things:* It's normal for people to forget their keys, but to forget they have a car is more likely to be indicative of Alzheimer's.

- *Personality changes:* Occasional bad moods are normal, but the personality of a person with Alzheimer's can change dramatically and become suspicious or fearful.

Alzheimer's disease begins slowly with mild forgetfulness that leads to problems finding the right word. Ever so gradually, it progresses to an inability to recognize objects, and ultimately, to an inability to use even the simplest of things, such as a hairbrush. This gradual degeneration often lasts more than 10 years.

People with mild dementia can usually live independently with only minor problems in work or social activities. As the dementia continues, patients may seem capable, but independent living becomes increasingly difficult. They may begin to dress carelessly and neglect work and family responsibilities, leave the stove or iron turned on, or become lost while away from home. As short-term memory falters, Alzheimer's patients can no longer perform everyday tasks such as zipping a zipper. Behavioral symptoms are also quite common, since the damage to the brain can cause a person to act in different or unpredictable ways. Some people become anxious or aggressive, while others engage in repetitive behavior. Other behavioral symptoms may include agitation, COMBATIVENESS, DELUSIONS, DEPRESSION, HALLUCINATIONS, INSOMNIA, and wandering.

As the dementia becomes severe, patients must be constantly supervised. Their language ability disintegrates, and they may string together unrelated words into meaningless sentences. Eventually the failing nervous system affects the entire body and they become completely incapacitated—even unable to eat. Death usually follows as the result of pneumonia or an infection.

Alzheimer's patients who have at least one other relative with the disease are categorized as familial. *Familial* does not necessarily mean that the disease is inherited; family members may have contracted the disease simply because they lived long enough to have developed it. If a person has Alzheimer's disease and no other family members

are known to have been affected, they are said to have sporadic Alzheimer's disease.

See also CAUSES OF ALZHEIMER'S DISEASE; DIAGNOSIS OF ALZHEIMER'S DISEASE; TREATMENT.

Alzheimer's disease, early onset   A rare form of Alzheimer's disease that occurs earlier in life than normally expected—usually before age 65. Early onset Alzheimer's disease affects about 60,000 Americans, appearing primarily during middle age, although the disease is known to have occurred in people as early as the middle 20s. About one person in every 1,000 develops Alzheimer's before the age of 65.

In some families around the world, early onset Alzheimer's strikes often enough to be given a name: early onset familial Alzheimer's disease. The disease has occurred in the 20s and 30s among two families in Belgium tracing back six or seven generations; a Japanese family has five members who developed the disease in middle age; a French-Canadian family has 23. In families descended from Germans who settled in the Volga River Valley in Russia in the 1800s, dozens of descendants have developed Alzheimer's disease in middle age.

Other than the unusually early appearance, the symptoms of early onset disease are similar to those of Alzheimer's disease that appears in older patients. However, some research suggests that people with the early onset form of the disease decline at a faster rate.

However, while the symptoms are the same, the early onset version can cause unique problems. Because people with the early onset form are usually still working and raising a family, problems related to the disease that appear on the job or at home may be mistakenly blamed on laziness or mental health problems. Patients with early onset Alzheimer's disease will eventually need to quit working, but many medical benefits and social support programs for Alzheimer's patients aren't offered for people under age 65. A younger person may need to get special permission to take advantage of these programs.

Early onset forms of the familial disease are more likely to be inherited in an autosomal dominant pattern of genetic transmission, which means it is easier to see a clear pattern of inheritance from parent to child. As many as half of all cases of early onset familial Alzheimer's are now known to be caused by a defect in one of three genes located on three different chromosomes: chromosomes 1, 14, or 21.

Mutations in genes known as presenilin-1 (PS1) and presenilin-2 (PS2) account for most cases of early onset inherited Alzheimer's disease. The defective genes, which are found on chromosome 14 and 1, respectively, appear to accelerate BETA AMYLOID plaque formation and APOPTOSIS, a natural process by which cells are programmed to self-destruct. If only one of the above mutations appears in one of the two copies of a gene inherited from the parents, the person will inevitably develop early onset Alzheimer's. However, the total known number of these cases is small (between 100 and 200 worldwide), and there is as yet no evidence that any of these mutations plays a major role in the more common, sporadic (nongenetic) form of late onset Alzheimer's.

Since the genes were first discovered in 1995, scientists have found that the mutated forms of the genes may cause Alzheimer's by boosting production of beta amyloid, a protein that creates the plaques found in the brains of Alzheimer's patients. Scientists believe that a buildup of beta amyloid damages cells, and that the presenilins also participate in cellular suicide, sending precise chemical messages to cells urging them to die. This mechanism of cell death begins in healthy people at around age 45. People with the mutated form of the presenilin gene are far more sensitive to these enzymes.

Genetic mutations in the genes that control AMYLOID-PRECURSOR PROTEIN (APP) found on chromosome 21 may also be a cause of early onset Alzheimer's. The genetic disease Down's syndrome, for example, overproduces beta amyloid precursor protein (APP), the source of beta amyloid, and almost always leads to early onset Alzheimer's.

See also CHROMOSOME 1; CHROMOSOME 14; CHROMOSOME 21; HEREDITY AND ALZHEIMER'S DISEASE.

Alzheimer's disease, late onset The most common form of Alzheimer's disease that occurs in people over age 65. The genetic form of this disease has been linked to a defective APOLIPOPROTEIN-4 GENE on CHROMOSOME 19, which contributes to the development of more than 60 percent of all late onset Alzheimer's cases, but that means 40 percent of cases are caused by something else. For this reason, scientists assume there must be other Alzheimer's susceptibility genes.

The apoE-4 gene was discovered by researchers who studied families in which many members developed the disease late in life, which suggested that there had to be a gene that the affected family members shared. Searching for this gene, they sifted through the DNA from these families and by 1992 had narrowed the search down to a region on chromosome 19. In the same laboratory, another group of researchers were looking for proteins that bind to BETA AMYLOID. One version of a protein called APOLIPOPROTEIN E (apoE) did bind to beta amyloid, and the gene that produced apoE was also on chromosome 19, in the same region of chromosome 19 as the Alzheimer's gene for which they had been searching. The two groups of scientists realized the apoE gene was identical to the gene they had been seeking.

The gene that produces apoE comes in three different forms—apoE-2, apoE-3, and apoE-4. Version apoE-4 is found in about 40 percent of all people with late onset Alzheimer's disease. This gene version is not limited to people whose families have a history of Alzheimer's, however. Patients with Alzheimer's who have no known family history of the disease are also more likely to have an apoE-4 gene.

Dozens of studies around the world have since confirmed that the apoE-4 version increases the risk of developing Alzheimer's disease. People who inherit two of the mutant apoE-4 genes (one from the mother and one from the father) are at least eight times more likely to develop Alzheimer's disease than those who have two of the more common E-3 versions. The least common allele, apoE-2, seems to lower the risk even more. For example, people with one E-2 and one E-3 gene have only one-fourth the risk of developing Alzheimer's as do people with two E-3 genes. People without apoE-4 have an estimated risk for developing Alzheimer's by age 85 of between 9 percent and 20 percent. In people with one copy of the gene, the risk is between 25 percent and 60 percent. In people with two copies, the risk ranges from 50 percent to 90 percent. Only 2 percent of the population carry two copies of the apoE-4 gene.

Many laboratories are now exploring what the apoE-4 protein product does, and many scientists think it has something to do with beta amyloid. Normally, the beta amyloid is soluble, but when the apoE-4 protein binds to it, the amyloid becomes insoluble. This could make it more likely to clump together in plaques. Studies of brain tissue suggest that apoE-4 does increase beta amyloid deposits, and that it directly regulates the protein from which beta amyloid is formed.

Other clues, however, point to TAU PROTEIN as pivotal. As the crosspiece in the microtubule, tau's function seems to be to stabilize the microtubule structure. One hypothesis suggests that the apoE-4 protein allows this structure to collapse, leading to the neurofibrillary tangles.

While still controversial, the apoE-4 hypothesis is an important new area of research. Now scientists are studying how tau and beta amyloid react with apolipoprotein in its several forms in living cells. Other experiments will attempt to determine the actions and role of the protein. Once scientists understand these processes, it will be easier to develop medicines that can affect the development of the disease.

The apoE-4 has other potential effects on Alzheimer's disease beyond its link to proteins. For example, scientists have discovered that Alzheimer's patients with the apoE-4 gene also have neurons with shorter dendrites (the branch-like extensions that receive messages from other neurons). Scientists think that the dendrites may have been cut by some unknown substance so that the neuron can't communicate as well with other neurons. Although this shortening is also found among people without the apoE-4 version, those who do have the apoE-4 version exhibit shortened dendrites 20 or 30 years earlier.

However, not everyone with the gene will develop Alzheimer's disease, and not everyone with the disease has the gene. A simple test for the presence of apoE-4 would result in too many false positives and false negatives, which is why it is not used as a diagnostic method.

Alzheimer's Disease and Related Dementias Research Act of 1986   A law signed by then president Ronald Reagan that establishes a council on Alzheimer's disease in the U.S. Department of Health and Human Services.

Alzheimer's Disease Assessment Scale-Cognitive Subscale (ADAS-Cog)   A test that is currently the most common standard for assessing the status of patients with Alzheimer's disease, and is considered to be the best brief exam for the study of language and memory skills. In this assessment, memory, orientation, language, and function are measured on a 70-point scale. The 11-part test takes 30 minutes to administer, and is more thorough than the BLESSED INFORMATION-MEMORY-CONCENTRATION TEST or the MINI-MENTAL STATUS EXAMINATION. The test is also used to help evaluate patient response in many clinical trials.

On the test, patients with Alzheimer's typically worsen six to nine points in the ADAS-Cog each year. An improvement of four points (a four-point decline in score) corresponds to a clinically significant reversal of symptoms of nearly half a year.

See also ASSESSMENT TOOLS.

Alzheimer's disease associated protein (ADAP)   A protein that seems to appear only in the tissue of people with Alzheimer's disease, found in both the brain and spinal fluid. The protein is concentrated in the part of the brain concerned with memory function—the cortex covering the front and side sections of the brain. If scientists can devise a test to detect the protein in the blood or spinal fluid, it may be possible to use this method of diagnosis on living patients.

Alzheimer's Disease Centers   A network of 32 government-funded specialty centers dedicated to research on Alzheimer's disease and educational programs for families, health professionals, and the community. The NATIONAL INSTITUTE ON AGING currently funds the Alzheimer's Disease Centers (ADC) at major U.S. medical institutions. Researchers at these centers are translating research into improved care and diagnosis for patients while focusing on finding a way to cure and prevent Alzheimer's disease. Center staff conduct basic, clinical, and behavioral research into the basic mechanisms of the disease, managing symptoms, and helping families cope with the effects of the disease.

Each of the 32 centers has its own unique areas of emphasis. Centers also have significant responsibilities to transfer information and train scientists and health care providers. All the centers are dedicated to providing a network for sharing new ideas as well as research results.

Currently, 27 ADC-affiliated satellite facilities offer diagnostic and treatment services and collect research data in underserved, rural, and minority communities. For patients and families affected by Alzheimer's disease, many centers offer diagnosis and medical management, information, opportunities for volunteers to participate in drug trials and research projects, and support groups and other special programs.

Alzheimer's Disease Education and Referral (ADEAR) Center

An organization established in 1990 by the NATIONAL INSTITUTE ON AGING to provide information about Alzheimer's disease, its impact on families and health professionals, and research into possible causes and cures. The idea was created by the NIA under the provisions of the ALZHEIMER'S DISEASE AND RELATED DEMENTIAS RESEARCH ACT of 1986.

The ADEAR Center offers information on current research efforts and findings related to Alzheimer's and also provides referrals to key resources, such as treatment centers, support groups, and family support services.

Consumers who call the center (at [800] 438-4380) can speak with an information specialist who can provide:

- answers to questions about Alzheimer's disease
- information about the latest research
- details of studies of new treatments
- publications about Alzheimer's disease and related disorders
- other groups to contact for more information, publications, and services

The center answers phones Monday through Friday, from 8:30 A.M. to 5:00 P.M. eastern time.

Alzheimer's Disease International

An umbrella group of 57 Alzheimer's disease associations throughout the world. Each member association is the national Alzheimer's association in its country, and supports people with dementia and their families. The ADI's key role is to build and strengthen Alzheimer's associations throughout the world, so they are better able to meet the needs of people with dementia. Most member associations are in developing countries where health and social services are limited.

The group was founded in 1984, and is registered as a not-for-profit organization in the United States. The ADI is also registered in the United Kingdom as a charity named Friends of ADI to enable deductible donations from United Kingdom taxpayers. The organization's office is based in London. For contact information, see Appendix I.

Alzheimer's Family Relief Program (AFRP)

A relief program offered by the AMERICAN HEALTH ASSISTANCE FOUNDATION (AHAF) to provide direct financial assistance and resources for the support of patients with Alzheimer's disease and their caregivers. AFRP has awarded grants totaling more than $1.5 million to patients and caregivers in 49 states since 1988. The program provides financial assistance up to $500 each to care for Alzheimer's patients, who can reapply every 90 days. Applications can be downloaded from the program's website at http://www.ahaf.org.

Emergency grants are provided for expenses such as short-term nursing care, home health care, respite care, ADULT DAY CARE, medications, medical or personal hygiene supplies, transportation, and other expenses. Grants aren't provided for paying nursing home fees.

Applications are funded based on established need and on a first-come, first-served basis. First-time applicants will receive priority treatment; repeat applicants are placed on a waiting list and are considered as funding becomes available.

To be eligible, the patient's liquid assets (including cash, bank accounts, money market accounts, stocks, bonds, and mutual funds) may not exceed

$10,000. Liquid assets don't include the patient's car or house. However, all of the patient's assets will be taken into consideration in determining the urgency of need. If the patient is dependent on a caregiver, the caregiver's assets must meet the eligibility requirements.

Applications must include a diagnosis from the patient's physician, health professional, or social worker before they are presented to the AFRP Review Committee for funding.

The extent to which assistance can be provided, as well as the number of patients who can be helped, is determined by the availability of funds. At times, it may be necessary to place an approved request on a waiting list until money becomes available.

Alzheimer Foundation of the South   A nonprofit organization dedicated to supporting scientific research aimed at finding a cure for Alzheimer's disease, while striving to educate the public in all aspects of the disease. The mission of the foundation is to support basic research intended to find treatments or preventions for Alzheimer's disease and related disorders and to enhance the quality of life and to preserve the dignity of patients through support and educational programs for the patients, families, and professional caregivers. For contact information, see Appendix I.

Alzheimer Society of Canada   A not-for-profit Canadian health organization that works together to form a nationwide network of services to help Canadians affected by Alzheimer's disease. For contact information, see Appendix I.

American Academy of Neurology (AAN)   A worldwide professional association of more than 17,000 neurologists and neuroscience professionals dedicated to providing the best possible care for patients with neurological disorders. The medical specialty society was established to advance the art and science of neurology, and to promote the best possible care for patients with neurological disorders by ensuring appropriate access to care, offering a variety of programs in clinical neurology and the basic neurosciences, and supporting clinical and basic research. For contact information, see Appendix I.

American Association for Geriatric Psychiatry
A national association representing GERIATRIC PSYCHIATRISTS, dedicated to promoting the mental health and well-being of older people and improving the care of those with late-life mental disorders. The association's mission is to enhance the knowledge and standard of practice in geriatric psychiatry through education and research, and to advocate for meeting the mental health needs of older Americans. For contact information, see Appendix I.

See also GERIATRIC PSYCHIATRY.

American Association of Homes and Services for the Aging (AAHSA)   A group of more than 5,600 not-for-profit nursing homes, continuing care retirement communities, assisted living and senior housing facilities, and community service organizations. Every day, AAHSA's members serve more than 1 million older persons across the country.

AAHSA represents the concerns of nonprofit organizations serving the elderly. It also strives to enhance the professionalism of practitioners and facilities through the Certification Program for Retirement Housing Professionals, the Continuing Care Accreditation Commission, conferences and programs, and publications representing current thinking in the long-term care and retirement housing fields.

Since its inception in 1961, AAHSA represented nonprofit approaches to caring for and serving the elderly. The majority of its charter members, like its members today, were not-for-profit organizations associated in various ways with religious denominations, fraternal groups, and other nonprofit sponsors, all committed to maintaining the dignity and respect of older persons. For contact information, see Appendix I.

American Geriatrics Society, The (AGS)   A national nonprofit association of geriatrics health care professionals, research scientists, and other concerned individuals dedicated to improving the health, independence, and quality of life of all older people. With an active membership of more than 6,000 health care professionals, the AGS has become a pivotal force in shaping attitudes, policies, and practices regarding health care for older people. Although historically members have been predominantly physicians, membership is open to anyone with an interest in geriatric health care, including nurses, researchers, medical educators, pharmacists, physician assistants, social workers, physical therapists, health care administrators, and others. The society was founded in 1942; beginning in 1979, the American Federation for Aging Research (AFAR) has held its annual meeting in conjunction with the AGS. For contact information, see Appendix I.

American Health Assistance Foundation (AHAF), The A nonprofit charitable organization dedicated to funding research on Alzheimer's disease, educating the public and providing emergency financial assistance to patients and their caregivers through the ALZHEIMER'S FAMILY RELIEF PROGRAM. The group offers a range of free publications. For contact information, see Appendix I.

American Society on Aging (ASA) A professional association that provides educational programming, publications, and state-of-the-art information and training resources for researchers, practitioners, educators, and policymakers concerned with aging.

The ASA Learning Center offers programs such as the Summer Series on Aging, web-enhanced teleconferences and computer-based training, and an on-line store and searchable database that provide a one-stop shop for education and training resources in aging. For contact information, see Appendix I.

amino acids The fundamental building blocks of proteins. The body uses amino acids as the basic substance from which to construct not only proteins, but also NEUROTRANSMITTERS. Individual amino acid molecules are linked together by chemical bonds to form short chains of peptides. In turn, hundreds of these chains of peptides (called polypeptides) are linked together to form a protein molecule. One protein differs from another in the way its amino acids are arranged.

A total of 20 different amino acids make up all the proteins found in the human body; 12 can be made within the body (these are known as nonessential amino acids). The other eight, called the essential amino acids, must be obtained from the diet, and can't be produced by the body. In addition, there are about 200 other amino acids not found in proteins but which play an important part in chemical reactions within cells.

Because animal sources usually provide a wider range of amino acids than do plant sources, people on a vegetarian diet must be especially careful that their selection of food includes all the essential amino acids.

Because the amino acids are responsible for producing neurotransmitters, some researchers believe that boosting the brain's supply of certain amino acids should also increase the production of neurotransmitters, which could affect cognition among Alzheimer's patients. Two amino acids have been singled out for particular study: tryptophan and TYROSINE. In fact, some research suggests that tyrosine appears to improve alertness and cognitive performance during stress. However, other scientists caution that simply increasing the pool of amino acids does not necessarily mean that more neurotransmitters will be produced.

amnesia Loss of the ability to memorize and recall stored information. In most cases of amnesia, the patient has problems storing information in long-term memory and recalling this information. There are many theories that explain the underlying mechanism of amnesia and many different causes, including brain damage from injury or disease. Anterograde amnesia is the loss of memory for events following trauma; retrograde amnesia is a loss of memory for events preceding the trauma. Some patients experience both types of amnesia.

Amnesia following trauma (such as a concussion) in areas of the brain concerned with memory function is known as traumatic amnesia. Degenerative disorders such as Alzhemier's disease or other types of DEMENTIA may also cause amnesia, as can infections such as encephalitis or a thiamine deficiency in alcoholics. Amnesia could also be caused by a brain tumor, STROKE, or a subarachnoid hemorrhage, or certain types of mental illness.

Transient global amnesia is a type of uncommon amnesia that refers to an abrupt loss of memory for a few seconds to a few hours without loss of consciousness or other impairment. During the amnesia period, the subject can't store new experiences and suffers a permanent memory gap for the period of time during the amnesic episode. There may also be loss of memory encompassing many years prior to the amnesia attack; this retrograde amnesia gradually disappears, although it leaves a permanent gap in memory that does not usually extend backward more than an hour before onset of the attack. These attacks, which may occur more than once, are believed to be caused by a temporary reduction in blood supply in certain brain areas. Sometimes, they act as a warning sign of an impending stroke.

amygdala   A region in the brain at the base of the temporal lobe whose primary function may be its responsibility to bring emotional content to memory. Sensory information from certain cortical areas enters the limbic system directly through the amygdala, an almond-shaped mass of gray matter deep inside each cerebral hemisphere.

Because the amygdala connects to the HIPPOCAMPUS, scientists believe that it may play a role in memory. While most now believe the amygdala does not itself process memory, scientists do believe that the amygdala is a source of emotions that imbue memory with meaning. For example, the remembrance of a memory or a whole stream of recollection often brings with it a burst of emotion—evidence that the amygdala is most likely involved.

amyloid   A protein deposit associated with tissue degeneration; amyloid is found in the brains of individuals with Alzheimer's disease.

See also AMYLOID PLAQUES; BETA AMYLOID.

amyloid plaques   Abnormal clusters of dead and dying nerve cells, other brain cells, and AMYLOID protein fragments. Amyloid plaques are one of the characteristic structural abnormalities found in the brains of individuals with Alzheimer's disease. Upon autopsy, the presence of amyloid plaques and NEUROFIBRILLARY TANGLES is used to positively diagnose Alzheimer's.

Amyloid plaques impede nerve cell function and cause nerve cell death in the brains of people with Alzheimer's disease. Although amyloid plaques are found in the brains of most individuals with Alzheimer's disease, it is not yet known whether plaques are a cause or a result of the disease process.

In Alzheimer's, plaques develop first in areas of the brain used for memory and other cognitive functions. They consist of largely insoluble deposits of BETA AMYLOID—a protein fragment snipped from a larger protein called AMYLOID-PRECURSOR PROTEIN (APP)—intermingled with portions of neurons and with other cells. Plaques are found in the spaces between the brain's nerve cells. There is evidence that amyloid deposits may be a central process in the disease.

Scientists know that changes in the structure of the APP protein can cause Alzheimer's, as shown in one inherited form of the disease that is caused by mutations in the gene containing instructions for making the APP protein.

amyloid-precursor protein (APP)   The parent protein from which BETA AMYLOID is derived, and which is found in the brain, heart, kidneys, lungs, spleen, and intestines. It is used by the body for unknown purposes.

APP is a large protein that protrudes through the neuron membrane, part inside and part outside the cell. While it is embedded in the membrane, enzymes snip it in two, creating a beta amyloid fragment. After the enzyme clips the APP, the resulting beta amyloid fragments then clump together into plaque deposits in the brain. Scientists don't know whether these deposits are caused by too much beta amyloid, or whether the enzymes that usually break it down are not functioning properly.

Several mutations have been identified on the APP gene, linking it closely to Alzheimer's disease. Scientists are looking at ways of stopping the abnormal process that triggers a damaging form of beta amyloid to splinter away from APP.

AMY plaque   A previously unidentified protein only recently discovered in the brains of people with Alzheimer's disease that may play a role in the onset or progression of the disease. AMY plaques resemble plaques made up of BETA AMY-LOID so closely that only with the use of highly sophisticated techniques are researchers able to detect them.

The new protein was found when scientists used a different method of detecting the plaques and tangles in brains with the disease. The staining and chemical dye methods that have been used in the past to label the plaques and tangles of Alzheimer's disease don't pick up this lesion. The new plaque and its protein were dubbed AMY plaque because an antibody called AMY117 was used in the laboratory to discover the new lesion.

AN-1792 This potential vaccine, which had been studied as a possible treatment for Alzheimer's disease, was abandoned in early 2002 when it caused serious brain inflammation among some study participants.

AN-1792 was designed to stimulate the immune system to recognize and attack the BETA AMYLOID plaques that are a hallmark of Alzheimer's brain abnormality. Amyloid plaques appear to slow down nerve cell function and kill cells in the brains of people with Alzheimer's. AN-1792 is a synthetic form of the naturally occurring beta amyloid protein.

Scientists at Elan Corporation developed the compound based on the theory that treatment with portions of beta amyloid might activate the immune system to produce its own antibodies to attack plaques in the brain.

Elan reported its first animal studies in July 1999, which showed that injections of AN-1792 prevented plaques in the brains of young mice genetically altered to develop characteristics of Alzheimer's. It also reduced existing plaques in older mice, and improved rodents' memory.

This led to the first human studies of AN-1792 in 2000 to assess safety and tolerability in people with mild to moderate Alzheimer's. A British trial of 80 participants and a U.S. study of 24 suggested that the vaccine was well tolerated in humans, and that some participants developed amyloid antibodies. Late in 2001, Elan began a small study in the United States and Europe to assess the drug's effectiveness, determine the best dosage, and build on the evi-dence of safety. This study enrolled about 375 people with mild to moderate Alzheimer's disease.

In January 2002, Elan and Wyeth-Ayerst Laboratories suspended the dosing schedule after four participants who had received multiple doses of AN-1792 developed symptoms of inflammation of the brain and spinal cord. When another 11 participants developed these symptoms by the end of February 2002, scientists on the independent Safety Monitoring Committee concluded that the trial should be stopped and that no one should be given further doses of AN-1792.

Researchers will continue to monitor the health of everyone who received AN-1792. Most individuals who experienced inflammation have shown improvement or recovered. The exact cause of the brain inflammation is not yet known.

angiography A type of diagnostic technique that enables blood vessels in the brain to be seen on X-ray film after an artery has been injected with a dye. Angiography can be used to help determine whether symptoms are caused by Alzheimer's disease or by a brain tumor or blocked artery. Carotid angiography sometimes is performed on patients suffering from transient ischemic attacks (brief symptoms of a stroke lasting less than 24 hours), to see whether there is a block or narrowing in one of the carotid arteries in the neck that supply blood to the brain.

Contrast dye is first injected through a fine catheter inserted into the carotid artery deep in the neck. Then skin and tissue around the artery are numbed with a local anesthetic, followed by a needle inserted through the skin into the artery; a long thin wire with a soft tip is inserted through the needle, the needle is removed, and the catheter is then threaded over the wire into the blood vessel. An X ray is used to guide the tip of the catheter into the vessel.

There are some risks involved with this procedure. While it is possible to experience an allergic reaction to the dye, new contrast agents have lowered the risk of a severe reaction to less than one in 80,000 exams. Blood vessels may be damaged at the puncture site, anywhere along the vessel during passage of the catheter, or at the dye injection site.

aniracetam   One of a class of drugs that some studies suggest may be capable of improving thinking, cognition, and memory. Its chemical structure is similar to PIRACETAM, a drug being studied in the treatment of Alzheimer's disease.

Studies suggest aniracetam stimulates the function of certain brain receptors. Research has found both long- and short-term memory improvement with aniracetam, but the drug is not approved for distribution in any country.

anomia   A type of APHASIA involving the inability to verbalize the names of people, objects, or places. It appears to relate to speech output, since patients usually have no problem comprehending when the object is named for them.

antacids   Nonprescription medications used for treating indigestion and ulcers, many of which contain large amounts of ALUMINUM compounds. Although aluminum has been implicated as a possible link to Alzheimer's disease, very little of the aluminum contained in antacids is normally absorbed. Antacids make the stomach more alkaline, and this prevents the absorption of most of the aluminum. Aluminum absorption is higher if antacids are taken with orange juice instead of water.

Although the recommended daily dose of some antacids may contain as much as 1,000 mg to 2,000 mg of aluminum, studies of people using antacids have shown that those exposed to high levels of aluminum over long periods are no more prone to Alzheimer's disease than other people.

anterior commissure   A collection of nerve cells that connects the brain's two hemispheres.

anterior communicating artery   A short artery located in the forebrain that connects the two arteries in the front of each cerebral hemisphere. Blockages often occur along this artery, which can cause a type of AMNESIA that may be confused with Alzheimer's disease.

antianxiety drugs   Medications that ease anxiety and are used to treat agitated, anxious patients with Alzheimer's disease. Although mild anxiety may be relieved with these drugs, they are often overused or used incorrectly. As a result, Alzheimer's patients may experience significant daytime sedation, dizziness, and falls.

Shorter-acting medications such as lorazepam (Ativan), buspirone (Buspar), ALPRAZOLAM (Xanax), and oxazepam (Serax), may be safer and easier to manage than longer-acting drugs such as diazepam (Valium) and chlordiazepoxide (Librium).

Other antianxiety drugs include flurazepam (Dalmane), quazepam (Doral), triazolam (Halcion), clonazepam (Klonopin), estazolam (ProSom), temazepam (Restoril), and clorazepate (Tranxene).

anticholinergic drugs   Medications that disrupt the transmission of ACETYLCHOLINE in the brain by blocking cholinergic receptors, preventing acetylcholine release or completely depleting neurons that use acetylcholine.

anticipatory grief   A deep sadness over an impending death that people may experience before a loved one actually dies. In the later stages of Alzheimer's disease, it may seem that the patient is no longer himself or herself, causing loved ones to grieve for the loss of the person they once knew. This is a type of anticipatory grief and should be recognized as a common reaction to a long-term illness like Alzheimer's.

anti-dementia drugs   See ACETYLCHOLINESTERASE INHIBITORS; DONEPEZIL; GALANTAMINE; RIVASTIGMINE; TACRINE.

anti-inflammatory drugs   See NONSTEROIDAL ANTI-INFLAMMATORY DRUGS.

antioxidants   Compounds that fight cell damage caused by FREE RADICALS, a rogue type of oxygen molecule that can attack cells throughout the body. Although free radicals serve important functions, such as helping the immune system fight off disease, at excessive levels they can cause problems. Research suggests that dying brain cells in patients with Alzheimer's disease may be linked to the excess production of free radicals.

Brain cells that produce a mutated form of BETA AMYLOID protein that causes the plaques in Alzheimer's also seem to produce more free radicals. At this point, it's unclear whether free radicals increase the amount of this harmful beta amyloid protein, or whether the protein boosts the levels of free radicals, but several studies have shown that antioxidants can interfere with the harmful effects of beta amyloid protein in tissue culture.

More important, there is growing research that antioxidants may help fight or prevent some of the brain cell damage in Alzheimer's that may be attributed to free radicals, thus slowing the progression of the disease. In particular, there is some evidence that vitamin C or vitamin E can slow down the course of Alzheimer's over several years.

This is exactly what two recent studies suggested. Eating foods rich in vitamins C and E may fend off Alzheimer's disease, according to two studies recently published in the *Journal of the American Medical Association.*

The first study questioned the diets of 815 Chicago residents aged 65 and older who initially had no symptoms of mental decline. After four years, 131 were diagnosed with Alzheimer's. After taking into consideration other factors that affect Alzheimer's risk, the researchers concluded that the people who reported eating the most vitamin E-rich foods had a 70 percent lower risk of developing the disease compared with those who ate the least dietary vitamin E. This study also suggested some protective benefit from vitamin C.

The second study in the Netherlands followed 5,395 people over age 55 for six years, during which time 146 people developed Alzheimer's. These researchers found that high amounts of vitamin C and E lowered the risk of Alzheimer's, even in people who had a gene variant linked to the disease. Taken together, the two studies suggest that antioxidant-rich foods—*but not vitamin supplements*—have a protective effect.

Other studies also found similar benefits in vitamins, some of which did seem to find a benefit with vitamin supplements. In a NATIONAL INSTITUTE OF AGING study, the antioxidant vitamin E delayed by six months progression of some symptoms of Alzheimer's disease. People in the mid- to late stages of Alzheimer's who took vitamin E at levels

70 times higher the recommended daily dose noticed some beneficial effects. At a dose of 2,000 I.U. daily, vitamin E was able to slow the expected rate of decline compared with patients who didn't take the vitamin.

Other studies also suggest that taking antioxidants (vitamins C and E) might significantly lower the risk of developing Alzheimer's. In one preliminary Massachusetts study, none of the 50 subjects who used either vitamin C or E developed Alzheimer's at follow-up studies.

Some scientists suspect that the beneficial effects of ESTROGEN in Alzheimer's disease and on the aging process in healthy women may be partly due to its antioxidant activity. And because soy has estrogen-like properties, some scientists suspect this substance might help protect against the disease, although at least one study reported more decline in mental function among older people who had a high intake of soy. Government studies of estrogen have not found it to have any benefits.

Other antioxidants, such as GINKGO BILOBA and PHOSPHATIDYLSERINE, melatonin, flavonoids (chemicals found in many plants, including tomatoes), and carotenoids (chemicals found in plants such as carrots) have been suggested to ease symptoms of Alzheimer's disease. Small studies of ginkgo did find slight improvement among patients with Alzheimer's who took the herb. Although German physicians have approval to use ginkgo to treat Alzheimer's, and it has been used for thousands of years in Chinese medicine, North American physicians disagree as to its benefits as a memory treatment.

According to several studies, eating plenty of dark-colored fruits and vegetables may slow brain aging. In one recent animal study, extracts taken from blueberries and strawberries reversed age-related decline in brain function. Tiny BLUEBERRIES may be the best anti-Alzheimer's antioxidants of all. When Tufts University researchers analyzed more than 40 fruits and vegetables, they found that raw blueberries contained the highest level of antioxidants (nearly 60 times the recommended daily levels)—more than blackberries, beets, spinach, and garlic. Animals fed an antioxidant-rich blueberry extract diet showed fewer age-related motor changes and outperformed their study counterparts on memory tests.

Some studies on wine have reported a lower risk, but have not been consistent. It might be that wine may increase even more the risk of developing Alzheimer's for people who carry the apoE-4 gene that has been linked to Alzheimer's while protecting people who don't carry the gene.

Side Effects

Supplements containing high doses of antioxidants can cause severe side effects including internal bleeding, and may be toxic in patients taking anticoagulant medication. No one should take these or any supplements without consulting a doctor. In addition, high doses of vitamin E are potentially harmful if combined with blood-thinning drugs.

It's safer to consume antioxidants as part of a healthy diet; antioxidants are found in

- fruits and vegetables (especially blueberries and yellow fruits and vegetables)
- brown rice
- whole grains
- meats
- eggs
- dairy products

antipsychotic drugs Drugs (also known as neuroleptics or major tranquilizers) that are very commonly used to treat a variety of behavior problems typical of patients with DEMENTIA, including restlessness, irritability and aggression, emotional instability, and loss of inhibitions. Experts believe that these drugs should be used in patients with Alzheimer's only as a last resort, after nondrug methods have failed.

All of these drugs can cause sedation or a variety of neurological side effects, such as Parkinson's-like tremors, abnormal movements of the mouth and tongue (dyskinesia), muscle spasms, and restlessness. The restlessness can be particularly confusing for caregivers, since it may seem as if the patient is getting worse rather than better; when this happens, doctors may be tempted to increase the drug further when in fact it should be decreased or stopped.

In the past few years there has been much more use of "atypical" antipsychotics quetiapine (Seroquel), risperidone (Risperdal), and olanzapine (Zyprexa). These seem to be quite effective in some patients in calming restlessness and have relatively fewer side effects than the older drugs, but this does not mean that there are no side effects. Olanzapine can cause weight gain, quetiapine can cause low blood pressure, and risperidone can cause sedation and unsteadiness. Because they are effective in relatively small doses, there is usually little advantage in increasing the dose.

These drugs are typically most useful when a person with dementia experiences hallucinations or delusions. However, Risperdal and Zyprexa may not be safe for patients diagnosed with LEWY BODY DEMENTIA who have visual hallucinations or behavior problems. For these patients, even small doses can produce serious side effects of over-sedation or neurological effects.

anxiety An unpleasant emotional state ranging from mild discomfort to intense fear that may be the result of an elevated level of arousal in the central nervous system. Anxiety is often one of the first signs of Alzheimer's disease, and may occur in as many as half of all patients.

Typically, periods of anxiety occur in late afternoon between 3 P.M. and 7 P.M.—a phenomenon known as SUNDOWNING, which is common not just among patients with Alzheimer's but any other of the dementias as well.

However, many behavioral problems in demented patients are not directly caused by cognitive decline, but instead may be attributed to other factors such as health, medication, and physical and social environment. Coexisting illnesses, impaired vision or hearing, medications, understimulation or overstimulation, lack of familiar cues in the environment, and lack of meaningful activities and social relationships can lead to anxiety as well.

The most common symptoms of anxiety center around the chest, including palpitations (forceful, irregular heartbeat), throbbing or stabbing pains, air hunger, feelings of tightness in the chest, and a tendency to hyperventilate. Other symptoms include headaches, neck spasms, back pain, and an inability to relax, together with restlessness, tremor, and a sense of tiredness. The symptoms of anxiety may include a feeling of impending doom in the absence of any particular threat. Other symptoms include dry mouth, feelings of distention, diarrhea, nausea, appetite change, swallowing problems, and belching.

apathy   Malaise or listlessness that is more common in Alzheimer's disease than DEPRESSION, although the two are often confused in these patients. Apathy responds to stimulants such as methylphenidate (Ritalin), rather than antidepressants. An apathetic patient lacks emotions, motivation, interest, and enthusiasm while a depressed patient is generally very sad, tearful, and hopeless.

aphasia   The loss of the ability to speak or understand spoken, written, or sign language as a result of damage to the corresponding nervous center in the brain. Aphasia is common in patients with Alzheimer's disease.

A person with aphasia might substitute one word for another close to it in meaning, such as saying "music" instead of "radio." Others might use a similar-sounding word ("hat" instead of "cat") or use a completely different word with no apparent link ("banana" instead of "horse").

Some Alzheimer's patients experience a combination of aphasia, constant verbal repetition, and ECHOLALIA (the involuntary repetition of words or phrases), which can make their speech hard to understand.

apoE gene testing   A test for the APOLIPOPROTEIN E (APOE) GENE that, when used with other tests, may help diagnose Alzheimer's disease in people with symptoms of DEMENTIA. However, the apoE test needs to be further evaluated before its use becomes more widespread in helping to diagnose Alzheimer's disease in people with symptoms of dementia. The apoE-4 gene is considered to be an inherited risk factor for Alzheimer's, but the mechanism by which it predisposes people to get Alzheimer's is not yet understood.

Three variations of the apoE gene have been identified—apoE-2, -3, and -4. Preliminary research indicates that the types of apoE genes a person inherits may also affect the age of onset of Alzheimer's. The apoE test can determine which types of apoE an individual has inherited. The apoE-4 is associated with late onset Alzheimer's.

Because the apoE test is commercially available, it is important for physicians to understand its limitations so they can best advise patients and families. The apoE test should not be part of a full diagnostic evaluation nor be used alone to diagnose Alzheimer's. ApoE testing should never be used to predict a person's risk of developing Alzheimer's disease in those without symptoms.

There are several reasons why this test should not be used to predict the risk of Alzheimer's. First, not everyone who carries the apoE-4 gene, which is a risk factor for Alzheimer's, goes on to develop the disease. At the same time, others who don't carry the gene may still develop Alzheimer's, so not having the apoE-4 gene doesn't mean a person is risk free. Since the apoE test can't be used for prediction, sharing test results may be unfairly alarming or comforting to people being tested.

Adequate counseling, education, and support should be provided when considering a diagnosis, including a discussion of the implications of the disease for patients and their families.

See also ALPHA-2-MACROGLOBULIN (A2M); HEREDITY AND ALZHEIMER'S DISEASE.

apolipoprotein E (apoE)   A protein whose main function is to transport CHOLESTEROL. The gene for this protein is on CHROMOSOME 19, and is referred to as the apoE gene. There are three forms of apoE: E-2, E-3, and E-4. ApoE-4 is associated with a higher risk for late onset Alzheimer's disease.

People without apoE-4 have an estimated risk of developing Alzheimer's by age 85 of between 9 percent and 20 percent. In people with one copy of the gene, the risk is between 25 percent and 60 percent. In people with two copies, the risk ranges from 50 percent to 90 percent. Only 2 percent of the population carry two copies of the apoE-4 gene.

See also APOE GENE TESTING; APOLIPOPROTEIN E-4 (apoE-4) GENE; HEREDITY AND ALZHEIMER'S DISEASE.

apolipoprotein E-4 (apoE-4) gene   A gene discovered in 1993 on CHROMOSOME 19, which appears in a particular form in families where Alzheimer's disease has developed at later ages.

The apoE lipoprotein is a part of the body's CHO-LESTEROL transport system.

Although there are three forms of apoE (2, 3, and 4), only apoE-4 is associated with late onset Alzheimer's cases and is considered to be a major risk factor for the disease. This gene is called a susceptibility gene, which means that people who carry it don't automatically develop Alzheimer's. This gene variation occurs in about 15 percent of the general population, but is found in half of those with late onset Alzheimer's. It is more than three times as common in Alzheimer's patients than in people without the disease.

People without apoE-4 have an estimated risk of developing Alzheimer's by age 85 of between 9 percent and 20 percent. In people with one copy of the gene, the risk is between 25 percent and 60 percent. In people with two copies, the risk ranges from 50 percent to 90 percent. Only 2 percent of the population carry two copies of the apoE-4 gene.

Experts think that other factors, such as diseases like DIABETES or atherosclerosis, boost the chance that the gene carrier will develop Alzheimer's. If they do, their brains appear to be more riddled with plaques and tangles than those of Alzheimer's patients who carry slightly different versions of the apoE gene. In addition, apoE-4 seems to have a broad impact on the health of nerve cells. For example, people who carry two copies of apoE-4 have more trouble recovering from strokes and head injuries, and are more likely to sustain brain damage during heart surgery.

Because not everyone with the gene goes on to develop Alzheimer's, and there is no cure, there is little benefit to being screened for the gene.

See also ALPHA-2-MACROGLOBULIN (AZM); APOE GENE TESTING; HEREDITY AND ALZHEIMER'S DISEASE.

apoptosis Programmed cell death. Apoptosis is an important part of brain development that may go awry in Alzheimer's disease, in which abnormal cellular death occurs in parts of the brain essential to learning, memory, attention, and judgment.

Normally, apoptosis is a kind of cell suicide that is an important way to eliminate unnecessary cells, maintain healthy tissues, and target cancer cells. However, a high level of apoptosis in the brain causes irreversible loss of brain function, since most neurons are irreplaceable.

A family of enzymes called caspases is important in the apoptosis process. Columbia University researchers found that BETA AMYLOID induced one particular caspase not only to start apoptosis, but also to kill cells. This study suggests that genetic or drug treatments that target this specific caspase might prevent the cell death associated with beta amyloid and Alzheimer's disease.

There are several other potential ways to prevent apoptosis. One of them involves an enzyme that maintains chromosome structure. Scientists have shown that under certain circumstances, this enzyme can block apoptosis and can decrease vulnerability to cell death triggered by beta amyloid.

appetite Alzheimer's disease affects the appetite, in addition to affecting how much and what type of food patients enjoys. For example, patients may develop a craving for sweets, since they have an altered sensitivity to salty or sweet tastes (usually becoming less sensitive). Patients also may experience changes in the sense of smell.

See also EATING PROBLEMS.

Area Agencies on Aging Groups located in communities across the country that offer services to help older adults remain in their home (if that is their preference) aided by services such as Meals-on-Wheels and homemaker assistance. By offering a range of options, AAAs make it possible for older individuals to choose the services and living arrangements that suit them best.

AAAs were established under the Older Americans Act (OAA) in 1973 to respond to the needs of Americans over age 60. The OAA also helps fund Native American aging programs, known as Title VI, to meet the unique needs of older American Indians, Aleuts, Eskimos, and Hawaiians.

The services available through AAA and Title VI agencies include information and access services, community-based services, in-home services, housing and elder rights. AAAs help

- locate services
- offer health insurance counseling

- provide care management (review an individual's social, psychological, and physical health challenges, resulting in a plan of care for services or treatment, if appropriate)

- provide transportation to critical destinations such as a doctor's office or the grocery store

- offer education and resources to enable caregivers to provide care for an older family member while maintaining his or her own quality of life

- provide retirement planning and education, focusing on pensions, health concerns, legal issues, and work and leisure

- employment services

- senior centers

- group meals served at senior centers, schools, and other sites to provide a nutritious meal in a social environment

- adult day care services

- Meals-on-Wheels

- homemakers (help with tasks essential to maintaining a household, such as food shopping and housekeeping)

- chore services (a step beyond homemaking, including minor home repairs, yard work, and general home maintenance)

- telephone reassurance (regular, prescheduled calls to homebound older adults to reduce isolation and provide a routine safety check)

- friendly visiting (periodic neighborly visits to homebound older adults to provide social contact and reassurance)

- energy assistance and weatherization (payment of fuel bills and home weatherization for low income people)

- emergency response systems (electronic devices which allow individuals to contact a response center in the case of an emergency, such as a fall)

- home health services (a variety of services including skilled nursing care, health monitoring, dispensing of medication, physical and other forms of therapy, and instructing individuals and family members about home care)

- personal care services (assistance with bathing, feeding, walking, and other daily activities)

- respite care (a break for family members from caregiving responsibilities for a short period of time)

- alternative community-based living facilities (a range of housing facilities that bridge the gap between independent living and nursing homes, such as assisted living and adult foster care)

- elder rights

- legal assistance

- elder abuse prevention programs

- ombudsmen services for complaint resolution

AAAs often serve as portals to care, assessing multiple service needs, determining eligibility, authorizing or purchasing services, and monitoring the appropriateness and cost-effectiveness of services. AAAs provide direct services and contract with local providers to furnish other services in the community. All AAAs and Title VI agencies support a range of home and community-based services, but these services vary across communities. While there is much consistency in the types of essential home and community-based services available across the country, these services are customized to reflect varying local needs and resources.

AAAs have more than 25 years' experience administering and coordinating services for older adults. And, as the population has changed over time—with people living longer but facing chronic illness and frailty—AAA services have evolved to meet these new and more challenging needs. AAAs coordinate the provision of low-cost, comprehensive, quality care to millions of older persons nationwide by helping them and their families navigate a complex system of services. In their local communities, these agencies strive to maximize service potential and avoid duplication of effort. They also collaborate with other groups to sponsor events of interest to older adults and their caregivers.

Aricept   See DONEPEZIL.

aromatherapy   The use of familiar smells may help patients with Alzheimer's disease stimulate their senses, stabilize mood swings, retrieve memories, alleviate depression, and modify sleep patterns.

Some experts believe that some fragrances can have a positive effect on mood and behavior, if used properly. While aromatherapy cannot stop the progression of Alzheimer's nor cure DEMENTIA, it does seem to be able to ease some common symptoms, making patients less anxious and lethargic, easing depression, and providing positive long-term memory associations and sensory stimulation.

Smell travels faster to the brain than any of the other senses, and can affect learning, memory, sexual attraction, and even buying habits. And in what may be an important benefit to Alzheimer's patients, the mental recall of smells is retained longer than any other sense. Still, a person's sense of smell can diminish through aging, or be completely lost after a traumatic head injury or stroke. Some scientists believe that some demented patients eventually lose their sense of smell altogether.

While scientists believe humans can identify about 10,000 different smells, they are only just starting to understand how the olfactory system works. Aromatherapy experts believe that the positive benefits of odors are derived from the botanical and chemical makeup of essential oils that are extracted from leaves, flowers, and fruit. These complex essential oils may include up to 100 constituents that, when combined, give each oil a unique aroma and therapeutic properties.

Many European Alzheimer's centers use lavender to ease symptoms among their patients. They believe the organic constituents extracted from the plant's flower during processing provide a calming, relaxing, decongestive, or cleansing effect among patients. Inhaling molecules of the essential oil allows these chemicals to pass through the mucous membrane in the nose to the bloodstream, which is why someone who has lost the sense of smell may still receive benefits from organic oils by inhaling them as well as through skin absorption.

Essential oils have been used since the ancient Egyptian times, when pharaohs would use the oils for religious rituals and as herbal remedies. Today's aromatherapy practitioners have created long lists of essential oils and their properties available in libraries, bookstores, and on the Internet. The oils are available in grocery stores, holistic health specialty shops, and other places that offer health-related products.

Essential oils may be used in several different ways, beginning with a simple method of slicing open a fresh fruit and letting the patient take in the fresh scent. Essential oils also can be used in electric heat diffusers; in spritzers or lotion dispensers; or placed on pillows or lamp rings. Oils may be placed on pillows, lamp rings, washcloths, tissues, or cotton balls, or diluted with a vegetable oil or lotion for massage.

The amount of oil that should be used depends on the room size, the number of patients, the strength of the oil, and the patient's sensitivity. Each patient responds differently to aromatherapy, so that what may help to ease one patient's anxiety might have no effect on another's.

Because essential oils are highly concentrated, a few drops usually are sufficient. Essential oils should never be applied directly to the skin; instead, the oils should be blended with lotion or water, or diffused into the air.

Aromatherapy should not be used as a room deodorizer, nor should synthetic or inorganic substances be used. These scents are not meant for therapeutic uses, and can cause more allergic reactions and problems from inhalation and skin contact.

Aromatherapy may be useful for patients in different stages of Alzheimer's disease. For patients in earlier stages, scents may spark reminiscence. Even those in later stages, whose sense of smell could be impaired, may benefit, although it might take some extra work.

artificial feeding Patients with advanced Alzheimer's disease sometimes find it impossible to eat and drink normally. If artificial food and fluids aren't provided, death from dehydration usually occurs in three to 14 days. Feeding tubes are often used in this situation, even though the benefits and risk of this therapy are not clear.

Using artificial feeding, patients can be kept alive for years by giving liquid nutrition and fluids through a catheter inserted into a vein, or via tubes inserted into the intestines or stomach. Such feeding must be carefully monitored to avoid digestive problems like vomiting, diarrhea, or pneumonia. Other risks include infection and bleeding when tubes are surgically implanted, and erosion and damage to the nasal passage, esophagus, stomach, or intestines.

In one recent study, Johns Hopkins researchers found that while the risks of tube feeding were substantial, there were no data to suggest that tube feeding was helpful. It did not appear to prevent ASPIRATION PNEUMONIA, prolong survival, reduce the risk of sores or infections, improve function, or keep the patient comfortable. In an article published in the *Journal of the American Medical Association* in 1999, the researchers concluded that hand feeding is the proper treatment for severely demented patients with eating problems.

According to the ALZHEIMER'S ASSOCIATION, if a severely and irreversibly demented patient rejects food and water by mouth, it is ethically permissible to withhold food and water artificially administered by vein or gastric tube. In 1999, the Alzheimer's Association's ethics advisory panel, made up of top ethicists from around the country, reviewed this position and continue to support it.

However, artificial feeding is often routine if patients have no living will stating that they don't want tube feeding or supplemental fluids. Even with a living will that stipulates no tube feeding, some nursing homes still require the procedure.

art therapy   A type of treatment using different forms of art that may help fight the depression often felt by people with Alzheimer's disease. In Britain, researchers discovered that patients who took part in art therapy became much more relaxed and sociable during the very first session, and their depression scores dropped markedly over the 10 weeks of the treatment.

Experts recommend that when engaging in art therapy, patients should:

- not be given childlike projects; crayons or anything else that might be demeaning should be avoided
- be encouraged to discuss the process, with creative storytelling or reminiscence

- be helped to begin the activity. If the patient is painting, the caregiver may need to start the brush movement.
- be given safe materials, avoiding sharp tools
- be given plenty of time to complete the art project. The person doesn't have to finish the project in one sitting.

aspartic acid   See VITAMINS.

aspiration pneumonia   A type of pneumonia that can occur in patients with Alzheimer's disease when food is inhaled into the lungs. In this condition, a patient inhales food or another substance that becomes lodged within the lungs. The substance then acts as a breeding ground for infection, which eventually leads to pneumonia. Aspiration pneumonia is a common cause of death among patients with Alzheimer's.

assessment tools   There are a number of tests that can be given to help diagnose Alzheimer's disease. Scientists are beginning to understand how certain abilities are linked with specific regions of the brain, so that a person's performance on a test measuring these abilities suggests' whether the associated areas of the brain are functioning properly.

Symptoms associated with Alzheimer's primarily affect thought processes, but there are often other behavioral or physical conditions that can make it hard to assess problems in one area of functioning. Symptoms also vary from person to person, and by how far the disease has progressed.

Current assessment tools are designed to evaluate several areas of function, including cognition, function, behavior, general physical health, and quality of life. Other tests measure very specific abilities, such as short-term or long-term memory, language, attention, abstract thought, and abilities of perception and orientation. Some of these tests are often part of the diagnostic workup for patients with dementia. The resulting pattern of strengths and weaknesses can offer useful information about the person's illness, and how the patient can best compensate for problems.

Full neuropsychological testing, which may take as long as four hours, may be useful for scientists trying to detect the earliest symptoms of Alzheimer's disease, track symptoms through the course of the disease, or measure the effects of experimental treatments.

Most assessment tools are designed to be completed either by the patient in the early stages of disease, the caregiver, or the patient's physician. Most often, a combination of tests should be used to evaluate the patient's overall condition.

For patients with Alzheimer's disease, no single test can simultaneously assess all areas of functioning. Typical neuropsychological tests may include assessments based on caregiver input, thinking ability, function, and overall performance.

Caregiver-based Tests

- Behavioral Pathology in Alzheimer's Disease Rating Scale (BEHAVE-AD)
- Neuropsychiatric Inventory (NPI)

Cognitive Tests

- Alzheimer's Disease Assessment Scale, cognitive subsection (ADAS-cog)
- Blessed Information-Memory-Concentration Test (BIMC)
- Clinical Dementia Rating Scale (CDR)
- Mini-Mental Status Examination (MMSE)

Functional Assessments

- Functional Assessment Questionnaire (FAQ)
- Instrumental Activities of Daily Living (IADL)
- Physical Self-Maintenance Scale (PSMS)
- Progressive Deterioration Scale (PDS)

Global Tests

- Clinical Global Impression of Change (CGIC)
- Clinical Interview-Based Impression (CIBI)
- Global Deterioration Scale (GDS)

assisted living   A special combination of housing, personalized supportive services, and health care designed to meet the needs of people typically in the early or middle stages of Alzheimer's disease who need help with ACTIVITIES OF DAILY LIVING. These residential settings maximize independence, but do not provide skilled nursing care. Assisted living may offer the same features as independent living communities, with the added assistance of personal care. It is designed to meet the individual needs of those requiring help with activities of daily living, who do not need the skilled medical care provided in a nursing home.

Assisted living residences, also called personal care, residential care, or domiciliary care, may be part of a retirement community, nursing home, elderly housing, or they may stand alone.

Assisted living residences may include anything ranging from a high-rise apartment complex to a converted Victorian home. Residences may be single homes or grouped with other residential options, such as independent living or nursing care; facilities usually have between 25 and 120 units. The goal of assisted living is to help the client continue to live as independently as possible.

Assisted living facilities may be operated by nonprofit or for-profit companies, and although regulations vary from state to state, some states require special staff certification and training. All residences must comply with local building codes and fire safety regulations. The exact definition will vary from state to state, and a few states do not license assisted living facilities. Generally regarded as one to two steps below skilled nursing in level of care.

Services

Services provided in assisted living residences usually include three meals a day served in a common dining area; housekeeping assistance; transportation; help with eating, bathing, dressing, toileting, and walking; access to health and medical services; 24-hour security; individual emergency call systems; exercise programs; medication management; laundry services; and social and recreational activities.

Costs

Costs vary with the type of residence, room size, and the range of services the resident needs, but daily basic fees range from $15 to $200. Many facilities charge a basic fee that covers all services; some facilities add on additional charges for special services. In addition, most assisted living residences charge a monthly rate, and a few residences require long-term arrangements.

The costs of care at these facilities are usually paid by the families or residents themselves; about 90 percent of the country's assisted living services are paid for with private funds, although some states have adopted Medicaid waiver programs.

Costs may be reimbursed if they are covered under health insurance or long-term care insurance. Some facilities also offer financial assistance programs, since government coverage for assisted living residences has been limited. Some state and local governments do offer subsidies for rent or services for low income elders; others may provide subsidies in the form of an additional payment for those who receive Supplemental Security Income (SSI) or Medicaid. Some states also use Medicaid waiver programs to help pay for assisted living services.

See also ASSISTED LIVING FEDERATION OF AMERICA.

Assisted Living Federation of America
An association that represents more than 7,000 for-profit and nonprofit providers of assisted living, CONTINU-ING CARE RETIREMENT COMMUNITIES, independent living, and other forms of housing and services. Founded in 1990 to support the assisted living industry and enhance the quality of life for the consumers it serves, ALFA broadened its membership in 1999 to embrace the full range of housing and care providers who share a consumer-focused philosophy of care. For contact information, see Appendix I.

See also ASSISTED LIVING.

association areas
A part of the brain that is not concerned with primary sensory processing, but that has a secondary role in integrating sensory information with other brain systems. Many scientists suspect that these areas play a large role in thinking and memory.

autoimmune disorders
The body's immune system protects against potentially harmful foreign invaders, but it can sometimes begin to attack its own tissues by mistake, producing antibodies to its own cells. This is called an autoimmune response, and it is responsible for many diseases, such as lupus and probably multiple sclerosis.

Many autoimmune disorders have been associated in one way or another with improper functioning of the immune system. Some experts speculate that certain changes in aging brain cells might trigger an autoimmune response that produces symptoms of Alzheimer's in vulnerable individuals. In fact, some anti-brain antibodies have been identified in the brains of those with Alzheimer's disease, but scientists aren't sure what this means since these antibodies also have been found in the brains of people without Alzheimer's disease. Even if changes are occurring in brain cells to trigger an autoimmune response, what originally set off these brain cell changes is not known.

autopsy
Examination of a body organ and tissue after death. An autopsy is often performed (upon request) to confirm a diagnosis of Alzheimer's disease. An autopsy usually provides the family with a definitive diagnosis as to whether or not the patient did indeed have Alzheimer's, which may be important to other family members, especially as scientists learn more about the genetics of Alzheimer's disease. An autopsy is vital for researchers, who need autopsy material to continue studies relating to the cause, treatment, and cure of Alzheimer's disease.

In cases where Alzheimer's disease is suspected, only the brain tissue needs to be examined; a complete autopsy is not necessary. The procedure can be performed in most mortuaries or hospitals. A complete autopsy usually costs several thousand dollars and is not reimbursed by insurance. However, Alzheimer Research Centers supported by the National Institutes of Health are able to provide an examination of the brain without charge to the family. These services are offered for patients with dementia, as well as healthy patients serving as controls, who are preenrolled in the research center's programs.

An autopsy is not disfiguring and does not interfere with a customary funeral or burial plans. Ideally, a family should decide whether they will want an autopsy well before the time of death. Brain tissue is most valuable when the mental abilities of the patient have been carefully studied before death, and when only a few hours have elapsed between death and the removal of brain tissue.

However, the Alzheimer's Association Medical and Scientific Advisory Board recommends that the body organs of a patient with Alzheimer's disease not be donated for transplant purposes.

The Baltimore Longitudinal Study of Aging (BLSA)   An ongoing study of one group of individuals to reveal how biology and behavior change as people get older. The BLSA began in 1958 as a small project involving a few men, but it now includes more than 1,200 men and women from ages 20 to 90 who undergo testing every two years. Participants return to the NATIONAL INSTITUTE OF AGING'S Gerontology Research Center in Baltimore, Maryland, to undergo tests of attention, problem solving, memory, personality, and other behavior. The BLSA is the longest-running study of human aging whose findings have influenced medical practice and the directions of aging research.

basal forebrain   An area in the deep region of the forebrain containing neurons that release the neurotransmitter ACETYLCHOLINE, typically found in much lower levels among patients with Alzheimer's disease. The basal forebrain includes the medial septum, which projects to the HIPPOCAMPUS; the band of Broca, which projects to the hippocampus and AMYGDALA; and the nucleus basalis of Meynert, which projects to the neocortex and amygdala. Damage to these structures of the brain is believed to contribute to the development of Alzheimer's.

basal ganglia   Clusters of nuclei deep within the cerebrum and the upper parts of the brain stem that play an important part in developing skills and habits, and that may also help coordinate thinking. Fibers pass from almost every region of the CEREBRAL CORTEX to the basal ganglia, and are then transmitted back to the supplementary motor area and premotor cortex of the frontal lobe.

bathing problems   Many people with Alzheimer's disease become frightened or resistant at bath time. DEPRESSION or illness may make patients lose interest in personal hygiene. A damaged hypothalamus (the body's "internal thermostat" regulator) could cause a changed sense of perception of hot and cold water temperature. BRAIN damage could also cause a different sensation of water. Patients with Alzheimer's may not be able to find the bathroom, or experience fears of falling or of water itself. Patients may be uncomfortable with the lack of privacy or unhappy about the disruption in their daily routine, they may forget why taking a bath is important, or feel humiliated by having to be reminded to take a bath.

Bathing may be easier if the caregiver can find the best time of day for the patient's bath and follow the patient's familiar bathing routines. Patients should be encouraged to do as much of the bathing themselves as possible. At first, verbal reminders to take a bath may be all that are needed. Eventually, CUES for each part of the process may become necessary.

behavioral neurologist   A physician who specializes in the diagnosis and treatment of behavioral and memory disorders caused by BRAIN disease. A typical neurological evaluation takes about one to two hours and involves testing for sensory and movement problems as well as a brief review of mental function. The neurologist may prescribe medications to treat the memory disorder or troublesome behavioral symptoms.

Behavioral Pathology in Alzheimer's Disease Rating Scale (BEHAVE-AD)   An ASSESSMENT TOOL used to evaluate possible Alzheimer's disease that provides a global rating of noncognitive symptoms. The test is designed for use in assessing the efficacy of prospective clinical drugs.

behavioral symptoms   Among patients with Alzheimer's disease, behavioral symptoms relate to action or emotion, such as WANDERING, DEPRESSION, ANXIETY, AGITATION, hostility, and sleep disturbances.

In the early stages of the disease, people with Alzheimer's may experience personality changes such as irritability, anxiety, or depression. As the disease progresses, other symptoms may appear, including sleep disturbances, DELUSIONS, HALLUCINATIONS, PACING, constant movement or restlessness, checking and rechecking, tearing movements, emotional distress, and cursing or threatening language.

Scientists are working to develop drugs that ease the behavioral symptoms of Alzheimer's disease.

behavioral treatment   Because problem behavior is a part of Alzheimer's disease, there are several kinds of effective treatments designed to help control behavior beginning with nondrug methods.

Behavior can be immediately affected by different lighting, color, and noise; dim lighting may make some people with Alzheimer's uneasy, and loud or erratic noise can exacerbate confusion and frustration. This is particularly apparent as evening approaches; in the SUNDOWNING effect, patients become more confused, restless, and agitated as day fades into night.

Ideally, patients should remain active for as long as possible, engaging in activities such as singing, playing music, painting, walking, playing with a pet, or reading. Behavior is best managed if established routines are maintained for bathing, dressing, cooking, cleaning, and laundry.

Once behavior deteriorates significantly, symptoms can be treated with medication: DONEPEZIL, RIVASTIGMINE, or GALANTAMINE; that are used to improve thinking and memory may also improve behavior. Several other drugs can treat problem behaviors, including antipsychotics such as HALOPERIDOL (Haldol); ANTIANXIETY DRUGS such ALPRAZOLAM (Xanax), buspirone (Buspar), or diazepam (Valium); or some of the newest antidepressants such as fluvoxamine (Prozac), nefazodone (Serzone), or paroxetine (Paxil).

benzodiazepines   Tranquilizers used to treat ANXIETY that may be effective in some patients with Alzheimer's disease. As many as half of all patients with Alzheimer's become anxious and may make demands for constant company and reassurance. Unfortunately, a paradoxical effect has been noted in Alzheimer's patients, in which the administration of benzodiazepines leads to increased confusion, disorientation, and ultimately, even greater agitation and anxiety.

Short-lived periods of anxiety, such as in response to a stressful event, may be helped by benzodiazepines. Continuous treatment in excess of two to four weeks is not a good idea because dependency can occur, making it difficult to stop the medication without withdrawal symptoms.

Benzodiazepines work by depressing BRAIN function, relieving anxiety, and promoting sleep, slowing down the activity of nerves that control many mental and physical functions.

The first benzodiazepine was marketed as an ANTIANXIETY DRUG in 1960 under the trade name Librium; three years later, its relative, Valium (diazepam), was introduced. The benzodiazepines are still widely used because they can relieve anxiety while being much less sedating and dangerous than barbiturates. Benzodiazepines can strengthen the sedating effects of ALCOHOL or barbiturates, and can also increase their depressant effects on important brain centers.

Side Effects

There are many different benzodiazepines, some with a short duration of action (lorazepam and oxazepam) and some with longer action such (chlordiazepoxide and diazepam). All of these drugs may cause excessive sedation, unsteadiness, and a tendency to fall, and they may worsen confusion and MEMORY deficits that are already present.

Major TRANQUILIZERS are often used for severe or persistent anxiety, but if taken for long periods these drugs can produce a side effect called TARDIVE DYSKINESIA—persistent involuntary chewing movements and facial grimacing. This may be irreversible, but is more likely to disappear if it is recognized early and the medication causing the problem stopped.

beta amyloid (beta-amyloid)   A specific type of small protein found normally in humans and animals, but that also appears in dense deposits called plaques in the BRAIN of a patient with Alzheimer's disease. Proteins are vital molecules that control all sorts of processes in the body. Amyloid protein occurs naturally in the brain, but as people age, too much of it in a form called beta amyloid builds up in the brain.

In the 1980s, scientists discovered that the Alzheimer's disease plaques were made primarily of the deposit of beta amyloid. In Alzheimer's patients, beta amyloid does not dissolve, as it does in healthy people, but instead accumulates into fibrils, which stick together to form the plaques. Therefore, the problem in Alzheimer's patients is not the presence of beta amyloid, but having too much of the substance or being unable to dispose of it normally.

The plaques and tangles caused by beta amyloid disrupt brain function by killing brain cells; as they die, they cannot be replaced, unlike other cells in the body, and symptoms of Alzheimer's appear. As more brain cells die, the brain cannot communicate with the body, eventually causing the body to shut down completely.

Scientists are just beginning to learn how beta amyloid is formed—and it starts with AMYLOID-PRECURSOR PROTEIN (APP), a large protein that protrudes through the neuron membrane, part inside and part outside the cell. While it is embedded in the membrane, enzymes snip it in two, creating a beta amyloid fragment. What happens to the beta amyloid segment once it separates from APP is less clear, although scientists do know that large amounts of the beta protein end up in Alzheimer's plaques in the brain. After the enzyme clips the APP, the resulting beta amyloid fragments then clump together in deposits. Scientists don't know whether these deposits are caused by too much beta amyloid, or whether the enzymes that usually break it down are not functioning properly.

Many studies have concentrated on how beta amyloid is processed, searching for abnormalities that could explain what goes wrong. Others are seeking clues in the environment surrounding the protein.

Some scientists are studying how beta amyloid affects nearby brain cells. In one study, cells in the HIPPOCAMPUS died when beta amyloid was added to the cell culture, which suggests that the protein is toxic to neurons. Another study suggested that when beta amyloid breaks into fragments, it releases toxic FREE RADICALS that attack neurons. Exactly how beta amyloid kills neurons is still unknown, but some scientists suspect that beta amyloid forms tiny channels in brain cell membranes that allow uncontrolled—and fatal—amounts of CALCIUM into the neuron. Still other studies suggest that beta amyloid interferes with potassium channels, which could also affect calcium levels. And some scientists think that beta amyloid may lower CHOLINE concentrations in neurons; since neurons need choline to produce ACETYLCHOLINE, this finding suggests a link between beta amyloid and the death of cholinergic neurons.

See also AMYLOID PLAQUES; TAU PROTEIN.

beta carotene (beta-carotene)   Preliminary studies suggest that levels of vitamin A and its precursor, beta carotene, may be significantly lower in people with Alzheimer's disease compared to healthy individuals, but the effects of supplementation have not been studied.

See also ANTIOXIDANTS.

beta secretase (beta-secretase)   An enzyme believed to be involved in the formation of BETA AMYLOID—fragments of protein that clump together to form the sticky plaques characteristic of Alzheimer's disease. Plaques begin to form in Alzheimer's when beta-secretase and a related enzyme called GAMMA SECRETASE snip a larger protein into the shorter fragment known as beta amyloid.

beta-secretase inhibitors   A substance that interferes with the enzyme BETA SECRETASE, blocking the production of BETA AMYLOID, a protein that collects into plaques in the BRAINS of people with Alzheimer's disease. Scientists believe these plaques kill brain cells and lead to the thought and memory problems common in Alzheimer's.

Binswanger's disease   An extremely rare form of DEMENTIA that may be confused with Alzheimer's disease. This condition is characterized by lesions in the white matter deep inside the brain, resulting in loss of memory, thinking, and learning. The disease is a slowly progressive condition for which there is no cure, often marked by strokes and partial recovery. Patients with this disorder usually die within five years after its onset.

In addition to memory and learning problems, patients with Binswanger's disease usually show signs of abnormal blood pressure, stroke, blood problems, mood disorders, disease of the large blood vessels in the neck, and disease of the heart valves. Other prominent features of the disease include urinary incontinence, difficulty walking, parkinsonian-like tremors, and depression. These symptoms, which tend to begin after the age of 60, are not always present in all patients and may sometimes appear only as a passing phase. Seizures may also be present.

There is no specific treatment for Binswanger's disease. Medications can be used to control high blood pressure, depression, abnormal heart rhythms, and low blood pressure.

biological markers   A component of a person's body, such as a protein or gene, that can be measured to determine whether the person has a particular disease. At one time or another scientists have studied more than 70 different substances in the blood, skin, and spinal fluid as possible biological markers for Alzheimer's disease.

If researchers could identify an accurate biological marker for Alzheimer's disease, the diagnosis of the disease in living patients would be much simpler. In addition, an effective biomarker would be helpful in predicting the onset of Alzheimer's, and monitoring its progression and response to treatment.

Several tests have already been marketed to clinicians, patients, and families concerned about Alzheimer's and also to people without symptoms curious about their own risk.

For inherited cases of EARLY ONSET ALZHEIMER'S DISEASE, it is now possible to test for mutations in the genes associated with this form of the disease: presenilin 1 (PS1) on CHROMOSOME 14, presenilin 2 (PS2) on CHROMOSOME 1, and AMYLOID PRECURSOR PROTEIN (APP) on CHROMOSOME 21. These relatively rare mutations are currently known to exist in only 120 families around the world. Experts believe that testing for these genes should be limited to those individuals with a family history of early onset Alzheimer's.

In all other cases of Alzheimer's disease, detecting an e4 version of the apoE gene on CHROMOSOME 19 can strengthen a diagnosis of Alzheimer's. However, some experts believe that apoE testing should be carried out only after doctors have already made a diagnosis of probable Alzheimer's. ApoE testing should not be used as a diagnostic test, and is not appropriate for people without symptoms, because it is not always accurate.

BRAIN scans that can detect brain shrinkage and slowed brain metabolism and blood flow are now being tested as possible biomarkers in the future.

Other biomarkers have not yet achieved wide acceptance among researchers and are not recommended for widespread use:

- skin test for amyloid deposits
- eye drop test (pupil dilation using tropicamide)
- testing for AD7C neuronal thread proteins
- blood test to measure levels of iron binding protein p97

Blessed Information-Memory-Concentration Test (BIMC)   An ASSESSMENT TOOL used to evaluate possible Alzheimer's disease that provides a quick test of thinking skills. The test, which takes about 10 minutes, assesses ACTIVITIES OF DAILY LIVING and memory/concentration/orientation.

blood pressure   Patients with high blood pressure may have as much as twice the risk of developing Alzheimer's disease as healthy people. A growing but not entirely consistent body of research points to a possible association between Alzheimer's and one or both of two major heart-disease risk factors—high blood pressure and high levels of CHOLESTEROL.

In one Finnish study published in the June 16, 2001, issue of the *British Medical Journal*, researchers looked at Alzheimer's levels in a group of 1,449 men and women who had been examined an average of 21 years earlier as part of an overall health study that included data on blood pressure and cholesterol levels. After examining the participants again in 1998, researchers found that 48 met the criteria for Alzheimer's disease. After analyzing the data, the researchers concluded that participants who had high cholesterol levels or high systolic blood pressure in middle age were about twice as likely to develop Alzheimer's disease as those who did not, even after accounting for age, weight, history of heart problems, and other factors. The risk was 3.5 times higher for those who had both high blood pressure *and* high cholesterol. There was no increased risk for people who had high diastolic pressure (the second of the two numbers in a blood pressure reading).

Studies in Sweden and Japan have found an association between Alzheimer's disease and high blood pressure, but the form of hypertension in these cases was diastolic, unlike the Finnish study.

Some experts think a link between high blood pressure and Alzheimer's makes sense since high systolic pressure could compromise blood flow to certain parts of the BRAIN; this could trigger production of more BETA AMYLOID proteins, one of the components that causes cell death in Alzheimer's.

blood tests There is no blood test that can definitely diagnose Alzheimer's disease, but these tests may be used to help rule out other medical conditions that cause DEMENTIA. This is why a series of blood tests is routinely requested to look for abnormalities associated with causes of dementia other than Alzheimer's disease, including assessments of electrolyte balance, thyroid function, liver function, syphilis infection, vitamin deficiencies, and autoimmune disorders.

Several new blood tests now in development may be used to predict the onset of dementing disease. One recent study found that elderly people with high levels of the amino acid HOMOCYSTEINE have nearly twice the risk of developing the disease. By testing for homocysteine and a harmful gene that doubles the risk of Alzheimer's, plus reviewing a patient's family history of longevity and the disease, it might be possible to accurately predict who is at risk.

Previous studies have shown people with Alzheimer's and other forms of dementia have higher levels of homocysteine in their blood than other people, but more recent studies have documented high levels in people years before they developed Alzheimer's.

Homocysteine levels can be lowered by getting more FOLIC ACID and related B vitamins, but scientists say more research is needed to show whether lowering homocysteine levels can ward off Alzheimer's. Researchers already know that elevated homocysteine levels can raise the risk of heart disease and STROKE, and stroke can increase the risk of dementia.

A different blood test now used on mice may one day predict Alzheimer's in humans long before symptoms appear, according to researchers at Washington University. The scientists used a simple blood test to track the buildup of neuron-killing BETA-AMYLOID protein associated with Alzheimer's disease in the brains of living mice. The new test uses an antibody that pulls the proteins into the blood to show researchers how the disease is developing in the BRAIN.

Although the test has not been used in humans (it may be 10 years before the test is available), experts say it is a potentially useful tool for detecting the disease 10 to 20 years before permanent damage occurs in the brain. The test also could be used to develop drugs that could stop or slow the progression of Alzheimer's disease.

Presently, the only way to diagnose the disease before death is to give MEMORY tests and neurological exams, but those methods are only helpful after brain cells start to die and symptoms appear.

In the studies of the new test, Washington University researchers studied mice genetically engineered to develop brain lesions and BEHAVIORAL SYMPTOMS similar to those of people with inherited Alzheimer's. The scientists injected middle-aged mice with an antibody that draws beta-amyloid protein out of the brain, and then compared the levels of beta amyloid in the mice's blood with samples taken before the antibody injection. When the scientists examined the brains of the mice, they found the amount of beta amyloid pulled into the blood was linked to the appearance of plaques and tangles that mark the beginning of Alzheimer's symptoms. If the test can be adapted for use in humans, it could be an effective screening method to warn people that they are at risk for developing the disease.

blood vessel theory of Alzheimer's disease   Some experts think that Alzheimer's disease may be caused by defects in blood vessels supplying blood to the BRAIN. Several studies have found that the protein BETA AMYLOID, the primary component of one of the brain lesions associated with Alzheimer's disease, seems to trigger blood vessels to constrict. The constriction is caused by the production of toxic FREE RADICALS as the beta amyloid interacts with certain cells on the blood vessels. This could increase the level of free radicals while decreasing blood flow to the brain. As oxygen and glucose levels drop and free radicals proliferate, brain cells can begin to die.

Scientists were able to prevent blood vessels from constricting by pretreating them with ANTIOXIDANTS (substances that eliminate free radicals). Studies in humans with Alzheimer's disease have failed to show the benefits of estrogen therapy. It is possible that antioxidants and estrogens are most effective before the onset of symptoms.

blueberries   A potent ANTIOXIDANT that may boost MEMORY performance. When Tufts University researchers analyzed more than 40 fruits and vegetables, they found that raw blueberries contained the highest level of antioxidants (nearly 60 times the recommended daily levels)—far more than blackberries, beets, spinach, and garlic.

Moreover, animals fed an antioxidant-rich blueberry extract diet showed fewer age-related motor changes and outperformed their study counterparts on memory tests.

board and care homes   A type of residential health care for elderly people and patients with Alzheimer's disease that involves more care than ASSISTED LIVING but less than would be available in a NURSING HOME. Also called personal-care homes or residential care facilities, board and care homes are often single-family houses in quiet, residential neighborhoods serving fewer than 10 residents.

The caregivers (usually two per home) are health-care aides, not registered nurses. Some board and care facilities provide 24-hour care for very frail seniors who don't need ongoing medical attention but might otherwise have to go to a nursing home. In the best situations, residents of board and care homes feel part of a family, eating in a dining room and enjoying social activities in the home. Board and care homes usually cost less than $1,000 a month.

brain   The jellylike major organ of the human nervous system that is part of a complex network of nerve cells and fibers responsible for controlling all the processes in the body. Sensations from nerves extending from the central nervous system to every other part of the body are received, sorted and interpreted by the brain.

The brain is split into two halves, called hemispheres—a left and a right—separated by a groove. The corpus callosum is a band of fibers that helps each half of the brain communicate with the other. Although the two halves look identical, they control different parts of the body. The left side of the brain controls the right side of the body, and the right brain controls the left side. This is because the nerves to each side of the body cross over at the top of the spinal cord. Although the two hemispheres are linked by the corpus callosum and share information, one half of the brain is always considered dominant. Right-handed people almost always have a dominant left hemisphere. Most left-handed people probably also have a dominant left hemisphere.

In addition, each half of the brain specializes in certain areas. The right hemisphere also controls painting, music, and creative activities, recognizing faces, shapes, and patterns, judging size and distance. It is also the seat of imagination, emotion, and insight.

The left hemisphere is the center of speech, reading and understanding language, understanding mathematics and performing calculations, and writing and language. It is the logical, problem-solving side of the brain. On each side of the brain are three main areas: the extension of the spinal cord deep within the brain called the brain stem, the cerebellum, and the cerebrum.

The brain stem controls basic body functions like heart rate and breathing that are responsible for life, and typically operates without any conscious control. It is made up of the midbrain, the medulla, and the pons.

Right behind the brain stem is a small apricot-sized cerebellum, responsible for controlling coordination and balance.

The largest area of the brain is the cerebrum, whose four sections completely wrap around the midbrain. It is this area that handles conscious and complicated jobs like thinking, speaking, and reading. The gray outer surface of the cerebrum, as wrinkled as a walnut, is the cerebral cortex. It is in the cortex that sensory messages are received and interpreted, and where all the brain's orders are sent. While its wrinkled surface doesn't take up much space within the skull, if it were flattened out the cerebral cortex would cover an average office desk.

Deep within the brain, in front of the brain stem, are a variety of structures of crucial importance in maintaining body functions, including the thalamus, hypothalamus, basal ganglia, and pituitary gland.

The four lobes of the brain are broad surface regions in each hemisphere that are named for the bones of the skull lying above them: the frontal, parietal, temporal, and occipital lobes. The frontal lobe is the seat of a person's personality, and the critical area for thought. Within the parietal lobe are areas that control pain, and sensations of itching, heat, and cold. It is the occipital lobe's job to interpret what a person sees.

The HIPPOCAMPUS is the part of the brain that is considered to be the gatekeeper of memory, and the part of the brain most often affected by Alzheimer's disease. A ridge along a fissure of the brain, it is one of the most ancient parts. A paired organ found on each side of the brain, it directly links nerve fibers involved in senses (touch, vision, sound, and smell) and the limbic system. Most researchers believe that the hippocampus and its interconnected neural structures register and temporarily hold new information, binding together the elements of environment, odors, and sounds that constitute a remembered episode. Research also suggests that the hippocampus also creates certain unconscious memories. This theory suggests that the role of the hippocampus in MEMORY is to relate different elements of experience.

Many scientists believe that the hippocampus is part of a large learning system that works in parallel with other forebrain learning systems.

See also BRAIN ATROPHY; BRAIN CELLS; BRAIN SCANS.

brain atrophy   Shrinking of the size of the BRAIN is a hallmark of patients with Alzheimer's disease. The shrinking of brain mass begins early in the disease, originating in the HIPPOCAMPUS, the part of the brain vital to learning and memory. Brain scans have shown that as brain atrophy continues, symptoms of Alzheimer's disease become more pronounced.

brain cells   There are two kinds of brain cells: neurons and glia. While most brain cells are glia (85 percent), it is the remaining 15 percent—the neurons—that make the brain the most important organ in the body.

Glial cells play a supportive role in the BRAIN, helping to remove waste products, supplying nutrients, and maintaining electrical balance. Neurons, on the other hand, control the body's emotions, activities, and the ability to think.

Neurons in the brain are structurally the same as nerve cells throughout the body, with a main cell body composed of a nucleus and cytoplasm. The nucleus contains the genetic material that allows a cell to reproduce; the cytoplasm provides energy for the cell. Neurons have very long extensions called axons; at the end of each axon are many branches that touch a neighboring neuron. This is what makes communication between neurons possible.

brain-derived neurotrophic factor   A substance that helps amplify nerve signals important in maintaining a healthy nervous system.

See also NERVE GROWTH FACTORS; NEUROTROPHIC FACTOR.

brain imaging   See BRAIN SCANS.

brain scans   An important group of diagnostic tests increasingly used as a tool to detect changes in

BRAIN anatomy and function. Brain scans can be used to rule out physical causes of DEMENTIA, such as a brain tumor. Recently, scientists have developed the first brain scan technique to image the earliest evidence of Alzheimer's disease in the living brain before the disorder begins attacking brain cells. Reported in the January 2002 issue of the *American Journal of Geriatric Psychiatry,* the newest technique will allow doctors to monitor the disease as it unfolds—speeding DIAGNOSIS, intervention, and new therapies for Alzheimer's.

Brain scans are generally divided into those that measure brain *structure* (such as CT and MRI scans) and those that measure brain *function* (such as PET and SPECT scans). The newest research technique pairs PET scanning with a new chemical marker called FDDNP to see for the first time the brain lesions that are the hallmark of Alzheimer's disease in a living patient.

In the new method, scientists inject a tracer molecule that zeroes in on the AMYLOID PLAQUES and tangles caused by Alzheimer's disease; they can then watch the molecule's progress on a PET scan.

When Alzheimer's disease strikes, the MEMORY center is the first location where plaques take root and destroy brain cells, so it's the first place where scientists must seek evidence of the disease. This noninvasive method can help doctors monitor new VACCINES and drugs designed to prevent and treat the brain damage caused by Alzheimer's disease.

Scientists discovered that PET scans of patients injected with FDDNP showed the presence of early brain lesions before the appearance of plaques that are believed to destroy brain cells. If experts' hypotheses about the lesions' role proves accurate, the technique could identify when medical intervention may still stave off or prevent the onset of disease.

In the study, the UCLA team detected high concentrations of FDDNP in the memory centers of nine Alzheimer's patients' brains. To verify their findings, the researchers performed a brain AUTOPSY after one of the patients died. The postmortem tissue showed FDDNP-stained lesions in the brain's memory centers confirming the results of the patient's PET scan.

Before UCLA's discovery, pathologists could make a definitive Alzheimer's diagnosis only by brain autopsy. As a result, physicians were able to treat Alzheimer's disease only after the disease has already caused apparent damage to the patient's memory. Furthermore, early clinical diagnostic methods produced accurate results only about half the time.

During the one-hour PET procedure, a technologist injects the FDDNP tracer molecule into the patient's arm after the patient enters the PET scanner. If lesions are present, the physician will see an accumulation of FDDNP in the brain's memory centers.

Functional Tests

Several types of brain scans can be used to measure brain function: positron emission tomography (PET) and single photon emission computed tomography (SPECT). Using these tools, researchers can "see" which areas of the brain are most active after injecting a substance into the bloodstream. Many scientists are using PET, SPECT, and some newer functional imaging methods to study how brain activity changes during disease. PET and SPECT are available at any hospital with a nuclear medicine division.

PET scan PET scans provide information about how the brain functions (instead of how it looks) by measuring the rate of sugar metabolism or blood flow in the brain. PET scans are designed to show the activity of brain cells in different regions of the brain by appearing as different colored areas. In Alzheimer's disease, brain activity is especially slow in the rear portion of the brain that is important for processing language and memories. PET scans may differentiate Alzheimer's disease from the normal effects of aging by revealing a drop in METABOLISM in one area of the brain that indicates decreased activity in that region.

PET scanning can also be used with an MRI to create three-dimensional images of the brain so that scientists can measure the rate at which various regions of the brain use, deposit, or metabolize certain chemicals. Researchers also are using advanced imaging techniques in combination with neuropsychological testing to study whether individuals at high genetic risk to develop Alzheimer's have detectable brain abnormalities.

In one three-year study, New York University medical school researchers could predict which healthy elderly men and women would develop memory impairment based on scans of their brains. The study shows that metabolic changes occur in particular regions of the brain years before there are any clinical signs of memory loss.

The study extended the use of PET scanning to identify in normal aging subjects the earliest metabolic abnormalities that may lead to the memory losses referred to as MILD COGNITIVE IMPAIRMENT (MCI), which carries a high risk for future Alzheimer's disease. Although PET scans allowed scientists to identify individuals at higher risk of memory impairment, they caution that it is still too early to apply the use of brain scans outside of a research setting.

The New York study followed a group of 48 healthy men and women between the ages of 60 and 80. At the beginning of the study, everyone scored within the normal range on a battery of tests typically used to detect early loss of memory and other mental skills. However, PET scans revealed a reduction in glucose metabolism in an area of the brain called the entorhinal cortex among 12 people. Three years later, 11 of these people had experienced MCI and one developed Alzheimer's disease. The individuals with normal PET scans did not show any signs of mental decline at the three-year follow-up. Moreover, among the group whose mental acuity declined, carriers of the APOLIPOPROTEIN E-4 gene, a biomarker linked to Alzheimer's, showed a big drop in brain metabolic activity over the course of the study. Such metabolic changes may account for the increased risk for Alzheimer's associated with the gene.

SPECT scan   This procedure measures blood flow in different areas of the brain and measures brain activity. SPECT is less expensive and more widely available than PET and is used more often in clinical settings. SPECT studies have also shown blood flow abnormalities in parts of the brains of patients with Alzheimer's disease.

This scan is a type of radionuclide scanning based on detecting radiation emitted by radioactive substances introduced into the body. Different radioactive substances are taken up in greater concentrations by different types of tissue, which gives a clearer picture of organ function than other scans.

The radioactive substance is swallowed or injected into the blood, where it builds up in the brain. Gamma radiation (similar to but shorter than X rays) is emitted from the brain, detected by a gamma camera, and used to produce an image that can be displayed on a screen. Using a principle similar to clinical trial scanning, cross-sectional images can be constructed by a computer from the radiation detected by a gamma camera rotating around the patient.

Structural Tests

Scans designed to reveal brain structure include computed tomography (CT or CAT) scans and magnetic resonance imaging (MRI). A number of researchers are working to improve early DIAGNOSIS of Alzheimer's by using these scans to measure changes in the size of certain brain regions known to be affected in the condition.

CT scan   A CT scan provides a picture of the anatomy of the brain by taking multiple X rays and reconstructing the image of the brain with a computer. CT scans are used in patients with DEMENTIA to rule out STROKE, tumor, or hydrocephalus. In the early stages of Alzheimer's disease, a CT scan may look normal because the changes in the brain occur at a microscopic level. However, in later stages, one of the memory centers of the brain known as the HIPPOCAMPUS may be smaller. Sometimes a contrast agent or dye is injected into a vein in the arm before the CT scan to obtain a more detailed picture of the brain's anatomy.

MRI scan   MRI scans provide a three-dimensional image using a strong magnetic field and radio frequency waves, rather than X rays, to provide pictures of the structure of the brain. As a result, MRIs are radiation-free and can also provide a more detailed picture of brain structures than CT. An MRI is better than CT scans in diagnosing some conditions, such as multiple sclerosis, but in the early stages of dementia both the MRI and the CT scan may look completely normal.

Nevertheless, although they are expensive, most experts prefer MRIs in helping with the diagnosis of Alzheimer's, especially in the later stages. MRIs can reveal brain tissue loss patterns typically seen in Alzheimer's, and can help differentiate

Alzheimer's from other types of dementia (especially frontal lobe dementia). Experts believe MRI will become an important tool for identifying patients who can benefit from treatment to delay or prevent the progression of the disease. Such tests should become available at any large hospital with high-resolution MRI capabilities.

The CT or MRI may be normal in patients with probable Alzheimer's disease (PRAD) and other dementias, especially in the early stages. However, a normal scan in this case only means that there is no evidence of a tumor, stroke, or other structural abnormality that could cause dementia—it does not mean that the brain is normal. The abnormalities of Alzheimer's disease are so small that they can't be detected by these scans in the initial stages of the disease.

brain waves Patterns of BRAIN activity traced on a sensitive electronic device called an ELECTROEN-CEPHALOGRAM. On an ongoing basis, even during sleep, electrical signals are constantly flashing over the brain; these signals can be detected and measured on an electroencephalogram. In some patients with Alzheimer's disease, this test reveals "slow waves." Although other diseases may evidence similar abnormalities, EEG data help distinguish a potential Alzheimer's patient from a severely depressed person whose brain waves would be normal.

Each brain cell produces a tiny electrical charge, and these charges together can be detected by sensors placed on the surface of the scalp. Because the tissues of the body conduct electricity well, metal sensors attached to the skin of the head can detect the signals passing from the brain through the muscles and skin. In an EEG, the electrical activity is recorded by placing small electrodes on the scalp; activity is magnified 1 million times and recorded as brain waves. These brain waves provide a picture of the activity going on under the surface, inside the brain. Electrical signals in the brain don't come steadily, but are produced in short bursts like a series of waves; the shape of the waves changes with the activity level of the brain.

Brain waves occur in various patterns, and so EEG activity can be used to determine whether a person is awake or in one of several sleep stages; EEG activity can also be used to evaluate coma or brain death. Waves are measured in up to 30 cycles per second; one cycle (or one hertz) is one complete oscillation. Brain-wave frequency is a measurement of oscillations per second; the more there are, the higher the frequency of the wave. Amplitude refers to half the height from the peak to the trough in a single oscillation.

calcium An element essential for a variety of bodily functions, such as neurotransmission and proper heart function. All cells use calcium to carry messages from outside of the cells to the inside, and from one component to another within the cells themselves. However, excessive levels of calcium in the BRAIN can disrupt communication in the brain, killing cells and possibly contributing to Alzheimer's disease.

Scientists speculate that as harmful amounts of a protein called BETA AMYLOID build up in the brain, it disrupts the channels that carry calcium, sodium, and potassium ions. These ions produce electric charges that must fire regularly if signals are to move from one nerve cell to the next. If the channels carrying the ions are damaged, the resulting imbalance can interfere with nerve function and communication.

Scientists believe that aging is associated with an increase in FREE RADICAL damage to specific proteins, including those that help cells regulate calcium. Normally, the amount of calcium in a cell at any one time is carefully regulated; calcium channels allow in certain amounts of calcium at certain times, other proteins store the calcium within the cell or remove it.

Too much calcium can kill a cell, and some neuroscientists suspect that in the end, a rise in calcium levels may be precisely what is killing neurons in Alzheimer's disease. According to one hypothesis, an abnormally high concentration of calcium inside a neuron is the final step in cell death. Perhaps an increase in calcium channels could allow an excess of calcium into the cell. Another possibility is that a defect develops in the structures that store calcium inside the cell or those that pump it out of the cell. Still another hypothesis suggests that calcium levels rise because chron-ically high levels of the neurotransmitter GLUTA-MATE disrupt energy METABOLISM, leading to a rise in calcium.

Glutamate triggers action in a neuron, stimulating the flow of calcium into the cell. If it is produced in higher-than-normal levels, it can overexcite a neuron, bringing in too much calcium. Even in normal levels, glutamate can be dangerous to a neuron if glucose levels are low. Therefore, a problem with glucose metabolism could allow glutamate to overexcite the cell, allowing an influx of calcium.

Another hypothesis involves the hormones called GLUCOCORTICOIDS that normally enhance the manufacture of glucose and reduce inflammation in the body. Studies in older animals showed that exposure to glucocorticoids contributed to neuron death and dysfunction in the HIPPOCAMPUS, a part of the brain important in learning and MEMORY. Several studies are currently exploring how glucocorticoids might lead to neuron death through their effect on glucose metabolism.

calcium channel blocker A drug that blocks the entry of calcium into cells, which could be helpful in the treatment of Alzheimer's disease, which features the excess accumulation of CALCIUM in BRAIN cells. Calcium channel blockers are used primarily in the treatment of certain heart conditions, but are now being studied as potential treatments for Alzheimer's disease. Scientists believe that calcium channel blockers such as NIMODIPINE prolong nerve cell survival by protecting against excessive levels of calcium.

California Verbal Learning Test (CVLT) A neuropsychological test that can be used to assess a patient's verbal MEMORY abilities. People with different types of BRAIN problems tend to make unique errors on this test.

In the test, the examiner reads aloud "Monday's shopping list," which contains 16 common words, each of which belongs to one of four categories (such as "fruits" or "herbs"). The patient must then recall as many of these items as possible, and the examiner records how many items the patient remembers over several trials. The examiner also records whether or not the subject is making use of category information. For example, if the four "fruit" items are apples, bananas, pears, and grapes, and the patient can only remember apples, bananas, and pears, if the patient guesses that the fourth term is another fruit (such as "cherries") then the patient has understood the category information in the list. If the subject guesses an unrelated word (such as "cat"), the patient wasn't able to understand the category information in the list.

Next, the examiner may read "Tuesday's shopping list" to see if the patient confuses the items from the two lists. Finally, after a 20-minute delay while the patient performs other tasks, the examiner again asks the patient to remember Monday's list.

The CVLT is a popular neuropsychological test of many aspects of verbal learning and memory. Patients with Alzheimer's disease tend to be unable to make use of category information and might recall: apples, bananas, grapes, and dogs.

calpain One of several BRAIN chemicals currently being studied for their role in MEMORY. Released by CALCIUM within neurons, calpain can alter PROTEINS and actually change the structure of nerve terminals, letting neurons communicate more easily with each other.

calsenilin A PROTEIN that helps regulate CALCIUM in BRAIN cells, and that counteracts the effects of a harmful protein produced by gene mutations causing an inherited form of early onset Alzheimer's disease. The discovery of calsenilins may open the door to preventing this genetic form of the disease.

This inherited form of Alzheimer's, which affects adults in their 30s and early 40s, is usually triggered by mutations in genes that produce a protein called PRESENILIN. Presenilin disrupts the proper handling of calcium inside brain cells, which can lead to neural changes associated with Alzheimer's.

Scientists found that calsenilin stabilized the presenilin signals that disrupt calcium in cells, which could lead to drug treatments to stop the advancement of early onset familial Alzheimer's disease.

Cambridge Neuropsychological Test Automated Battery (CANTAB) A test that is used to assess cognitive deficits in patients with Alzheimer's disease. The test, which consists of 13 interrelated computerized tests of MEMORY, attention, and EXECUTIVE FUNCTION, is administered using a touch-sensitive screen from a personal computer. The tests are highly sensitive in the early detection and routine screening of Alzheimer's disease.

See also ASSESSMENT TOOLS.

Canada It is estimated that 83,200 Canadians age 65 and over are expected to develop DEMENTIA in 2001, and that 50,500 of them will be women. About 238,000 Canadians over 65 have Alzheimer's disease. By 2011, new cases of dementia are expected to reach 111,600 per year. By 2031, more than three-quarters of a million Canadians are expected to have Alzheimer's disease and related dementias. One in 20 Canadians over age 65 is affected by Alzheimer's disease, which rises to one in 100 between ages 65 and 74, one in 14 between ages 75 to 84, and up to one in four over age 85. Approximately $5.5 billion (Canadian) a year is spent on patients with Alzheimer's disease and related dementias.

See also ALZHEIMER SOCIETY OF CANADA.

caregivers The primary person in charge of caring for an individual with Alzheimer's disease, usually a family member or a designated health care professional. More than 23 percent of all U.S. households contain a caregiver for the elderly, which means there are an estimated 22 million caregiving households nationwide. The average caregiver is 46 years old, and 73 percent of them are women.

Taking care of a family member with Alzheimer's has a profound impact on families. In fact, more than 80 percent of caregivers report high levels of stress, and nearly half say they suffer from depression. Yet many caregivers don't recognize their needs, fail to do anything about them, or don't know where to get help.

Because too much stress can be harmful to caregivers and the patient with Alzheimer's, it's important to recognize stress and learn how to reduce it. Warning signs of stress buildup in caregivers include

- anger
- anxiety
- concentration problems
- denial
- depression
- exhaustion
- health problems
- irritability
- sleeplessness
- social withdrawal

care planning   A written action plan containing strategies for delivering care that address the specific needs or problems of a person with Alzheimer's disease. An action plan might include exploring the type and cost of available health care providers and facilities in the community, where and with whom the patient will live, and any preferences regarding treatment and care, including end-of-life wishes. As part of the care planning, the patient should complete an ADVANCE DIRECTIVE and durable power of attorney.

carnitine   The shortened name for acetyl-L-carnitine, a scavenger of FREE RADICALS that is also involved in the growth of BRAIN cells, in addition to being structurally similar to the brain chemical ACETYLCHOLINE.

Alzheimer's disease is associated with lower levels of acetylcholine in the brain, and a key ingredient of acetylcholine is the amino acid CHOLINE. But for some reason, taking supplements of choline doesn't stop the progression of Alzheimer's. However, carnitine (another combination of amino acids) has shown some promise as a potential Alzheimer's treatment.

A few small studies have suggested that carnitine slows cognitive deterioration in people with Alzheimer's disease. For example, in a 1995 study, University of Pittsburgh researchers divided 12 people with Alzheimer's into two groups, five of whom took a placebo and seven of whom took 3,000 mg of carnitine daily for a year. Compared with the placebo group, those taking carnitine showed significantly less mental deterioration based on the Mini-Mental Status test and the ALZHEIMER'S DISEASE ASSESSMENT SCALE.

However, study results sometimes conflict. For example, one trial suggests that this supplement may help prevent the progression of Alzheimer's in the early stages of the disease, but that it may worsen symptoms in later stages of the disease.

For these reasons, many experts believe that use of this supplement for Alzheimer's should be avoided until more information is available. Reported side effects include increased appetite, body odor, and rashes.

catastrophic reactions   Emotionally intense responses to trivial events that may involve sudden mood changes, crying, verbal abuse, or physical violence. Catastrophic behaviors are typical of patients with Alzheimer's disease and may be a response to overstimulation in the environment. They usually happen when an event overwhelms an individual's ability to think or react.

CAT scans   See BRAIN SCANS.

causes of Alzheimer's disease   Most scientists believe that there is not one simple underlying cause of Alzheimer's disease, but instead a number of culprits that may interact to trigger the disease. It may be that several factors must occur in combination to cause Alzheimer's disease, even though no single factor is sufficient by itself. In fact, the number of risk factors and abnormalities at the anatomical, cellular, and molecular levels supports the idea that a variety of mechanisms may contribute to Alzheimer's. There is no compelling evidence that these mechanisms are mutually exclusive. In some patients, a particular mechanism may play a major role, while in others it may not.

In Alzheimer's, progressive degeneration of cells occurs in many areas of the BRAIN, including the nuclei basalis, HIPPOCAMPUS, AMYGDALA, ENTORHINAL CORTEX, and eventually the high-order association cortex of the temporal, frontal, and parietal regions. The brain cell damage and loss of brain density disable several brain systems essential to learning and retrieval of memories.

Many types of DEMENTIA are caused by the degeneration of brain cells, which lose their ability to communicate and then die. Scientists aren't sure what triggers this brain cell degeneration commonly found in Alzheimer's. There are at least five major theories about the cause of Alzheimer's, including chemical, genetic, viral, environmental, and autoimmune problems.

The hallmarks of Alzheimer's include deposits of a protein called BETA AMYLOID in plaques and blood vessel walls, as well as the appearance of NEUROFIBRILLARY TANGLES and loss of neurons. These changes greatly impair the function of neurotransmitter systems. At the same time, lower levels of ACETYLCHOLINE are typical in Alzheimer's patients, and have been associated with deficits in learning and MEMORY. Alzheimer's patients also have low levels of other neurotransmitters, including serotonin, norepinephrine, and somatostatin; these changes may contribute to the typical behavioral problems in Alzheimer's. Other biochemical evidence suggests that inflammation or the harmful effects of FREE RADICALS play a role in the development of Alzheimer's.

Chemical Causes

For the past 20 years scientists have been tracking down the elusive causes of Alzheimer's amidst the billions of cells in the brain. Within and among the extensive connections between brain cells flicker dozens of chemical messengers (NEUROTRANSMITTERS, hormones, and GROWTH FACTORS) that connect each brain cell with others in a vast communications network throughout the brain. If scientists can understand the underlying causes of

the disease, it will be easier to diagnose, treat, prevent, and cure Alzheimer's.

Brain cells need certain nutrients to grow, and one of the important nutrients is called nerve growth factor (NGF). Experiments on rats have shown that NGF promoted growth of new synaptic connections in a part of the brain called the hippocampus; scientists suspect that a drop in NGF might contribute to the development of Alzheimer's.

One of the earliest potential causes of the disease that scientists uncovered was the result of research into NEUROTRANSMITTERS—the chemicals that relay messages between brain cells. Neurotransmitters are located at the tip of an axon (the long tubelike extensions of neurons). When electrical impulses pass along the axon, chemicals fire in a burst of energy, travel across the tiny space between neurons called the synapse, and attach to a receptor in the membrane of the next neuron. Then, the neurotransmitters either break down or return to the first neuron, while the next neuron relays the message.

In the mid 1970s, scientists discovered that a neurotransmitter called acetylcholine, important in the formation of memories, was deficient in people with Alzheimer's disease. Typically, acetylcholine is found in highest amounts in the hippocampus and CEREBRAL CORTEX—brain regions devastated by Alzheimer's disease. Since that early discovery, which was one of the first to link Alzheimer's disease with biochemical changes in the brain, acetylcholine has been the focus of hundreds of studies. Scientists have found that levels fall somewhat in normal aging but plunge by about 90 percent in people with Alzheimer's disease; the decline of this chemical has been linked to memory impairment.

Other neurotransmitters have also been implicated in Alzheimer's disease. For example, serotonin, somatostatin, and noradrenaline levels are lower than normal in some Alzheimer's patients, and deficits in these substances may contribute to sensory disturbances, depression, sleep disturbance, aggressive behavior, and neuron death. Most neurotransmitter research, however, continues to focus on acetylcholine because of its steep decline in Alzheimer's disease and its close ties to memory formation and reasoning.

Once the message carried by a neurotransmitter has crossed the synapse it passes into another territory, where neuroscientists are beginning to find more clues to Alzheimer's disease. The gateways to this new territory are the receptors, coil-shaped proteins embedded in neuron membranes. They interest Alzheimer's researchers because the molecules have chemical bonds with molecules of fat (phospholipids) lying next to them in the membrane; several abnormal phospholipids have been detected in neurons affected by Alzheimer's disease. These abnormalities might change the behavior of neighboring receptors and garble the message as it passes from neuron to neuron.

Researchers also have uncovered several types of receptors for acetylcholine and are now exploring their different effects on message transmission. It may be that the shapes and actions of the receptors themselves play a role in Alzheimer's.

However, the receptor is just the starting point for the cell's communications system. When a neurotransmitter binds to a receptor, it triggers a cascade of biochemical interactions that relay the message to the neuron's nucleus, where it activates certain genes, or to the end of the axon, where it passes to other cells. This message system involves a number of proteins, and abnormalities in these proteins or dysfunction at the relay points could block or garble the message. So could other events and processes in the cell, such as problems with the system that turns food into energy (METABOLISM).

Mutant Proteins

For nearly a century scientists have wondered which of the brain lesions associated with Alzheimer's causes the disease—the plaques that clutter up the empty spaces between nerve cells or the stringy tangles that erupt from within those cells. In the mid-1980s, researchers discovered a class of sticky proteins called BETA AMYLOID in the plaques of Alzheimer's patients that turned out to be one of the most important proteins in the development of Alzheimer's disease.

A short time later, four research teams found the gene that makes the protein; beta amyloid is a fragment of a much larger protein called AMYLOID-PRECURSOR PROTEIN (APP), which is involved in cell membrane function and is found in the brain, heart, kidneys, lungs, spleen, and intestines. Scientists discovered that the plaques typical of Alzheimer's disease are created when an enzyme snips APP apart at a specific place and then leaves the beta amyloid fragments in brain tissue, where they clump together in abnormal deposits.

Beta amyloid protein is produced by cells throughout the body, but it's found in large amounts in the brain. While the normal function of beta amyloid is unknown, scientists do know it occurs in two lengths, and that in the brain the slightly longer version is more likely to clump into plaques.

For some reason, in Alzheimer's disease the brain identifies the tiny broken bits of beta amyloid as foreign, and immune cells try to clear them away using FREE RADICALS of oxygen. The chronic inflammation that results progressively injures nearby nerve cells.

Researchers are intrigued by beta amyloid plaques because they occur early in the disease, before there is any damage to surrounding brain cells, and 10 to 20 years before symptoms develop.

While plaques are made of beta amyloid clumps, the tangles are made of another kind of protein called tau. Scientists know that TAU PROTEIN plays a critical role in the brain. In healthy neurons, the internal support structure for nerve cells (called microtubules) is shaped like train rails, with long parallel tracks joined by crosspieces that function like rungs of a ladder to hold the tracks apart. These crosspieces are made of tau protein. Microtubules are essential to healthy cells, since they carry nutrients from the body of the cells down to the ends of axons.

In cells affected by Alzheimer's, the tau that normally forms the crosspieces between microtubules begins to twist, like two threads wound around each other, until the entire microtubule collapses and becomes hopelessly entangled. Eventually, the entangled axons shrivel and die.

Together, beta amyloid and tau form the plaques and tangles that have been the hallmarks of the disease since it was first described in 1907 by Alois Alzheimer. Scientists disagree about whether it's the sticky plaques of beta amyloid in the brain or the tangles of tau protein inside brain nerve fibers that play a more central role in the destruction of brain cells. While tangles of tau have been found in the brain of people with Alzheimer's, many scientists believed that tangles were probably a secondary part of the disease. Most Alzheimer's researchers have focused attention on beta amyloid as the substance that kills brain cells.

Others think the mutant protein plaques and tangles are really a marker left by nerve cells killed by some other cause. The key question scientists need to resolve is the relationship between beta amyloid and tau. It's also important to discover if these substances are the triggers of the disease, or merely the byproduct of some neurological process gone terribly awry.

What scientists do know is that the higher the levels of beta amyloid in brain tissue, the more severe the DEMENTIA.

Having identified beta amyloid and tau, researchers are now trying to find out more details about how these proteins function, and what happens when they malfunction. Some ideas about their functions may come from studies of certain genes.

Alzheimer's Genes

Every cell in the body contains 23 pairs of chromosomes, and each chromosome features DNA, a large double-stranded molecule that contains genes that direct the manufacture of every enzyme, hormone, growth factor, and other proteins in the body.

Genes are made up of four chemicals arranged in various patterns. Each gene has a different sequence of chemicals, and each one directs the manufacture of a different protein. Even slight alterations in the DNA code of a gene can produce a faulty protein, which can lead to cell malfunction and disease.

Genetic research has turned up evidence of a link between Alzheimer's disease and genes on seven chromosomes—1, 3, 10, 12, 14, 19, and 21. So far, four genes have been definitely associated with Alzheimer's:

- amyloid precursor protein (APP) on chromosome 21
- apolipoprotein E (apo-E) on chromosome 19

- presenilin 1 (PS1) on chromosome 14
- presenilin 2 (PS2) on chromosome 1

Of these four genes and their protein products, three are associated with highly aggressive, early onset familial forms of Alzheimer's disease (APP, PS1, and PS2) and represent a very small subset of patients. The exception is the protein apoE, which exists in three variants, apoE-2, apoE-3 and apoE-4. Inheriting one or two copies of the apoE-4 version of the gene increases the risk of developing Alzheimer's. However, apoE-4 inheritance is only a risk factor for Alzheimer's; its presence alone is not a guarantee that the disease will develop.

Late Onset Alzheimer's

Late onset Alzheimer's disease (the most common form) has been linked to the apoE-4 gene on chromosome 19. The apoE-4 gene was discovered by researchers who studied families in which many members developed the disease late in life, which suggested that there had to be a gene that the affected family members shared. Searching for this gene, they sifted through the DNA from these families and by 1992 had narrowed the search down to a region on chromosome 19. In the same laboratory, another group of researchers were looking for proteins that bind to beta amyloid. One version of a protein called apolipoproteinE (apoE) did bind to beta amyloid and the gene that produced apoE was also on chromosome 19, in the same region of chromosome 19 as the Alzheimer's gene for which they had been searching. The two groups of scientists realized the apoE gene was identical to the gene they had been seeking.

The gene that produces apoE comes in three different forms—apoE-2, apoE-3, and apoE-4. Version apoE-4 is found in about 40 percent of all people with late onset Alzheimer's disease. This gene version is not limited to people whose families have a history of Alzheimer's, however. Patients with Alzheimer's who have no known family history of the disease are also more likely to have an apoE-4 gene.

Dozens of studies around the world have since confirmed that the apoE-4 version increases the risk of developing Alzheimer's disease. People who inherit two of the mutant apoE-4 genes (one from the mother and one from the father) are at least eight times more likely to develop Alzheimer's disease than those who have two of the more common E-3 versions. The least common allele, apoE-2, seems to lower the risk even more. For example, people with one E-2 and one E-3 gene have only one-fourth the risk of developing Alzheimer's as do people with two E-3 genes. People without apoE-4 have an estimated risk for developing Alzheimer's by age 85 of between 9 percent and 20 percent. In people with one copy of the gene, the risk is between 25 percent and 60 percent. In people with two copies, the risk ranges from 50 percent to 90 percent. Only 2 percent of the population carry two copies of the apoE-4 gene.

Many laboratories are now exploring what the apoE-4 protein product does, and many scientists think it has something to do with beta amyloid. Normally, the beta amyloid is soluble, but when the apoE-4 protein binds to it, the amyloid becomes insoluble. This could make it more likely to clump together in plaques. Studies of brain tissue suggest that apoE-4 does increase beta amyloid deposits, and that it directly regulates the protein from which beta amyloid is formed.

Other clues, however, point to tau as the pivotal protein. As the crosspiece in the microtubule, tau's function seems to be to stabilize the microtubule structure. One hypothesis suggests that the apoE-4 protein allows this structure to collapse, leading to the neurofibrillary tangles.

While still controversial and far from proven, the apoE-4 hypotheses is an important new area of research. Now scientists are studying how tau and beta amyloid react with apolipoprotein in its several forms in living cells. Other experiments will attempt to determine the actions and role of the protein. Once scientists understand these processes, it will be easier to develop medicines that can affect the development of the disease.

The apoE-4 has other potential effects on Alzheimer's disease beyond its link to proteins. For example, scientists have discovered that Alzheimer's patients with the apoE-4 gene also have neurons with shorter dendrites (the branchlike extensions that receive messages from other neurons). Scientists think that the dendrites may have been cut by

some unknown substance so that the neuron can't communicate as well with other neurons. Although this shortening is also found among people without the apoE-4 version, those who do have the apoE-4 version exhibit shortened dendrites 20 or 30 years earlier.

It is important to remember, however, that not everyone with the gene will develop Alzheimer's disease, and not everyone with the disease has the gene. A simple test for the presence of apoE-4 would result in too many false positives and false negatives, which is why it is not used as a diagnostic method.

The risk of late onset Alzheimer's has also been linked to a gene on chromosome 3 by three separate research studies. It is believed that a gene in this area may be responsible for the condition by altering beta amyloid levels.

Early Onset Alzheimer's Disease

Several genes also have been linked to the much less common early onset Alzheimer's disease. Alzheimer's strikes early and fairly often in these families, who are found throughout the world often enough to be singled out as having a separate form of the disease.

Six or seven generations of one Belgian family have had some members who developed Alzheimer's disease in their 30s and 40s. A Japanese family has five members who developed the disease in middle age; a British family, eight; a Hispanic family, 12; a French-Canadian family, 23. Descendants of a group of German families who settled in the Volga River valley in Russia in the 1800s count dozens of members who developed Alzheimer's disease in middle age.

By studying DNA of these early onset families, researchers have found a mutation in one gene on chromosome 21 that is common to a few of the families, and another recently identified gene on chromosome 14 that affects a much larger proportion of early onset families.

The gene on chromosome 21 occurs less often in people with early onset familial Alzheimer's disease (FAD) than the chromosome 14 gene. The chromosome 21 gene carries the code for a mutated form of the amyloid precursor protein, APP, the parent protein for beta amyloid. The discovery of this gene supports the theory that beta amyloid plays a role in Alzheimer's disease, although the mutation occurs in only about 5 percent of early onset families. The chromosome 21 gene is also the gene involved in Down syndrome; since people with Down syndrome have an extra version of chromosome 21, as they grow older they almost always develop plaques and tangles like those found in Alzheimer's disease.

There are likely more genes involved in early onset Alzheimer's. For example, the Volga Germans share neither the PRESENILIN 1 chromosome 14 nor the chromosome 21 abnormality.

Most researchers believe that Alzheimer's is related to several genes, and that other conditions may be required for the disease to develop. One of these conditions may be a problem with the metabolism of sugar (glucose).

Metabolism

Brain activity requires energy, which is produced as neurons metabolize glucose and oxygen. Measuring the amount of glucose metabolism can reveal how active the brain is. Glucose metabolism declines dramatically as neurons degenerate and die. Brain scans have revealed differences in brain activity between a normal brain and a brain affected by Alzheimer's disease, but experts don't know whether the drop in metabolism causes neurons to degenerate or whether metabolism slows as a result of neurons' degeneration.

Scientists can track brain metabolism by a type of BRAIN SCAN called positron emission tomography (PET). PET scans can reveal which areas of the brain are active, which is translated into multicolor images: red and orange for areas of high activity, yellow for medium, blue and black for little or none. By deciphering these patterns, Alzheimer's researchers can chart the progress of the disease.

As blood carries glucose through the capillaries, specialized transporter molecules capture the glucose and move it into the neurons. One recent study found that levels of two of these transporter molecules (GLUT1 and GLUT3) were low in the cerebral cortex of people with Alzheimer's disease. This could be one reason why glucose metabolism drops in Alzheimer's—there aren't enough transporter molecules to capture the glucose, and move it into cells.

The condition of the capillaries could also affect the transport of glucose, as capillary walls thicken with deposits of minerals, cholesterol, and amyloid.

Once inside the cell, glucose moves into the mitochondria, where it is metabolized into energy by the action of enzymes, proteins, and oxygen. Any problem with any of these ingredients could have a profound effect on metabolism. For example, studies have found that the enzyme cytochrome oxidase is produced at lower levels in cells affected by Alzheimer's. Since its decline matches the declines in glucose metabolism, it may play a role in the disease.

While the problem in glucose metabolism is not yet fully understood, its results are devastating. Since neurons are completely dependent on glucose, when glucose metabolism fails, neurons can't produce as much acetylcholine as normal cells, which may be one reason this neurotransmitter declines in Alzheimer's. And neurons having metabolic problems react abnormally to a neurotransmitter called GLUTAMATE, which triggers a deadly flood of CALCIUM, which can kill the cell.

Environment

It's clear that genetic and biological factors are important in the development of Alzheimer's disease, but environmental factors could also contribute to its development. One of the most publicized and controversial hypotheses is that aluminum deposits in the brain might be linked to Alzheimer's. Aluminum became a suspect when researchers found traces of this metal in the brains of Alzheimer's patients. Many studies since then have either not been able to confirm this or have had questionable results. While aluminum is found in higher amounts than normal in some autopsy studies of Alzheimer's patients, it doesn't occur in all. Further, it may be that the aluminum found in some studies didn't originate in the brain tissue at all, but came from the special substances used in the laboratory to study brain tissue.

Aluminum is a common element in the Earth's crust and is found in small amounts in numerous household products and in many foods, so some experts worried that aluminum in the diet or absorbed in other ways could be a factor in

Alzheimer's. One study found that people who used antiperspirants and antacids containing aluminum had a higher risk of developing Alzheimer's. Others have also reported an association between aluminum exposure and Alzheimer's disease. On the other hand, various studies have found that groups of people exposed to high levels of aluminum do not have an increased risk. Moreover, aluminum in cooking utensils does not get into food and the aluminum that does occur naturally in some foods, such as potatoes, is not absorbed well by the body. So far, scientists have concluded that they don't know whether exposure to aluminum plays a role in Alzheimer's disease.

Zinc is another compound that has been implicated in Alzheimer's disease. Some autopsies found low levels of zinc in the brains of Alzheimer's disease patients, especially in the HIPPOCAMPUS. On the other hand, a recent study suggests that too much zinc might trigger beta amyloid to form plaques in the brain.

Toxins in foods have come under suspicion in a few cases of dementia, since two amino acids found in seeds of certain legumes in Africa, India, and Guam may cause neurological damage. Both enhance the action of the neurotransmitter glutamate, which is also linked to Alzheimer's disease. In Canada, an outbreak of a brain disorder much like Alzheimer's occurred among people who had eaten mussels contaminated with DEMOIC ACID. This chemical, like the legume amino acids, also stimulates glutamate.

While these toxins may not be a common cause of dementia, they could eventually shed some light on the mechanisms that lead to neuron degeneration.

Viral/Bacterial Causes

Some neurological diseases have been linked to a slow virus, which lurks in the body for decades before being stimulated into action. While no specific "Alzheimer's virus" has ever been found, scientists suspect that people with a genetic susceptibility to Alzheimer's may be vulnerable to certain viruses, particularly under circumstances when the immune system is weakened.

In one study, the risk for Alzheimer's was very high in people with both the apoE-4 gene variety and evidence of herpes virus (HSV) 1, a form of herpes that causes cold sores. Those with only one of these factors had normal risk. Furthermore, research is finding that parts of the HSV1 protein strongly resemble beta amyloid and, in laboratory studies, have even have been observed to kill brain cells and develop sticky plaques. Most Americans are infected during childhood with HSV-1. (Herpes simplex virus 2 (HSV-2), also known as genital herpes, is transmitted by sexual contact.) Most people who are exposed to HSV-1 do not develop Alzheimer's; it appears that only those genetically disposed to Alzheimer's are more likely to develop the disease if they are exposed to herpes.

Another suspected germ link is *Chlamydia pneumoniae,* a bacterium that causes respiratory infections. Researchers have found evidence of it in parts of the brain affected by late onset Alzheimer's, but not in unaffected parts. Scientists don't know whether the presence of the bacterium is the result of Alzheimer's disease or a cause.

Autoimmune Theories

A person's immune system fights off infection from bacteria, viruses, and other threats to general health. If this system breaks down, a person's immune system can attack its own tissue. Scientists suspect that if an aging person's immune system attacks the brain, it could cause Alzheimer's symptoms.

Celebrex   See CELECOXIB.

celecoxib (Celebrex)   A NONSTEROIDAL ANTI-INFLAMMATORY DRUG (NSAID) that eases pain and lessens inflammation by interfering with the production of prostaglandins. Considerable evidence suggests that inflammation may play a role in the degenerative process of Alzheimer's disease, and the use of NSAIDs may ease symptoms or prevent the development of the disease.

Celecoxib is one of two NSAIDs being studied in a randomized trial that is assessing the drugs' ability to delay or prevent the onset of Alzheimer's. The study found no benefit, and side effects (including stroke) were significant in the Celebrex group.

While some experts have hoped that celecoxib is gentler on the stomach than some NSAIDs, there's no proof that it is better tolerated than older, cheaper painkillers, say government scientific advisers.

Center for Health Care Law, The   A nonprofit, public-interest law firm established by the NATIONAL ASSOCIATION FOR HOME HEALTH CARE in 1987 to help protect the rights of the elderly, disabled, handicapped, and chronically ill who require health care services. The center intervenes on behalf of these people by filing lawsuits against MEDICARE, MEDICAID, health maintenance organizations, and private insurance companies when necessary.

While concentrating on matters that significantly affect the home health industry and patients, the center also is available to help individual members who require expert, specialized legal assistance. Since 1987, the center has helped thousands of individual agencies with legal problems related to third-party payments, licensure, risk management, employment law, and business planning.

For contact information see Appendix I.

cerebellum   A small, two-lobed wrinkled BRAIN structure that may be responsible for coordinating thinking in addition to maintaining movement, balance and muscle coordination. The arrangement of nerve cells in the cerebellum is different from other parts of the brain; here, the cells are positioned with mathematical precision, much like an electrical writing diagram. In Alzheimer's disease, the area of the cerebellum usually remains intact.

cerebral cortex   The wrinkly gray outer layer of the BRAIN in which thought processes take place. The gray covering that makes up the cerebral cortex actually consists of the cell bodies of nerve cells (neurons); underneath lies the "white matter," formed of the axons of these neurons. In Alzheimer's disease, nerve cells in the cerebral cortex degenerate and die.

The surface of the cortex is wrinkled because the brain has grown at a faster rate than the skull, and so the surface of the brain must fold to fit inside the skull. The cerebral cortex is divided into right and left halves which are mirror images of each other. In most cases, structures which appear on the left side have a matching structure on the right. In general, sensory and movement information from the left side of the body is processed in the right hemisphere, and vice versa.

The cortex is often divided into large regions, called lobes, based on function and anatomical structure. These include the frontal lobes, the parietal lobes, the occipital lobes, and the temporal lobes.

cerebral hemispheres   The two divisions of the cerebrum, labeled left and right, that are separated by a deep groove called the cerebral fissure. The left hemisphere controls the right side of the body, and the right hemisphere controls the left, because of a crossing of the nerve fibers in the medulla. In most people, the left hemisphere area controls speech, and areas in the right control spatial perceptions.

cevimeline (Evoxac)   A drug currently approved for the treatment of dry mouth in Sjögren's syndrome has been shown to reduce levels of BETA AMYLOID in the cerebral spinal fluid of patients with Alzheimer's disease. Cevimeline is the first drug ever shown to have such an effect in human patients.

Beta amyloid is a protein that builds up in the BRAIN and forms the plaques that are a hallmark of Alzheimer's. Cevimeline works by blocking production of beta amyloid.

The drug was tested in 19 patients with Alzheimer's and found to reduce beta amyloid levels by 22 percent in 14 patients. The drug is now in a Phase II trial that will assess its effects on cognitive status and long-term disease progression.

chemical theories of Alzheimer's disease   Many scientists are studying how chemicals may affect the nervous system, and how that may contribute to the dysfunction or death of brain cells typically seen in Alzheimer's disease. These harmful effects could be caused by low levels of chemicals called

NEUROTRANSMITTERS; from a decrease in growth-promoting factors in the brain, or from toxic levels of chemicals that accumulate in the brain.

Biochemical growth factors Some researchers believe that in Alzheimer's disease, nerve cells die either because there is a drop in the level of growth-promoting factors that maintain the functioning of brain cells, or because there is a spontaneous increase in factors that are toxic to brain cells.

Other researchers are studying whether changes or an imbalance in the metabolism of certain elements (such as CALCIUM) in brain cells may be part of the process that triggers cells to degenerate and die.

Neurotransmitters Chemicals called neurotransmitters enable brain cells to communicate with each other. Patients with Alzheimer's disease have lower levels of several neurotransmitters that affect intellectual functioning and behavior. For example, low levels of the neurotransmitter ACETYLCHOLINE have been found in patients with Alzheimer's. In addition, scientists discovered that drugs that lower acetylcholine levels in the brain can cause reversible memory problems. These findings have led to a number of studies assessing the effect of drugs that raise levels of acetylcholine, such as lecithin, CHOLINE, PHYSOSTIGMINE, DEPRENYL, and TACRINE, used alone or in different combinations with one another. In some of these studies, a few patients seem to show minor improvement over a brief period of time, but those improvements are usually slight, and not usually in significant ACTIVITIES OF DAILY LIVING. Of these drugs, tacrine (Cognex), has been studied extensively. Early studies indicated that tacrine appeared to have a slightly positive effect on patient functioning, but assessment by a skilled observer showed no overall improvement. More recent studies with DONEPEZIL, RIVASTIGMINE, and GALATAMINE have shown significant improvement in activities of daily living.

Toxic chemical excesses Although some researchers have found increased levels of ALUMINUM, mercury, or other metals in the brains of patients with Alzheimer's disease, others have not. And while some investigators have hypothesized that aluminum may play a role in the genesis of Alzheimer's disease, most have regarded aluminum as an effect of the disorder rather than its cause. Research continues in an effort to better understand this link and to determine whether the chemical deposits are a cause or a result of the disease.

Children of Aging Parents (CAPS) A nonprofit charitable organization whose mission is to provide the nation's nearly 23 million caregivers of the elderly with reliable information, referrals, and support, and to heighten public awareness that the health of the family caregivers is essential to quality care of the nation's growing elderly population.

CAPS writes, collects, and disseminates fact sheets and publishes a bimonthly newsletter with news and advice for caregivers. The organization arranges conferences and workshops and shares new product information. CAPS refers caregivers to appropriate groups anywhere in the country and encourages the formation of new, CAPS-affiliated groups.

The group was started in Levittown, Pennsylvania, in 1977 when a small band of neighbors who were caring for their elderly parents began to share their problems and feelings; three years later, CAPS was established as a nonprofit organization. For contact information see Appendix I.

chlamydia pneumonia A type of pneumonia caused by the chlamydia bacteria, the disease commonly occurs in children and young adults. While this type of pneumonia is generally mild and rarely requires hospitalization when appropriately treated, some research suggests there may be long-term complications. (Chlamydia pneumonia is not caused by the organism *Chlamydia trachomatis*, which causes a sexually transmitted disease, although the two are related.)

Some studies have revealed *C. pneumoniae* in areas of the brain affected by Alzheimer's disease but not in other areas. In one 1998 study, the bacteria were found in postmortem brain samples of 17 out of 19 people with Alzheimer's disease, but were found in only one out of 19 people who had died of other causes. Scientists suspect that the damaging plaques and tangles typically found in Alzheimer's disease may form in response to infection with *C. pneumoniae,* which may live in a person's cells for decades, causing a slow, chronic immune response. Since *Chlamydia pneumoniae* triggers a strong inflammatory response at sites of infection, this bacterium may be a major component to the inflammatory process in the brain, a well-documented characteristic of late onset Alzheimer's.

However, there may be other factors that act in relationship with *C. pneumoniae.* The bacterium is extremely common, yet not everyone who is infected also gets Alzheimer's. This is why some scientists suspect there may be unidentified genetic factors working in relationship with *C. pneumoniae,* such as APOLIPOPROTEIN E, a protein used to transport fat in the body. Each person's DNA contains some combination of two of five different types of apolipoprotein E; while the APOE-4 version occurs in 13 percent to 15 percent of the general population, it is found in 60 percent of Alzheimer's patients. Some scientists think that apoE-4 may act together with *C. pneumoniae* infection to cause Alzheimer's.

cholesterol   High levels of "good" cholesterol in the blood may serve as a marker for those at risk for Alzheimer's disease, although experts aren't sure if cholesterol is a direct cause. Early research had suggested cholesterol may play a role in the development of brain plaques and tangles characteristic of Alzheimer's disease. More recent studies have found that patients with high cholesterol may have as much as twice the risk of developing Alzheimer's disease as healthy people. A growing but not entirely consistent body of research points to a possible association between Alzheimer's and one or both of two major heart-disease risk factors—high levels of cholesterol and high blood pressure.

In one Finnish study published in the June 16, 2001, issue of the *British Medical Journal,* researchers looked at Alzheimer's levels in a group of 1,449 men and women who had been examined twice in 20 years as part of a study that included data on blood pressure and cholesterol levels. Researchers concluded that participants who had high choles-

terol levels or high systolic blood pressure in middle age were about twice as likely to develop Alzheimer's disease as those who did not, even after accounting for age, weight, history of heart problems, and other factors. The risk was 3.5 times higher for those who had both high blood pressure *and* high cholesterol. There was no increased risk for people who had high diastolic pressure (the second of the two numbers in a blood pressure reading).

Earlier research has supported these conclusions. One study of African Americans in Baltimore found an association between Alzheimer's and cholesterol levels, while studies at the University of Massachusetts and Loyola University concluded that people who were treated with statin drugs to lower cholesterol also were less likely to develop Alzheimer's. In fact, patients who took these cholesterol-lowering medications were about 70 percent less likely to have dementia compared to people who had no diagnosis of high cholesterol or exposure to other cholesterol-lowering medications. A new study is assessing the effects of statins on mild to moderate Alzheimer's.

Brain cells affected by Alzheimer's often show an increase in levels of a protein called BETA AMYLOID. As the levels of beta amyloid rise, the proteins eventually get deposited into plaques in the brain that are the hallmark of advanced Alzheimer's disease. Scientists suspect that high levels of cholesterol in the brain may be linked to problems with processing the amyloid protein that gets deposited in the brain and leads to plaques. In one study, researchers found that the men with higher levels of "good" cholesterol (HDL) had more plaques and tangles in their brain in both midlife and old age. This was surprising since HDL was considered to be helpful, and higher levels of HDL reduce a person's risk of heart disease.

There appears to be no link between total cholesterol levels and plaques, although some studies have found an association with levels of "bad" (LDL) cholesterol and plaques.

See also CHOLESTEROL-LOWERING DRUGS.

cholesterol-lowering drugs   Recent research shows that medications called statins, taken to lower a person's cholesterol level, may also ward off Alzheimer's disease. High cholesterol levels appear to harm the brain and lead to mental decline and Alzheimer's disease, and in one recent study, researchers found that older women who took statins (Lipitor, Zocor, and Mevacor) had less mental impairment than nonusers.

However, the study was not designed to test the drugs' effects on mental sharpness, so scientists cautioned that more work is needed to determine whether statins really can lower the risk of getting Alzheimer's.

The study also was limited to data primarily from white women suffering from heart disease, so it is not clear whether the results would apply to nonwhite women or men, or anyone without heart disease.

Previous research on cholesterol and Alzheimer's has been mixed. High cholesterol can narrow the arteries and raise the risk of heart disease, and some researchers think high cholesterol may also affect brain arteries and promote the clumping of a protein called BETA AMYLOID, thought to damage the brain in Alzheimer's.

In the study of 1,037 postmenopausal women with heart disease at an average age of 71, scientists tested the effects of hormone supplements on their hearts. It included data on cholesterol levels and statin use. The women were subjected to tests of their memory, attention, and language. None of the participants were taking Alzheimer's drugs or had been diagnosed with DEMENTIA.

Women with the highest overall cholesterol readings (235 to 432) faced a 77 percent higher risk of having cognitive impairment, compared with those with lower levels. A similar risk was found in women with the highest levels of the artery-clogging LDL (bad cholesterol) at levels between 145 to 347.

Among women who used statin drugs, just 37 women (6 percent) had cognitive impairment, compared with 42 (9 percent) nonusers.

Women whose total and LDL cholesterol levels declined during the four years by using statins or from other means were about half as likely to have cognitive impairment as those whose levels increased.

choline   A natural substance required by the body that is an essential component of ACETYL-CHOLINE, a chemical messenger that brain cells use to communicate with each other, especially in parts of the brain important for thought, memory, and judgment. Acetylcholine is a critical neurotransmitter in the process of forming memories, and it is the neurotransmitter commonly lacking in regions devastated by Alzheimer's disease. When brain cells are damaged by Alzheimer's disease, they produce less acetylcholine, which disrupts communication in the brain.

See also CHOLINE ACETYLTRANSFERASE.

choline acetyltransferase   An enzyme that controls the production of ACETYLCHOLINE that appears to be depleted in the brains of individuals with Alzheimer's disease.

cholinergic   A term that refers to those neurons that use ACETYLCHOLINE as a neurotransmitter.

cholinergic drugs   See CHOLINESTERASE INHIBITORS.

cholinergic hypothesis of Alzheimer's disease The theory that suggests there is a link between memory loss and the decrease in activity of CHOLINE ACETYLTRANSFERASE (ChAT) in the brains of patients with Alzheimer's disease.

ChAT is a crucial ingredient in the chemical process that produces ACETYLCHOLINE, a neurontransmitter linked to learning and memory that is present in abnormally low levels in Alzheimer's. There has been a link between this change in neurochemical activity and changes in memory loss and the physical appearance of Alzheimer's brains (especially in the number of plaques).

Researchers have found a loss of nerve cells in a part of the base of the brain called the nucleus basalis; some patients with classical Alzheimer's have been shown to have lost as many as 90 percent of these cells. The nucleus basalis is a major site of cholinergic neurons in the brain; its projections reach a number of brain areas associated with learning and memory.

cholinergic system The system of nerve cells that uses ACETYLCHOLINE as its neurotransmitter, and that is damaged in the brains of individuals with Alzheimer's disease.

See also CHOLINERGIC HYPOTHESIS OF ALZHEIMER'S DISEASE.

cholinesterase An enzyme that breaks down ACETYLCHOLINE, a chemical important in learning and memory that is deficient in the brain of patients with Alzheimer's disease.

cholinesterase inhibitors Drugs used to treat Alzheimer's disease by blocking the action of CHOLINESTERASE, an enzyme that normally breaks down and cleans up excess ACETYLCHOLINE. By stopping cholinesterase from breaking down acetylcholine, these drugs boost the levels of acetylcholine in the brain. Higher levels of acetylcholine improve cell-to-cell communication and may compensate for the loss of functioning brain cells.

Because acetylcholine levels are abnormally low in people with Alzheimer's, cholinesterase inhibitors are used to treat Alzheimer's disease. Cholinesterase inhibitors are able to contribute to modest improvements in thinking and reasoning, memory and daily activities in between 30 percent and 50 percent of patients. The drugs cannot slow or reverse the progression of the disease, however.

TACRINE (Cognex) was the first cholinesterase inhibitor approved for use in Alzheimer's patients. Many research subjects given tacrine showed some improvement in symptoms and some were able to resume normal activity and personal care. Not all patients respond to tacrine, however, and side effects included higher levels of liver enzymes. Within the past few years, other compounds less toxic than tacrine have become available for clinical use, including DONEPEZIL, RIVASTIGMINE, and GALANTAMINE.

Responses to these four drugs vary from one patient to the next for reasons that are not well understood. If one drug has no effect, a physician may try another, although up to half of all patients show no improvement with any of the four drugs.

Side Effects

All of these drugs may cause side effects including nausea and vomiting, loss of appetite, and diarrhea. Tacrine may trigger liver damage. Some patients taking rivastigmine lose weight. Donepezil can cause sleep problems.

cholinomimetic agents Any compound that activates cholinergic receptors, such as arecoline, nicotine, or muscarine.

chromosome An H-shaped structure inside the cell nucleus made up of tightly coiled strands of genes. Each person has 46 chromosomes (23 from each parent) containing genes that serve as the blueprint for the development of a human being. Mutations of these genes can lead to specific diseases or conditions. So far, scientists have linked the risk of developing Alzheimer's disease with genes on chromosomes 1, 14, 19, and 21.

The first Alzheimer's gene was found in 1991, when John Hardy at St. Mary's Hospital Medical School in London and colleagues showed that mutations in the gene for the AMYLOID PRECURSOR PROTEIN (APP) on CHROMOSOME 21 cause Alzheimer's disease in some families. This discovery provided a direct link to the BETA AMYLOID protein found in the plaques that stud Alzheimer's victims' brains. But this mutant gene only accounts for between 2 percent and 3 percent of familial Alzheimer's cases.

Next, scientists discovered a genetic risk factor on CHROMOSOME 19. While this gene does not cause Alzheimer's in everyone who inherits it, its presence does increase the risk for developing the late onset form of Alzheimer's.

In 1995, a Canadian research team discovered an Alzheimer's-linked gene on CHROMOSOME 14 (presinilin 1). The S182 gene causes 70 percent to 80 percent of early onset familial Alzheimer's.

Just months after the S182 gene discovery, a group of geneticists in Seattle, Washington, uncovered a gene on CHROMOSOME 1 that encodes the protein STM2, similar to S182. The search for the STM2 gene stemmed from the fact that a handful of Alzheimer's-carrying families in the Seattle study did not show a mutation on either chromosome 14 or chromosome 21. A mutation in STM2 was a common trait for a group of families who descend from ethnic Germans living in Russia in the 18th and 19th centuries. The protein is presenilin 2.

In 2000, three groups of scientists identified CHROMOSOME 10 as the site of a major risk factor for the development of late onset Alzheimer's.

Currently, scientists are studying the interrelationship between the various genes (particularly the mutation on chromosome 21), and how environmental factors could affect a person's susceptibility to Alzheimer's.

See also HEREDITY; CAUSES OF ALZHEIMER'S; CHROMOSOME 1; CHROMOSOME 12; CHROMOSOME 14.

chromosome 1   A mutation of a gene on this chromosome (called STM2) has been linked to EARLY ONSET ALZHEIMER'S DISEASE. This gene abnormality is fairly rare and is found primarily in descendants of Germans who immigrated to an area near the Volga River in Russia in the 18th century, and then came to the United States early in the 20th century. The early onset form of Alzheimer's caused by the defect on chromosome 1 is not as common as the late onset form of Alzheimer's, which occurs in people over age 65.

The gene on chromosome 1 is quite similar to a different gene on CHROMOSOME 14 that also is linked to early onset Alzheimer's, but that affects a different group of families.

Discovering what the gene's presenilin 2 does and how presenilin 2 changes when the gene mutates, may mean it is possible to develop new drugs that could help all Alzheimer's patients. The discovery of this gene gave researchers an important new clue toward a better understanding of what causes the formation of BETA AMYLOID, a toxic substance found in the brains of patients with Alzheimer's. Determining the function of the proteins associated with all the Alzheimer's genes should help researchers develop a drug to slow or stop the disease process.

See also CHROMOSOME 10; CHROMOSOME 14; CHROMOSOME 19; CHROMOSOME 21; HEREDITY.

chromosome 10   This chromosome appears to harbor a gene (or genes) that could be a powerful risk factor for the development of late onset Alzheimer's disease, the most common form of the condition. Scientists believe that the Alzheimer's gene in this region could be as influential as the APOLIPOPROTEIN E (APOE) GENE on CHROMOSOME 19. Although scientists have not yet located the actual gene, they suspect that its variant could (like the early onset Alzheimer's genes APP and the PRESENILINS) cause disease directly rather than merely increase vulnerability.

Researchers at the Mayo Clinic in Jacksonville, Florida, found a relationship between the level of BETA AMYLOID in the blood of Alzheimer's patients and a region on chromosome 10. Corroborating these findings, another team at Washington University School of Medicine in St. Louis, Missouri, reported how that genetic region had been seen in hundreds of pairs of siblings who had Alzheimer's disease. A third team at Harvard Medical School focused on another gene (insulin degrading enzyme) found in more than 400 families with Alzheimer's disease, which is also located on chromosome 10. This gene is believed to help degrade the Alzheimer's disease-causing beta amyloid.

In yet another study, 325 first-degree relatives of 189 Alzheimer's patients were studied for more than 11 years. Researchers found that those relatives who had a previously identified risk factor (the APOE-4 gene) and a specific form of a gene on chromosome 10 had a 16 times greater risk of developing Alzheimer's disease. More research is needed to identify the function of this gene on chromosome 10 and exactly how it increases risk.

The Washington University School of Medicine researchers found a part of chromosome 10 that appeared to be a "major risk factor" in the development of late onset Alzheimer's by studying more than 400 siblings who developed the condition after age 64. The researchers concluded that a part of chromosome 10 was linked to Alzheimer's after analyzing 16 different chromosomal regions. The risk seemed to be independent of the risk associated with another Alzheimer's-related gene mutation (apoE-4).

Mayo Clinic scientists found a relationship between beta amyloid levels in Alzheimer's patients and an area on chromosome 10. High beta amyloid levels are a risk factor for Alzheimer's; this type of protein is found clogging brain plaques characteristic of the disease. Mayo scientists believe that the area on chromosome 10 increased the risk for Alzheimer's by increasing beta amyloid levels.

See also CHROMOSOME 1; CHROMOSOME 12; CHROMOSOME 14; CHROMOSOME 19; CHROMOSOME 21.

chromosome 12 Location of the gene A2M (alfa-2-macroglobulin) that, when defective, may make people who inherit it more susceptible to Alzheimer's disease. The gene was discovered by researchers at Massachusetts General Hospital and the Harvard School of Public Health, who found that patients with late onset Alzheimer's were more likely to have a mutation in this gene than were siblings who had not developed the disease. Although the defective gene doesn't always cause Alzheimer's, its presence increases the risk of developing the disease.

The A2M gene controls the activity of enzymes that break down other proteins, and has been known to interact with a nerve cell receptor called LRP. Two important clues led researchers to wonder whether mutations in A2M might be associated with Alzheimer's risk. First, two proteins known to be involved with Alzheimer's—the AMYLOID PRECURSOR PROTEIN (APP) and APOLIPOPROTEIN E (apoE) also interact with this nerve cell receptor. Second, cell culture studies have shown that A2M helps break down and remove the protein fragment BETA AMYLOID, the major component of the plaques found in the brain of Alzheimer's patients. Scientists believe that Alzheimer's may be caused by a failure in the process of the breakdown and removal of beta amyloid. A flawed A2M gene may fail to help brain synapses function properly.

Scientists believe that the key event triggering Alzheimer's is the buildup of amyloid plaques made up of toxic deposits of insoluble beta amyloid protein fragments inside the brain. It could be that the A2M, apoE, and LRP proteins are involved in a sensitive, balanced system that breaks down beta amyloid and removes it from brain cells.

If A2M-2 interfered with this system, or if a variant of apoE blocked the usual breakdown process, beta amyloid plaques could form and clog the synapses, slowing nerve signals and preventing the release of growth factors that keep cells healthy.

The risk of developing Alzheimer's disease conferred by the A2M-2 mutation seems to be the same as the risk conferred by the gene variant apoE-4. However, people who carry both variants don't seem to be at higher risk. Although apoE-4 appears to affect the age at which symptoms appear, A2M-2 doesn't affect age of onset.

chromosome 14 Location of a gene that, when abnormal (identified as S182), has been linked to some cases of inherited early onset Alzheimer's disease. This gene mutation (PRESENILIN 1) causes 80 percent of all cases of inherited Alzheimer's. This mutant gene was identified in 1995 by a Canadian research team.

Each human being has 46 chromosomes (23 from each parent) containing genes that serve as the blueprint for the development of a human being. Mutations of these genes, such as the S182, can lead to specific diseases or conditions.

chromosome 19 One of the 46 human chromosomes that, when it contains a gene mutation called APOE-4, appears to serve as a risk factor for Alzheimer's disease. The apoE-4 gene variation occurs in only about 15 percent of the general population, yet is found in half of those with late onset Alzheimer's. It is more than three times as common in Alzheimer's patients than in people without the disease. Although people with this so-called "e-4 type" gene appear to be more susceptible to the disease, the presence of this gene mutation alone does not guarantee the disease will occur.

Each human being has 46 chromosomes (23 from each parent) containing genes that serve as the blueprint for the development of a human being. Mutations of these genes, such as the apoE-4, can lead to specific diseases or conditions.

chromosome 21 The smallest chromosome in the human genome, and the chromosome on which the first gene mutation linked to Alzheimer's disease was found. Each human being has 46 chromosomes (23 from each parent); each chromosome contains genes that serve as the blueprint for the development of a human being.

Identified in 1991, the gene on this chromosome linked to Alzheimer's codes for the AMYLOID PRECURSOR PROTEIN (APP), the source of a protein (BETA AMYLOID) that is found in the plaques common in the brain of Alzheimer's patients. Mutations in this gene cause Alzheimer's in some families, although this mutant APP gene accounts for only 2 percent to 3 percent of inherited Alzheimer's.

Chromosome 21, which has only 225 genes, is also linked to DOWN SYNDROME. Down syndrome is caused by the presence of three copies of genes on chromosome 21 instead of two. Virtually every person with Down syndrome will also develop Alzheimer's disease by age 60.

circadian rhythm A biological cycle or rhythm pattern that recurs about once every 24 hours, such as the adult sleep-wake cycle. People with Alzheimer's disease often experience disturbances in circadian rhythm, which affects body functions such as sleep cycles, temperature, alertness, and hormone production. This can lead to impaired sleep and nocturnal restlessness.

In addition, researchers have found that patients with Alzheimer's disease tend to have abnormal circadian rhythms that correlate with the severity of the Alzheimer's symptoms. Patients with Alzheimer's consistently have a higher percentage of activity in the evening, and show greater temperature fluctuations, than do healthy subjects. According to researchers, this pattern suggests that the circadian abnormalities progress together with cognitive and functional deterioration. Scientists suspect that the problems with regulating temperature may be caused by the neurofibrillary tangles common in Alzheimer's patients. This is especially true if tangles form in the hypothalamus, which (among other functions) regulates body temperature.

Dutch and Japanese scientists have found that patients with Alzheimer's disease who received two hours of bright light therapy for a month experienced improvements in sleep and in body temperature.

circulatory disorders Heart problems, high blood pressure, or stroke can restrict the oxygen available to brain cells by reducing blood flow.

Even people who feel fine may have a buildup of plaque in their arteries (a condition known as atherosclerosis), which can eventually limit the oxygen supply to the brain, causing loss of memory and thinking problems.

One recent study found that men with high blood pressure in midlife are much more likely to have trouble thinking and remembering things when they are old, according to at least one study involving 3,735 Japanese-American men who were enrolled in a heart study in the 1960s and tracked through the early 1990s. Their ability to remember, think abstractly, make judgments, and concentrate was measured when the men were 78. Men with high systolic blood pressure (the first of the two numbers in a blood-pressure reading) during midlife were almost 2.5 times more likely to have poor cognitive function in old age than men with low systolic blood pressure. In fact, the higher the blood pressure in midlife, the greater the likelihood of trouble thinking and remembering in old age. For every 10-point increase in systolic blood pressure, there was a 9 percent increase in the risk of poor cognitive function later.

Brain scans performed on the patients suggested that many of them suffered tiny silent strokes that cause no symptoms but can permanently impair thinking. High blood pressure may also damage the brain in some ways that aren't clear to doctors.

Clinical Dementia Rating Scale A clinical assessment developed at Washington University designed to characterize subjects from normal function through various stages of DEMENTIA. The rating of 0.5 represents very mild Alzheimer's disease.

Clock Draw test A simple ASSESSMENT TOOL best used in combination with other cognitive tests that can assess cognitive or visuospatial problems. There are slightly different versions of the test, but the basic idea is that a subject is asked to draw the face of a clock with all the numbers and is then asked to draw the hands to indicate a certain time.

coenzyme Q10 Also known as ubiquinone, this is a naturally occurring ANTIOXIDANT that is needed for human cell reactions to take place; some people believe coenzyme Q10 can improve the symptoms of Alzheimer's disease. Antioxidants are compounds that fight cell damage caused by FREE RADICALS, a rogue type of oxygen molecule that can attack cells throughout the body.

CoQ10 may also protect against other brain diseases associated with aging and the slowdown in mitochondrial function. In Alzheimer's disease, mitochondrial function seems to be impaired, so in one study researchers gave CoQ10 (along with iron and vitamin B_6) to patients with the disease. In this study, reported in the British medical journal *Lancet,* the antioxidant appeared to prevent the progression of Alzheimer's by up to two years.

However, not much is known about its safety. Because of dosage concerns and nonregulation in manufacturing, experts recommend that patients talk to a neurologist before treating themselves with coenzyme Q10.

Cognex   See TACRINE.

cognitive abilities   Mental abilities such as judgment, MEMORY, learning, comprehension, and reasoning. Alzheimer's disease causes gradual worsening of these cognitive abilities.

cognitive screening exam   See ASSESSMENT TOOLS.

combativeness   One type of behavioral symptom that becomes common in patients with Alzheimer's disease as the condition progresses. The combativeness may include angry words and agitation, and may lead to physical violence. Often, patients become combative simply as a result of frustration, especially if they feel they are being pressured to do something they do not want to do.

Combativeness can appear in many forms—either verbally lashing out or physically pushing or hitting caregivers. Patients trying to get dressed but having trouble pulling on a pair of slacks may get so frustrated that they begin to lash out at anyone nearby. Patients who become frightened by water running into the sink may roughly push aside a caregiver.

There may be a variety of reasons for the combativeness. Patients may simply be too tired or overmedicated; they may be in pain or overstimulated by noise or clutter. An unfamiliar environment can sometimes trigger combativeness, or the patient may simply be reacting to a caregiver's own frustration or anger.

Preventing Combativeness
Episodes of combativeness may be avoided by watching for frustration during ACTIVITIES OF DAILY LIVING such as dressing or eating. Caregivers should always try to respond to combativeness calmly, without getting angry and certainly without striking back at the patient. Raising the voice in response to a combative attitude by the patient will only worsen the problem. Caregivers should always keep in mind the level of abilities of the patient, and not expect more than the person can handle. Caregivers should always distract, never argue, and not insist that a patient perform a particular task if it is causing frustration. For example, if a patient is getting frustrated at trying to put an arm through a sleeve, the caregiver should distract with another activity, such as putting on shoes, or moving to another room for a break.

Clear communication is important in avoiding combativeness. Caregivers should always speak in slow, clear, short, and simple sentences. Comments should be repeated as often as necessary, together with a lot of reminders.

Patients should be encouraged to make limited choices—having too many decisions to make about what to eat or wear might be too overwhelming. Each task should be broken down into small steps so that the patient can slowly complete one step at a time.

Some caregivers have found that pets, such as dogs or cats—or even stuffed animals—have a calming effect on the person. If a dog or cat seems too unpredictable, a tank of fish may be sufficient.

Handling Combativeness
It may be helpful for caregivers to identify early signs of agitation, which may be preceded by fidgeting, flushing, restlessness, or signs of frustration.

If the patient seems so combative that physical violence may be a real risk, the caregiver should step back away from the person, but if the patient starts to do something dangerous (such as run into traffic or bolt from the house) then gentle restraint will be necessary. However, unless the situation is truly serious, any sort of physical restraint should be avoided, because fighting with the patient will likely only worsen the feelings of anxiety and frustration.

communication problems Most people have had problems remembering a word or name from time to time, but for patients with Alzheimer's disease the ability to recall or correctly apply the words they want to use is often lost. As the DEMENTIA worsens, the patient will have more and more problems with communication, which can cause a great deal of embarrassment and frustration. Typically in Alzheimer's disease, communication problems include not just forgetting words, but substituting one word for another; for example, the person may say "Look out the mirror" when he or she means "Look out the window."

A person with Alzheimer's who may still be able to communicate with one individual at a time may still have trouble holding a conversation in a group. As the person's attention span becomes shorter and the ability to focus and concentrate is gradually lost, following the thread of a conversation becomes more difficult. The noise, interruptions, and separate conversations that occur when a group of people are talking together are too confusing for a patient with Alzheimer's. As a result, many patients begin to withdraw in social situations. This withdrawal can be very subtle, and the primary caregiver may be the only person who notices at first. Withdrawing isn't the only way that cognitive problems can surface. Some patients in a group may make remarks that have nothing to do with the topic of conversation. Still others will embark on a running commentary so that no one else can speak. Eventually, the patient with Alzheimer's may try to avoid social encounters altogether.

Other communication problems include repeating questions over and over, since someone who can't remember information will not remember the answer to a previous question. In some cases, repeated questions aren't used as a means of eliciting information as much as obtaining reassurance. For example, a repeated question of "Is it time to go?" may simply reflect the patient's concern about being late for an appointment.

concentration The loss of concentration and lack of ability to pay attention is one of the early signs of Alzheimer's disease.

See also SYMPTOMS OF ALZHEIMER'S DISEASE.

conservator In some states, the guardian who manages an individual's assets.

conservatorship A court proceeding to appoint a manager for the financial affairs or the personal care of a patient who is either physically or mentally unable to handle either or both.

continuing care retirement communities Residential campuses that provide a continuum of care from private units to assisted living, and then skilled nursing care, all in one location. These communities are designed to offer active seniors an independent lifestyle while also providing assisted living services and on-site intermediate or skilled nursing care if necessary.

These retirement communities usually offer a variety of residential services including a maintained apartment, townhouse, or cottage, cleaning and laundry service, meals in common dining areas, grounds maintenance, security, and social, recreational, and cultural programs.

Health care services include personal care and help with daily activities, nursing care, rehabilitation, respite and hospice care, and Alzheimer's and special care.

These types of retirement communities offer a wide variety of contracts and fees ranging from unlimited long-term nursing care for little or no increase in monthly fees to a specified amount of health care beyond which additional fees are incurred. Some communities require residents to purchase long-term care insurance before acceptance.

Monthly fees usually include meals, transportation, cleaning services, unit maintenance, laundry, utilities, organized social activities, emergency call monitoring, and security.

Some states strictly regulate continuing care retirement communities, but others do not. Some communities may choose to be accredited by the Continuing Care Accreditation Commission (CCAC), a private nonprofit organization that reviews finances, governance, and administration, resident health and wellness, and resident life of these specialized care facilities.

coordination   One of the symptoms of Alzheimer's disease is visibly impaired coordination, including slowing of movements, halting gait, and reduced sense of balance.

cortisol   A stress hormone produced by the adrenal glands that, in sustained high levels, might actually hasten degeneration of the HIPPOCAMPUS, the seahorse-shaped part of the brain vital to learning and memory. The hippocampus is a part of the brain that is particularly vulnerable to stress and stress hormones. Some researchers have reported that high cortisol levels are linked to the development of Alzheimer's disease.

Studies show that prolonged depression or stress leads to elevated levels of cortisol and a smaller hippocampus. While cortisol levels normally fluctuate throughout the day, they often soar when a person is faced with a stressful situation. Studies have shown that this stress also affects memory. For example, researchers reported in the April 2000 issue of *Nature Neuroscience* that people taking cortisone pills (which change into cortisol in the body) were not as good at remembering a list of words as people taking placebo pills.

However, researchers haven't yet determined what role cortisol definitely plays in Alzheimer's disease, since studies show that while all people with Alzheimer's have hippocampal damage, their cortisol levels vary. In general, however, patients with Alzheimer's have higher levels of cortisol. In addition, preliminary findings suggest that the higher the cortisol levels, the more likely memory and other functions are to decline.

Researchers also suspect that stress may be a risk factor for the development of Alzheimer's. Chronic exposure of the brain to toxic levels of cortisol is a cause of brain degeneration. Cortisol damages nerve cells in and around the hippocampus. As these cells die, critical neurotransmitters are depleted, damaging other cells in the system, eventually damaging cells in the cortex. As the

cells attempt to react to the growing damage, they overproduce proteins which become the tangles and plaques that are the hallmark of Alzheimer's disease.

More recently, several studies have shown that individuals who have been subjected to significant trauma have a hippocampus that is between 15 percent and 25 percent smaller than normal.

If cortisol toxicity caused by extreme or chronic stress does lead to Alzheimer's disease, lifestyle changes could help prevent the condition.

COX-II inhibitors (Vioxx, Celebrex, Mobic)   A new type of NONSTEROIDAL ANTI-INFLAMMATORY DRUG (sometimes called "super aspirin") that may help protect against the development of Alzheimer's disease. These drugs block coenzyme-2 (COX-II), a substance that may regulate specific inflammatory factors involved in Alzheimer's.

These drugs do not appear to have such negative effects on the intestinal lining as standard NSAIDs like ibuprofen. Long-term use of older NSAIDs can cause bleeding and ulcers in the gastrointestinal tract. For this reason, no one should take NSAIDs for protection against Alzheimer's disease without the recommendation of a physician.

CELECOXIB (Celebrex), rofecoxib (Vioxx), and meloxicam (Mobic) are currently approved in the United States.

Creutzfeldt-Jakob disease (CJD)   This rare, fatal brain disease causes memory impairment, behavior change, and ultimately, dementia, and strikes about 250 Americans each year. About 10 percent of patients with CJD have symptoms similar to Alzheimer's disease, but an accurate differentiation between the two can usually be made with ELECTROENCEPHALOGRAM (EEG) testing and an analysis of cerebrospinal fluid. CJD is usually distinguished from other dementias by its rapid course—it takes only months from onset of symptoms until death.

There are three varieties of this brain-wasting disease: sporadic, acquired, and hereditary. Most experts believe all three versions are caused by a transmissible infectious particle called a PRION, a misshapen protein that alters the shape of other proteins, causing cavities in the brain. All three varieties of CJD are considered infectious but not contagious. It is not possible to get the condition during contact such as hugging, kissing, or sexual intercourse.

Types of CJD

Acquired CJD This version of the condition includes both iatrogenic CJD (contamination with infected tissue via medical procedures) or variant CJD, which is linked directly to eating meat from cattle infected with bovine spongiform encephalopathy (mad cow disease). At least 80 people in Europe have died from vCJD since the mid-1990s. Mad cow disease was first diagnosed in Britain; cases also have been reported in France, Italy, Germany, and Spain. It is estimated that about a million pounds of contaminated beef may have entered the human food chain, and experts estimate this could result in up to 136,000 cases of vCJD in humans. Because of its long incubation period, it may be years before the toll of vCJD can be determined. VCJD is actually much rarer than classic CJD. As of January 1, 1999, this disease had killed 39 people in Britain and one in France. As of June 2001, there were more than 100 cases of variant CJD in Britain, and no increase in the incidence of variant CJD between 1994 and 1997 in that country. Experts caution there could be more cases if the incubation period is very long, but without knowing the exact route of the infection, or who is most at risk and why, it is currently impossible to predict how many more cases of variant CJD there will be.

No known cases of new-variant CJD in cattle or humans have been found in the United States. Medically induced CJD is transmitted during medical procedures by exposure to brain or nervous system tissue, including eye tissue and spinal cord fluid.

Sporadic CJD This variety accounts for at least 85 percent of all cases in the United States, but is not linked to eating meat. It occurs in patients who have no known risk for the disease, appearing suddenly, usually affecting people over age 50. Its course is usually measured in months, although it can last up to two years.

Hereditary The inherited form of the disease occurs in people with a family history for the condition and who test positive for the genetic mutation in their prions. This version of the condition affects younger people and accounts for between 10 percent and 15 percent of all cases.

Symptoms

The first symptoms of CJD include a sudden, progressive memory loss, with insomnia, mental deterioration, personality changes, bizarre behavior, visual distortions, hallucinations, and thinking problems. It progresses rapidly with involuntary movements, weakness in the limbs, and blindness. Patients soon lose the ability to communicate and lapse into a coma.

Although scientists believe that the disease incubates over many years before causing symptoms, patients typically live only a few months to a year after symptoms appear.

Diagnosis

Doctors use a series of tests (including a very specific pattern on brain scans) to diagnose the condition. The diagnosis can't be confirmed beyond doubt until autopsy. The accuracy of a diagnosis varies depending on the form of the disease. A correct diagnosis may be possible only after death when a postmortem has been performed.

In inherited cases of CJD, a diagnosis depends on analyzing symptoms and genetic testing. Iatrogenic CJD is diagnosed on the basis of symptoms developing in someone with a relevant exposure, for example, in someone who has been given human growth hormone. The diagnosis of variant CJD is very difficult, but brain scanning, using magnetic resonance imaging (MRI), and tonsil biopsy may be useful.

Treatment

There is no treatment beyond treating symptoms with medications for the spasms, seizures, and stiffness. There are a number of drugs that can relieve symptoms and make the patient more comfortable, including valproate and clonazepam for jerking movements.

cues Giving a person with Alzheimer's disease visual cues can be an important way to communicate nonverbally. Caregivers should look directly at the patient with a smile as a way of maintaining attention. Visible gestures and other types of body language can also help reinforce verbal messages.

cyclo-oxygenase 2 (COX II) A substance that may regulate specific inflammatory factors involved in Alzheimer's disease. COX-II INHIBITORS (Vioxx, Celebrex, Mobic) are a new type of NONSTEROIDAL ANTI-INFLAMMATORY DRUG that block the coenzyme.

cytochrome oxidase (CO) An enzyme in the mitochondria of a cell that is a key part of the cellular energy production process. Many patients with Alzheimer's disease appear to have inherited a high level of a mutant form of this enzyme.

Previous studies had shown that children of mothers with Alzheimer's disease were more likely to get the disease than children of fathers with the condition—a hallmark of mitochondrial inheritance. Mitochondria with these CO mutations had poor energy production and high levels of oxygen FREE RADICALS (the damaging molecules produced by incomplete energy generation). Free radicals damage cell membranes and have been linked in the death of brain cells common among Alzheimer's patients.

In addition, reduced CO activity leads to an increase in the direct precursor of AMYLOID PRECURSOR PROTEIN (APP).

dapsone An anti-inflammatory drug that has been used for decades in the treatment of leprosy, and is now being tested for use in Alzheimer's disease. Research sites have been established in Brazil, Israel, Poland, and South Africa with trials involving more than 300 Alzheimer's patients.

Current medications only ease symptoms in some patients, but don't stop the underlying brain cell death associated with the disease. Prior studies support the use of dapsone for people suffering from DEMENTIA. In 1992, 3,792 Japanese leprosy patients were monitored for dementia after using dapsone for five years. The study found that those patients who were taking dapsone had a 37 percent lower prevalence of developing dementia compared with those who were not taking the drug.

However, other studies question the effect of dapsone on Alzheimer's. One study found the dementia rate of patients with tuberculoid leprosy is similar to that of patients with lepromatous leprosy, although the latter group took more dapsone.

Side effects include back, leg, and stomach pains, unusual tiredness or weakness, difficulty breathing, loss of appetite, dryness or peeling of skin, and sore throat. The Canadian Phase I clinical study was stopped due to unexplained problems with blood samples from healthy volunteers. Previous studies in other countries have not reported such adverse effects, and the Canadian experience has not affected the ongoing international Phase II trials of the drug.

day care See ADULT DAY SERVICES.

death The most common causes of death in patients with Alzheimer's disease are from infec-tions and not eating. The course of the disease varies from person to person; some people have the disease for only the last five years of life, while others may have it for as many as 20 years. Most people with Alzheimer's die within seven years of a diagnosis.

dehydroepiandrosterone (DHEA) One of the four most common steroid hormones in the body that may play a role in cognition. Produced mainly in the adrenal gland, DHEA is the precursor hormone to testosterone and estrogen. Because nerve degeneration occurs most often when DHEA levels are low, some researchers suspect that DHEA may protect brain cells against Alzheimer's disease and other forms of DEMENTIA. Because patients with Alzheimer's have only half as much DHEA as their same-aged colleagues without the disease, studies are looking into the possibility of using this drug to enhance COGNITIVE ABILITIES of patients. DHEA has been shown to improve long-term MEMORY in mice.

However, critics point out that DHEA may raise the risk of prostate or endometrial cancer, or that it could make cancer grow faster in someone who already has the disease.

delirium A group of symptoms temporarily impairing mental function characterized by a clouding of consciousness with a reduced capacity to focus and sustain attention. The individual suffering from delirium has a decreased ability to pay attention to what's going on around him, and is often highly disruptive. Delirium usually begins abruptly and is worse at night, either because of disturbed sleep or because the dark and quiet make visual illusions more common.

The total duration is usually brief, ranging from hours to days, but can be serious if the condition is not identified and treated, which is why it is essential to recognize the difference between DEMENTIA and delirium. It is most common among the very old.

Delirium is usually reversible once the underlying condition is recognized and treated. Patients require calm and clear communication, sufficient lighting, appropriate seclusion, and familiar attendants. It is important to maintain fluids and nutrition; tranquilizers are often necessary to treat restlessness.

delusions   A false idea that is firmly believed and strongly maintained in spite of contradictory proof or evidence. Delusions are common symptoms in Alzheimer's disease.

Because of MEMORY problems, a person with DEMENTIA may sometimes become suspicious and may accuse someone of stealing when something has been mislaid. However, as the disease progresses, suspicions begin to worsen and patients may develop distorted ideas about what is actually happening. Patients may become convinced that others want to harm them, and no amount of evidence to the contrary will persuade them otherwise.

Common delusions that people with Alzheimer's have are

- Their partner is being unfaithful.
- Their partner or close relative has been replaced by an impostor.
- Their home is not their own.
- Their food is being poisoned.
- Others are spying on them.

Delusions are the result of the changes that are occurring in the BRAIN, although sometimes these ideas may be the result of HALLUCINATIONS.

Arguing with a delusional patient is not helpful. CAREGIVERS should try to reassure patients and distract them with other activities. Medication can sometimes be helpful, particularly if the person is becoming aggressive. This type of medication needs to be reviewed regularly.

dementia   A general term for a group of serious symptoms caused by changes in brain function that leads to a loss in at least two areas of intellectual function, such as language, MEMORY, visual and spatial abilities, reasoning, and judgment. The problems must be severe enough to interfere with a person's daily functioning. Dementia affects more than 4 million Americans, about half of whom are demented as a result of Alzheimer's disease.

Dementia is not a disease itself, but describes symptoms that may accompany certain diseases or conditions. Dementia is irreversible when caused by disease or injury, but may be treatable when caused by drugs, alcohol, hormone or vitamin imbalances, or DEPRESSION.

Symptoms
Dementia affects many areas of intellectual function, and may include changes in personality, mood, and behavior. However, in the beginning a patient may experience problems in only one area, such as

- repeatedly asking the same questions
- getting lost in familiar places
- being unable to follow directions
- getting disoriented
- neglecting personal safety, hygiene, and nutrition.

Cause
Dementia can be caused by an infectious process (such as in CREUTZFELDT-JAKOB DISEASE), by an unknown problem, as in Alzheimer's disease, or by reduced blood flow to the BRAIN. Other treatable causes of dementia may include high fever, dehydration, vitamin deficiency and poor nutrition, reactions to medicines, thyroid problems, or a minor head injury.

In addition, emotional problems in the elderly can be mistaken for dementia. Feeling sad, lonely, worried, or bored may be more common for older people facing retirement or coping with the death of a spouse, relative, or friend, and these changes may trigger episodes of confusion or forgetfulness.

The two most common forms of dementia in older people are Alzheimer's disease and multi-infarct dementia (or vascular dementia). These types of dementia are irreversible and can't be cured. In Alzheimer's disease, nerve cell changes in certain parts of the brain result in the death of a large number of cells. Symptoms of Alzheimer's disease begin slowly and become steadily worse. As the disease progresses, symptoms range from mild forgetfulness to serious impairments in thinking, judgment, and the ability to perform daily activities. Eventually, patients may need total care.

Patients with multi-infarct dementia experience a series of small STROKES or changes in the brain's blood supply that may destroy brain tissue. The location in the brain where the small strokes occur determines the symptoms and seriousness of the problem. Symptoms that begin suddenly may be a sign of this kind of dementia. People with multi-infarct dementia are likely to show signs of improvement or remain stable for long periods of time, but then quickly develop new symptoms if more small strokes occur. Often, multi-infarct dementia is caused by high blood pressure.

Alzheimer's disease and multi-infarct dementia often occur together, which makes it difficult to diagnose either one specifically. Scientists once thought that multi-infarct dementia caused most cases of irreversible mental impairment, but today experts think most older people with irreversible dementia have Alzheimer's disease.

Other types of medical conditions that cause dementia include

- Parkinson's disease; Lewy body dementia
- PICK'S DISEASE
- CREUTZFELDT-JAKOB DISEASE
- Korsakoff's syndrome
- AIDS
- brain tumors
- hydrocephalus (fluid on the brain)
- head injuries

Treatment

Even if the doctor diagnoses an irreversible form of dementia, it is still possible to treat the patient's symptoms and help the family cope. A person with dementia should be under the care of a neurolo-gist, psychiatrist, family doctor, internist, or geriatrician. The doctor can treat the patient's physical and behavioral problems and answer the many questions that the person or family may have.

Antipsychotic drugs can ease agitation, anxiety, and aggression. Keeping a familiar routine, encouraging social and physical activity, and maintaining a safe environment can help the patient remain comfortable.

In cases where the underlying cause of dementia is untreatable, it may eventually be necessary to place the person in a health facility providing care on a 24-hour basis.

dementia-capable Health care workers who are skilled in working with people with DEMENTIA and their caregivers, knowledgeable about the kinds of services that may help them, and aware of which agencies and individuals provide such services.

dementia-specific Services that are provided specifically for people with DEMENTIA.

demoic acid A chemical that is found in some shellfish, which also stimulates a neurotransmitter called GLUTAMATE that is normally involved in learning and memory. Glutamate is also linked to the development of Alzheimer's disease. Some scientists believe that chronically high levels of the neurotransmitter glutamate may disrupt metabolism in the cell, leading to its ultimate destruction.

In Canada, an outbreak of a neurological disorder similar to Alzheimer's occurred among people who had eaten mussels contaminated with demoic acid.

dental care Taking care of the teeth can be difficult for a patient with Alzheimer's disease, although it is very important to keep patients comfortable and healthy. Patients may have trouble brushing because they forget what to do with the toothpaste or how to rinse. As the disease progresses, patients may totally forget why dental care is important and neglect their teeth.

Dental problems can be dangerous in patients with Alzheimer's, since they can choke if they can't chew properly due to tooth disorders. Moreover, dental problems can interfere with good nutrition or cause such severe pain from cavities that the person can't communicate. If good dental hygiene is ignored, the patient may experience significant tooth problems later, when treatment could become more difficult. Good tooth care also can help maintain the patient's appearance and comfort despite the progression of their disease.

Even healthy older people often have dental problems that cause pain or make it hard to chew, swallow, and speak. These problems are even more likely in someone who has forgotten how to use a toothbrush or keep dentures clean.

What Caregivers Can Do

Brushing may be difficult if the patient cannot understand or accept help from others. CAREGIVERS should provide simple yet specific tooth brushing instructions that break the process down into a step-by-step series of commands.

Patients with Alzheimer's may forget how to brush and floss, so it may also help if the caregiver demonstrates correct tooth brushing techniques for the patient. Caregivers should encourage patients to brush, guiding them through each step of the process or demonstrating by brushing their own teeth at the same time.

Caregivers who must brush the patient's teeth should gently place the toothbrush in the person's mouth at a 45-degree angle so the gum tissue can be massaged as the teeth are cleaned. A spoon or another brush can be used to help pull the cheek sideways to reveal the area being brushed.

Patients should brush the teeth at least twice a day for two minutes, if possible, with the last brushing after the evening meal and evening liquid medication. If the person seems agitated or uncooperative, caregivers may want to postpone brushing until later in the day, or try brushing fewer times a day.

Many caregivers have found that a soft-bristle children's toothbrush works better than a hard-bristle adult's brush; a long-handled or angled brush may work well for caregivers who must brush a patient's teeth. Patients who have trouble spitting may need to have the gel wiped from the mouth.

To protect tooth surfaces from decay, caregivers should encourage patients to use a fluoride rinse or gel as well as a fluoride toothpaste. Although fluoride rinses can be bought without prescription, stannous fluoride gels require a prescription. Most dentists recommend dental floss, although caregivers and patients may find it frustrating to use.

Patients may find it easier to use a toothbrush if a ball, bicycle handlebar grip, or aluminum foil is attached to the end of the handle. Alternatively, a Velcro strap around the patient's hand and attached to the toothbrush may help. Electric toothbrushes are probably not a good idea, since they may confuse a person with Alzheimer's or cause safety problems.

Dentures require special care. They should fit properly and be rinsed with plain water after mealtimes to remove food particles. Dentures should be cleaned with a hard-bristle brush, and they should soak in a cleanser or mouthwash overnight. In the later stages, patients may not be able to wear full or partial dentures.

As the patient's condition deteriorates, patients may refuse to brush their teeth at all, or may become uncooperative at the dentist's office, which may force the caregiver to assume complete responsibility for toothbrushing.

Because there is a direct relationship between diet and good dental health, it is usually a good idea to limit or eliminate sugary foods such as candy, cookies, cakes, and soft drinks. This is even more important for those who are particularly attracted to sweet foods, as many patients are. Many patients become obsessed with food, and some between-meal sugary snacks can lead to tooth problems. If caregivers do provide sugary foods, they should be given along with regular meals, so that the patient can brush teeth or at least rinse the mouth with water afterward.

Seeing a Dentist

A dentist should be consulted soon after a patient is diagnosed with Alzheimer's, before the condition has progressed. Local dental associations should list names of dentists qualified to work with elderly patients. Some general dentists are familiar with the illnesses and conditions of older people and have often spent extensive time working in nursing homes.

Although healthy people visit the dentist twice a year, a patient with Alzheimer's should see a dentist more often for regular cleanings so as to prevent tooth decay and gum problems. Since the patient may not brush as effectively as in the past, and because it can be hard for caregivers to brush someone else's teeth well, these extra visits can be important.

By working with a dentist to treat dental problems soon after the diagnosis of Alzheimer's, the patient can avoid having extensive dental work in end-stage disease.

Some medications used to treat Alzheimer's may cause oral symptoms. Caregivers should discuss with the dentist how these medications might affect teeth, gums, and mouth, including blood thinners, antidepressants, antianxiety agents, antihistamines, diuretics, and blood pressure pills.

For example, many medications cause dry mouth by reducing the production of saliva, which acts as a buffer against tooth decay. As the mouth dries, the likelihood of tooth decay and gum problems increases. If patients complain of dry mouth, they should drink periodically throughout the day, or use "artificial saliva" (available at drugstores and pharmacies). Since alcohol can contribute to a dry mouth, some experts suggest using mouth rinses that are low in alcohol, or adding water to mouth rinses that contain alcohol.

deprenyl   See SELEGILINE.

depression   An unrelenting, pervading sense of sadness or despair common in as many as half of all patients with Alzheimer's disease, especially in the early stages of the condition.

Temporary episodes of depression are a perfectly normal response upon learning the diagnosis of Alzheimer's disease. Depression also may be triggered by having to leave home because of declining mental abilities, feeling unproductive, or the effects of medications. However, other cases of depression in patients with Alzheimer's are related to significant changes in BRAIN chemistry. Typically, depression is the result of a collision between genetics, biochemistry, and psychological factors. The physiological basis of depression may be found

in neurons in the part of the brain responsible for human emotions centered in the hypothalamus, a cherry-sized structure that controls basic functions such as thirst, hunger, sleep, sexual desire, and body temperature. It is a part of the brain often affected by Alzheimer's as well.

Each nerve cell in the brain is separated by tiny gaps called SYNAPSES; neurons communicate by sending chemical messengers across these gaps to a receptor on the other side. Each neurotransmitter has a special shape that helps it fit exactly into a corresponding receptor like a key into an ignition switch. When the neurotransmitter "key" is inserted into its matching receptor's "ignition," the cell receiving the transmitter may then fire an action potential—the electrical impulse that travels down the axon to release its own transmitter to the next neuron.

Once the message is sent, the neurotransmitter is either absorbed into the cell, or burned up by enzymes patrolling the gap.

When there are abnormally low levels of certain neurotransmitters, messages can't get across the gaps, and communication in the brain slows down. It appears that depression occurs if there isn't enough of these neurotransmitters circulating in the brain, or if the neurotransmitters can't fit into the receptors for some reason.

While there are as many as 100 different kinds of neurotransmitters, norepinephrine, dopamine, and serotonin seem to be of particular importance in depression. The pathways for these neurotransmitters reach deep into many of the parts of the brain responsible for functions that are affected in depression, such as sleep, appetite, mood, and sexual interest.

Scientists aren't sure whether depression is directly related to abnormal levels of these transmitters, or whether these neurotransmitters affect yet another neurotransmitter that is even more directly involved in depression. It is clear that neurotransmitters are related to depression because medications that boost their levels also ease depression. However, some of the newer antidepressants do not affect the levels of all of these neurotransmitters, while they still relieve depression, and other drugs (such as cocaine) that *do* interfere with neurotransmitter level do *not* affect depression.

Moreover, antidepressants can raise neurotransmitter levels almost immediately, but depression does not improve until weeks after drug treatment begins. For these reasons, depression appears to be far more than a simple problem with the amount of neurotransmitters in the synaptic cleft. It is probably influenced by a complex interplay of receptor "ignition" responses and the release of the neurotransmitter "keys"—and probably not just by the number of keys affected, but also the quality and availability of the receptor "ignitions."

Depressive symptoms appear in about 15 percent of people over age 65, with major depression affecting 3 percent in this age group. Experts estimate that between 11 percent and 50 percent of people with Alzheimer's also have depression.

Symptoms

Symptoms include restlessness, feelings of hopelessness, suicidal thoughts, concentration problems, withdrawal, lack of interest or pleasure in activities that were once enjoyed, sleep problems, appetite change, lethargy, and extreme fatigue.

Diagnosis

A team of researchers led by the National Institutes of Mental Health (NIMH) has developed the first diagnostic criteria to characterize the depression that commonly occurs in Alzheimer's disease, a milestone experts hope will result in better recognition and treatment of depression in these patients. While doctors know that depression occurs in Alzheimer's patients, the lack of diagnostic criteria has meant that too many patients are not diagnosed or properly treated.

Treatment

In the early stages of Alzheimer's, support groups, education about the disease, and counseling can help the patient deal with the diagnosis. Caregivers also need to keep reassuring the patient in the early stages of the disease that he or she can still have some control over life by participating in decisions made for the future.

Medication may help the person suffering from depression brought on by Alzheimer's. Some experts believe that disease progression may even be delayed by using both an antidepressant and an Alzheimer's drug such as DONEPEZIL. The newer antidepressants known as SELECTIVE SEROTONIN REUPTAKE INHIBITORS (SSRIs) (such as Prozac or Zoloft) may be particularly effective in relieving depression, irritability, and restlessness associated with Alzheimer's.

It is important to understand the difference between depression and APATHY, since the two are often confused; according to one study, apathy is more common than depression in patients with Alzheimer's. Apathy responds to stimulants, such as methylphenidate (Ritalin), rather than antidepressants. An apathetic patient lacks emotions, motivation, interest, and enthusiasm while a depressed patient is generally very sad, tearful, and hopeless.

There are some indications that in some people, depression may be a risk factor for the development of Alzheimer's—or a very early symptom. In these patients, depressive symptoms appear before the memory problems or behavior changes of Alzheimer's. Their relatives may notice slight changes in personality; as the depression persists over the next few years despite medication, the symptoms eventually deepen into full-blown Alzheimer's.

diabetes   Patients with diabetes have almost double the risk of developing Alzheimer's disease or DEMENTIA as does the non-diabetic population. Several long-term studies, including the Atherosclerosis Risk in Communities (ARIC) study and the Framingham Heart Study, have shown that Alzheimer's disease, cognitive impairment, and vascular dementia are more common in people with type 2 diabetes.

Researchers suggest that both high blood sugar and insulin resistance, (both underlying conditions found in type 2 diabetes) may speed up a patient's decline in thinking abilities. For example, high concentrations of sugar in the blood can lead to the development of blood vessel abnormalities that may affect the brain and the ability to think clearly.

While the cause of diabetes-related cognitive impairment is not fully understood, several studies suggest that insulin resistance may be a contributing factor to the condition.

Researchers are currently studying whether drugs that treat insulin resistance can have an effect on cognitive performance in patients with type 2 diabetes. Together with diet and exercise, the drug Avandia helps improve blood sugar control.

See also INSULIN-DEGRADING ENZYME (IDE).

diagnosis of Alzheimer's disease Alzheimer's disease is a complex illness characterized by a range of gradual, subtle changes that make it hard to diagnose. Because of the many other disorders that can be confused with Alzheimer's, a comprehensive clinical evaluation is essential to arrive at a correct diagnosis.

While there is no single test that can determine if someone has Alzheimer's disease, an early diagnosis is important since medication and care options are most effective in those with mild to moderate Alzheimer's.

Of course, the only definite way to diagnose Alzheimer's disease is at autopsy, although doctors at specialized centers can correctly diagnose the disease 80 percent to 90 percent of the time by conducting physical and neuropsychological testing with CAREGIVER input.

The ALZHEIMER'S ASSOCIATION has developed a list of 10 warning signs to help differentiate Alzheimer's from normal aging. Individuals who have several of the following symptoms should see a doctor for a complete exam:

1. Memory loss that affects job skills
2. Problems in performing familiar tasks
3. Problems with language
4. Getting lost in familiar places
5. Problems with judgment
6. Problems with abstract thinking
7. Misplacing items
8. Change in mood or behavior
9. Personality change
10. Loss of initiative

People who are worried about memory problems should see a doctor, who may recommend a thorough physical, neurological, and psychiatric evaluation if the problem seems serious. Often, the diagnosis will involve a primary care physician together with a psychiatrist or neurologist.

Typically, a doctor will first ask 10 simple questions to determine if the person knows who and where he is. In addition, tests of visual memory may help diagnose the condition. Visual memory is the ability to remember and reproduce geometric patterns. People with Alzheimer's begin to lose immediate visual memory sooner than is expected in normal aging, and long before other symptoms of DEMENTIA are noticeable. One way to test visual memory is to have a patient draw the face of a clock with the hands pointing to a certain hour.

A complete medical examination for memory loss may include gathering information about the person's medical history, including use of prescription and over-the-counter medicines, DIET, past medical problems, and general health. Because a correct diagnosis depends on recalling these details accurately, the doctor also may ask a family member for information about the person.

In addition to the detailed history, the doctor will probably order several tests, including a complete physical and neurological examination, a psychological assessment and laboratory tests. Information from the medical history and any test results help the doctor rule out other possible causes of the person's symptoms. For example, thyroid gland problems, drug reactions, DEPRESSION, brain tumors, and blood vessel disease in the brain can cause Alzheimer's-like symptoms. Once these tests are completed, a diagnosis of Alzheimer's disease can be made with about 90 percent accuracy.

Many things can cause dementia, which is a decline in intellectual ability severe enough to interfere with a person's daily routine. It is important to identify the actual cause of the dementia in order for the person to receive the proper care. Although the onset of Alzheimer's disease symptoms cannot yet be stopped or reversed, an early diagnosis gives people with the disease a greater chance of benefiting from existing and experimental treatments.

The following tests include some of the information the doctor may need to make a diagnosis:

Medical history The doctor may ask about the person's general health and past medical problems. He or she will want to know about any problems the person has carrying out daily activities. The doctor may want to speak with the person's family or friends to get more information.

Basic medical tests Tests of blood and urine may be done to help the doctor eliminate other possible diseases. In some cases, testing a small amount of spinal fluid also may help. In addition, scientists are busy trying to develop a test to diagnose Alzheimer's that will be easy and accurate.

Neuropsychological tests Tests of memory, problem solving, vision, motor coordination, attention, counting, and language will help the doctor pinpoint specific problems and may provide the only evidence of dementia, especially in the early stages.

Psychiatric evaluation These tests can assess mood and other emotional factors that could mimic dementia or may accompany Alzheimer's disease.

Brain scans Several types of brain scans, including computerized tomography (CT) scan, magnetic resonance imaging (MRI) scan, or a positron emission tomography (PET) scan, can be used to take a picture of the brain. In the early stages of Alzheimer's, brain changes won't show up on most scans, but these tests can be used to help rule out some other disorders that mimic Alzheimer's. In later stages, however, scans may begin to show changes in the brain, such as shrunken brain tissue with widened tissue indentations and enlarged cerebral fluid-filled chambers.

See also ASSESSMENT TOOLS.

diet A healthy diet with low fat intake may reduce the risk of developing Alzheimer's disease, according to research. Studies also suggest that a high-fat diet during early and mid-adulthood may be associated with an increased risk of developing Alzheimer's, especially in people with a marker called the APOE-4 GENE. In a retrospective study that examined food eaten by 304 men and women (72 with Alzheimer's disease and 232 healthy individuals), researchers found that people with the apoE-4 gene who also ate the most fat were seven times more likely to develop Alzheimer's than people with the marker who ate lower fat diets. In a separate 2000 study of Americans between the ages of 40 and 50, those who carried the apoE-4 gene and whose diet consisted of 40 percent fat calories had 29 times the risk for Alzheimer's compared to non-apoE-4 carriers on the same high-fat diet.

Some population studies have reported an association between low-fat diets and a lower incidence in Alzheimer's. For example, in China and Nigeria, where fat intake is low, the risk of developing Alzheimer's is 1 percent at age of 65 compared to 5 percent in the United States. In the Netherlands, researchers reported an association between DEMENTIA and diets high in total fat, saturated fat, and cholesterol.

Getting lots of ANTIOXIDANTS in the diet may also be important in lowering the risk of Alzheimer's. Antioxidants are substances that protect the body from the harmful effects of FREE RADICALS (molecules that can cause cellular damage within the body and have been blamed for heart disease and some types of cancer). A recent study involving more than 5,000 Dutch participants over the age of 55 suggests that a diet high in antioxidants may reduce the risk of developing Alzheimer's disease by as much as 25 percent. Antioxidants identified as beneficial in the study group were beta-carotene, vitamin C, and vitamin E, which are found in many fresh fruits and vegetables.

See also DOCOSAHEXAENOIC ACID (DHA).

dimethylaminoethanol (DMAE) A naturally occurring nutrient found in some types of seafood and in the human BRAIN that may improve MEMORY and learning. It is believed to improve the brain's production of ACETYLCHOLINE, which plays an important part in memory. Patients with Alzheimer's disease have abnormally low levels of acetylcholine.

Drugs such as TACRINE and danazol, and supplements such as HUPERZINE A, are all used to treat Alzheimer's disease based on their ability to increase acetylcholine levels. Because DMAE is also thought to increase acetylcholine, some studies have tested its effectiveness for the same purpose. However, there is no real evidence as yet that it works.

A double-blind placebo-controlled study involving 27 patients with Alzheimer's disease tested DMAE as a treatment. Thirteen participants received DMAE, but six of them had to drop out because of side effects such as drowsiness, increased confusion, and elevated blood pressure. In those completing the trial, no differences were seen between the treatment group and those taking placebo. Likewise, an open trial enrolling 14 patients found no improvement in either memory or cognitive function. Researchers did note improvements in symptoms of depression, but in the absence of a placebo group this observation means little.

Overdoses of DMAE can cause insomnia, headache, or muscle tension. While no serious side effects have been reported, it may deepen the depression phase in manic-depression patients.

disorientation A cognitive disability in which the senses of time, direction, and recognition become difficult to distinguish. Disorientation is a common symptom of Alzheimer's disease.

docosahexaenoic acid (DHA) An omega-3 fatty acid that is found in lower amounts among patients with Alzheimer's disease. Scientists have already found DHA can reduce the risk of heart disease, depression, and attention deficit disorder. It's concentrated in fatty fish (the fattier the better) such as salmon and tuna, fish oils, and omega-3-enriched eggs.

Canadian researchers who discovered that people with Alzheimer's have lower levels of DHA in their blood aren't sure if more DHA in the diet would prevent the disease. The low levels in Alzheimer's patients could be a signal of the disease as easily as it could be a cause.

Until researchers know more, experts believe that it's a good idea to increase consumption of fish to at least two servings a week, or four omega-3-enriched eggs a week. Eating fish may help to prevent Alzheimer's, but even if it doesn't, it's a healthy diet choice anyway.

The recommended daily allowance of omega-3 fatty acids (of which DHA is one) for people aged 25 to 49 is 1.5 grams a day.

doctor visits Because visiting the doctor can be stressful for a moderately disabled patient with Alzheimer's disease, the office staff should be informed of the person's situation before the visit.

Because a patient's attention span is short, the time spent sitting in the waiting room should be limited. Waiting in an empty room is usually preferable to the main (and usually crowded) waiting room. Appointment times should be based on the person's daily routine when function is best, or when the office is less crowded or noisy.

A patient with Alzheimer's should never be left alone in a waiting room; if necessary, a third person may go along to drive and help keep the person occupied. Extra reassurance is often important for the person with Alzheimer's, who is away from the familiar environment. While waiting, caregivers can provide nutritious snacks to appease hunger if the wait is long, or distract the person with a deck of cards or a magazine.

donepezil (Aricept) A new drug approved for the treatment of mild to moderate Alzheimer's disease that has helped some patients by improving thinking, general function, and behavior. The drug works by boosting the levels of ACETYLCHOLINE, a chemical important in learning and MEMORY. Acetylcholine levels have been found to be much lower than normal among patients with Alzheimer's.

Because animal tests suggest that it might also make a difference in less serious memory disorders, the National Institute on Aging is studying the feasibility of using Aricept for people with mild cognitive impairment.

Although this drug helps slow the progression of Alzheimer's in some patients, it doesn't work for everyone and it doesn't cure the disease in anyone. All of these drugs are most effective if taken early in the disease when there are more functioning brain cells capable of producing acetylcholine. After the disease progresses and too many acetylcholine-producing cells die, its effectiveness lessens.

The drug is available in 5 mg or 10 mg tablets. Although many patients can tolerate Aricept, it can cause diarrhea and vomiting, nausea, nightmares, sleep disturbances, fatigue, and anorexia. These are mild in most cases and usually last from one to three weeks, declining with continued use of the drug.

Do Not Resuscitate orders   A legal directive by a physician that instructs hospital staff not to try to help a patient whose heart has stopped or who has stopped breathing.

A patient can request a DNR order either by filling out an ADVANCE DIRECTIVE form or by telling the doctor that cardiopulmonary resuscitation (CPR) should not be performed. DNR orders are accepted by doctors and hospitals in all states.

Down syndrome   A genetic abnormality characterized by abnormal facial features and delayed intellectual and language development that is caused by an extra copy of all or part of CHROMOSOME 21. Most individuals with Down syndrome develop Alzheimer's disease at a young age—usually by the late 40s or early 50s. Nearly every person with Down syndrome who lives to the age of 60 will develop DEMENTIA.

Scientists suspect people with Down syndrome are vulnerable to Alzheimer's because they produce too much BETA AMYLOID protein—the major component of plaques. The gene for the protein that produces beta amyloid is found on CHROMOSOME 21 and Down syndrome patients have an extra copy of this chromosome. It's likely that the overproduction of beta amyloid ultimately leads to its buildup in the brain in the form of plaques.

Psychologists recommend that individuals with Down syndrome take a baseline test of cognitive function at age 30 and periodically thereafter, to check for the development of Alzheimer's. If the tests show deterioration, further tests must be made to rule out diseases which present similar symptoms.

dressing   Choosing and wearing clothing is a personal, private activity that may become difficult for patients with Alzheimer's disease. Patients who need help should be given tactful, sensitive assistance so that they can continue to make their own choices for as long as they can.

Because people with Alzheimer's will take longer to process information than they used to do, this will affect their ability to make choices; it will likely take much longer to help patients dress. Patients should be encouraged to dress themselves for as long as possible.

Many patients find it helpful if CAREGIVERS lay out clothes in the order they will put them on, gently reminding patients which garment goes on next, or handing them appropriate clothing as needed. Dirty clothes should be promptly removed, since this will help prevent patients from putting dirty clothes back on.

As the disease progresses and patients become more confused, caregivers should give instructions in very short steps, such as: "Now put your foot into the sock." If a patient makes a mistake, such as putting something on backward, quiet correction will keep disruption to a minimum.

The room should be warm as the patient gets dressed. Because the patient may no longer be able to articulate if they are too hot or too cold, it may make sense to provide several layers of thin clothing rather than one thick layer. A morning and evening routine can be very helpful. Patients may prefer to get completely dressed on top before beginning on the bottom. Patients who resist a caregiver's efforts to help may be best handled by leaving them for a while instead of insisting, which can trigger AGITATION.

People with Alzheimer's should still be treated with personal dignity, so caregivers should allow patients to choose what they wear. However, because too many options can be confusing, it is better to make suggestions one at a time. When buying clothes for patients with Alzheimer's, look for items that are washable and don't need much ironing, that are easy to put on and take off. Shoes with laces may be difficult for someone with DEMENTIA to manage, so well-fitting slip-ons may help the person to remain independent a little longer. Slippers should not be worn for more than a few hours because they do not offer enough support to the feet.

Because patients may be reluctant to undress, or refuse to change their clothes, it may help for caregivers to remove dirty clothing and substitute clean clothing when patients get washed or take a bath. Patients may be willing to change if someone comes to visit. As long as it does no harm, it is probably better to accept bizarre clothing or clothing that is out of place rather than having a confrontation. If a person is determined to wear a hat in bed, for example, caregivers should try when possible to respect the choice.

driving Driving is a complex activity that requires quick reactions, memory of traffic laws, good thinking skills, and the ability to make split-second decisions. For all of these reasons, the person with Alzheimer's disease will find it difficult (if not impossible) to drive safely. Unfortunately, the patient may not recognize at first that changes in thinking and sensory skills impair driving abilities.

Drivers with Alzheimer's disease have a substantially increased rate of accidents and driving performance errors, according to a number of research studies. Because they pose a significant traffic safety risk, they should be advised not to drive by health care providers.

Results from studies conducted at Johns Hopkins University and at the National Institute on Aging (NIA) support the belief that people should not be allowed to drive after a diagnosis of Alzheimer's disease. In the Hopkins study, more than 40 percent of patients studied had been in an accident after a diagnosis of the disease. Of these, 11 percent had caused accidents themselves; 44 percent had routinely gotten lost, and 75 percent continually drove below the speed limit. Studies found that even those with early Alzheimer's had markedly impaired driving skills. A separate Swedish study found that over half of elderly people involved in fatal accidents had some degree of neurological damage. In some states, such as California, a physician must report a diagnosis of Alzheimer's disease to the health department, which then reports it to the Department of Motor Vehicles. That agency then may revoke the person's license.

drug treatments There are two kinds of medications that are used in the treatment of Alzheimer's disease—drugs to treat cognitive problems and medications used to control problem behaviors. In addition, more than a dozen new medications are now in research trials in hopes of final approval by the U.S. Food and Drug Administration.

Cognitive Treatments

There are four medications that have been currently approved for treating cognitive problems common in mild to moderate Alzheimer's, all of which work primarily by interfering with the breakdown of ACETYLCHOLINE, a neurotransmitter that occurs in abnormally low levels in patients with Alzheimer's. These medications all belong to a class of drugs known as cholinesterase inhibitors, which means they interfere with the breakdown of acetylcholine.

Acetylcholine is a chemical messenger in the BRAIN that appears to be important in proper functioning of brain cells involved in MEMORY, thought, and judgment. Acetylcholine is released by one brain cell to help send a message to another cell; once a message is received, enzymes including ACETYLCHOLINESTERASE break down acetylcholine for reuse. In patients with Alzheimer's, the cells that use acetylcholine are damaged or destroyed, which lowers the levels of acetylcholine.

A CHOLINESTERASE INHIBITOR is designed to stop the activity of acetylcholinesterase. By slowing down the metabolic breakdown of acetylcholine, more of the brain chemical is available to enhance cell communication.

Although these drugs do not affect the underlying disease process, they may temporarily stabilize or delay worsening of memory problems. However, not all patients respond to these drugs.

Four medications have been approved to treat loss of memory and decline in abilities such as thinking and reasoning: TACRINE (Cognex), available by prescription since 1993; DONEPEZIL (Aricept), available since 1996; RIVASTIGMINE (Exelon), approved in 2000, and GALANTAMINE (Reminyl), approved in 2001. All these drugs work by increasing the brain's supply of acetylcholine. Galantamine also appears to stimulate the release of acetylcholine and affects the way some of the brain's receptors on message-receiving nerve cells respond to acetylcholine.

Although these can help slow the progression of Alzheimer's, they don't cure the disease. All of these drugs are most effective if taken early in the disease when there are more functioning brain cells to produce acetylcholine. After too many acetylcholine-producing cells die, the drug no longer works.

These drugs are approved for treatment of mild to moderate Alzheimer's and may not be as useful for people in more advanced stages. Currently, there is no known way to predict whether or not a patient will benefit from any of them. Because of this uncertainty, doctors and patients' families must weigh the potential benefits, risks, and costs associated with their use.

Side Effects

Tacrine is very rarely prescribed because of side effects including possible liver damage. Donepezil, rivastigmine, and galantamine are all fairly well tolerated by most people with Alzheimer's disease.

Any cholinesterase inhibitor may cause nausea, vomiting, loss of appetite, and increased frequency of bowel movements. Scientists do not believe that combining any of these drugs would be more helpful, and would probably cause more side effects.

Behavioral Treatments

Patients with Alzheimer's may experience a range of problem behaviors such as AGITATION and COMBATIVENESS that may respond to some types of drugs. Although experts don't recommend widespread use of these drugs, neuroleptic drugs have been found to be better than placebo in controlling ANXIETY, SUSPICIOUSNESS, uncooperativeness and HALLUCINATIONS.

In general, experts recommend that these drugs be used only if symptoms of psychosis or significant agitation interfere with patient management. On the other hand, REPETITIVE BEHAVIORS such as aimless WANDERING, PACING, or SHOUTING don't usually respond to drugs. Neuroleptic medications also don't work very well in improving self care, or SOCIAL WITHDRAWAL, and they may cause unpleasant side effects such as sedation or falls. In general, most experts recommend that drugs to control behavior should be used only as a last resort.

durable power of attorney A legal document that allows an individual (the principal) an opportunity to authorize an agent (usually a trusted family member or friend) to make legal decisions when the patient is no longer able to do so. Durable power of attorney (DPA) forms are available at most office supply stores.

There are two types of DPA available, one for financial affairs and one for health care decisions. The DPA for Health Care is a legal document that allows a patient to appoint an agent to make all decisions regarding health care, including choices regarding health care providers, medical treatment, and, in the later stages of the disease, end-of-life decisions. It would include the patient's wishes about whether or not to use tube feeding or a ventilator, for example. It isn't necessary to have a DPA for health care completed by an attorney, but it requires the signature of the patient and a witness; it does not usually require notarization.

The DPA for Property provides for the management of personal property and finances by a designated agent, who would have virtually complete control of the patient's income and assets. The DPA for property doesn't include precise directives about how the agent should use the income for the patient's behalf.

The DPA for Property is extremely important in the future planning for someone with Alzheimer's disease, since it names the person responsible for paying for the patient's future care. For these reasons, an attorney should be consulted when negotiating the profoundly important financial decisions of a DPA for Property. A DPA for Property requires signatures of the patient, a witness, and a notary.

dysphasia A term used to describe a problem with the ability to select words (and/or to comprehend and read). Expressive dysphasia involves a difficulty in saying what the patient wants to say. Receptive dysphasia refers to a problem in understanding and processing what the patient hears or reads.

early onset Alzheimer's disease See ALZHEIMER'S DISEASE, EARLY ONSET; CAUSES OF ALZHEIMER'S DISEASE.

eating problems Many patients with Alzheimer's disease have problems with eating either too much or not enough, forgetting how to swallow, or forgetting whether a meal has been served at all. Others have lost the ability to tell whether food is too hot or too cold. Weight loss and the gradual inability to swallow are associated with an increased risk of death among patients with Alzheimer's. Weight gain, however, is linked to a lower risk of dying.

Mouth sores, poor-fitting dentures, gum disease, or a dry mouth may make it hard for a patient with Alzheimer's to eat. Diabetes, intestinal, or cardiac problems might lead to loss of appetite. Constipation or depression can also decrease appetite. Agitation may interfere with the ability to sit still long enough to eat an entire meal.

Sometimes a patient wants to eat constantly, which can lead to an unhealthy weight gain. There could be several different reasons why the Alzheimer's patient overeats. Patients with Alzheimer's may not have the capacity to realize that they are not really hungry. Emotional factors can also cause patients to overeat. Food may provide security, lessen anxiety, or make patients feel in control. Side effects of some medications also may cause the patient to feel hungry most of the time. Sometimes patients are just bored and have nothing to do except eat. Depression is another potential factor in the desire to eat constantly. Memory loss could also be a possible cause of this behavior, since patients may not remember that they just ate. In extreme cases, it may be necessary to lock up foods in the cupboard.

There are many factors that explain why a person with Alzheimer's disease won't eat. Dental problems such as ill-fitting dentures, sores in the mouth, or an infected tooth may make eating painful. Anxiety or confusion can also cause an Alzheimer's patient not to eat. If patients cannot see food clearly, they may not want to eat. Some medications (such as antidepressants) may lessen appetite. Memory loss is another key factor in this behavior. The patient may have forgotten how to use a knife or fork, or may have forgotten that eating is important for health.

Caregivers should first make sure there are no dental problems. Patients should be encouraged to wear glasses during mealtimes if poor vision is a suspected cause of appetite problems. The patient should eat during a calm period, without any distractions or loud noises.

If memory loss is part of the problem, the patient may mimic caregivers who go through the actions of eating. Finger foods, or single foods at mealtime, may make the patient more likely to eat by easing the feeling of being overwhelmed.

Patients should not be rushed through a meal. Food and beverages should be alternated to keep the throat from becoming dry.

In later stages of Alzheimer's disease, some patients have trouble chewing or swallowing and are at risk of choking. They may forget to chew at all and swallow their food whole, or have lost muscle control. Another common symptom of the later stages of Alzheimer's is drooling, which is most likely caused by weak muscles, medications, or food being held in the mouth and not swallowed.

In the later stages of Alzheimer's disease, patients should be given food that requires little or no chewing, such as soup, cottage cheese, mashed potatoes, applesauce, scrambled eggs, pudding, yogurt, or milk shakes. If the Alzheimer's patient has lost sensation in the mouth, the caregiver should gently move the person's chin to trigger chewing. Lightly stroking the throat can remind a patient to swallow. Food should be all the same texture; cereal in milk would be a bad choice, since the combination of solid and liquid could confuse the patient, who might not then know whether to chew or swallow. Bedridden patients should eat sitting up to prevent choking. Nutritional supplements may need to be included in the patient's diet. However, straws in liquids should not be used if the patient has a swallowing problem, which could cause the patient to breathe the liquid into the lungs. Aspiration can easily lead to pneumonia.

echolalia The meaningless, persistent, verbal repetition of words or sounds (often with a mocking, mumbling, staccato tone) that often appears in Alzheimer's disease.

economics of Alzheimer's disease The costs of Alzheimer's disease in the United States—including costs of diagnosis, treatment, nursing home care, informal care, and lost wages—is estimated to be more than $100 billion each year. The federal government covers about $4.4 billion of this cost, and the states provide another $4.1 billion. Much of the remaining costs are borne by patients and their families.

education Statistically, the more education a person has, the less likely that person will develop Alzheimer's disease. While it's not clear whether education can actually prevent plaques and tangles from forming, there is substantial evidence that schooling does postpone MEMORY problems.

It could be that education may help the BRAIN's nerve cells produce more and better connections, giving the brain more of a reserve from which to draw when the network of brain cells begins to fade.

Eldepryl See SELEGILINE.

elder abuse At least a half million seniors in domestic settings were abused and/or neglected,

or experienced self neglect during 1996, according to the National Center on Elder Abuse for the Administration for Children and Families and the Administration on Aging. Many experts agree that 4 percent of elders age 65 and over in this country are abused or neglected at any given time. Depending on the study, only one in five to one in 14 cases is reported to authorities. Most abusers are family members.

Physical abuse includes sexual assault such as rape or fondling, and other acts such as beating, slapping, shoving, or kicking of an elderly person. Psychological abuse includes verbal harassment, threats, or other forms of intimidation directed toward an elder, such as the threat of institutionalization as a punishment.

Financial abuse includes the stealing or misuse of property or other assets belonging to an elder, such as a house, bank account, pension funds, or Social Security payments.

"Neglect" is the failure to provide an elder with basic necessities such as adequate food, shelter, medical treatment, or personal care.

Outright physical abuse often takes place within families in which there is a history of violence, including child abuse and spouse abuse, or a history of drug abuse or mental illness. In some cases, elder physical abuse is a retaliation for earlier child abuse.

Financial abuse usually occurs within situations where the elder person is exploited by an unscrupulous relative or other caregiver who sees an opportunity to take advantage of the elder's vulnerability. Financial abuse is often connected with substance abuse and the need to support an abuser's drug habits.

Neglect often occurs in situations where the caregiver is unaware of the full needs of the elder, or too stressed to meet those needs. In some cases, the caregiver could do better but simply chooses not to take sufficient responsibility for the elder's care.

Psychological abuse is sometimes the result of stress, but is often used in combination with other types of abuse to control the behavior of an elder.

Eldercare Locator A nationwide directory assistance service designed to help older people and caregivers locate local support resources that enable older Americans to remain independent in their own homes. It can also help caregivers find ways to take a break from their daily caregiving responsibilities.

Each Eldercare phone representative is a trained professional with access to an extensive list of referral services that lend support to seniors, including information on meals, home care transportation, housing alternatives, home repair, recreation, social activities, and legal and other community services. The Eldercare Locator can provide names and phone numbers of organizations at any location in the country. The Eldercare Locator can be reached toll-free at (800) 677-1116, Monday through Friday, from 9 A.M. to 8 P.M. EST. Callers should provide the Eldercare Locator staff with either the name of the county and city or the zip code of the person requiring assistance, together with a description of the situation.

In addition, an on-line version of the Eldercare Locator provides users with 24-hour access to community assistance resources for seniors at http://www.eldercare.gov. The website will initially provide consumers with basic contact information about elder service agencies in the state and local area requested by zip code. The website will gradually expand to provide links to the full range of services now available by telephone.

Founded in 1991, Eldercare Locator is a service of the U.S. Administration on Aging (AoA) and the National Association of Area Agencies on Aging that provides state and local information on home care, assisted-living programs, and nursing homes. The average number of calls increased 15.3 percent from 9,043 each month in 2000, to 10,425 each month in 2001. For contact information see Appendix I.

elder law attorney An attorney who specializes in the legal problems of older adults. An elder law attorney might handle general estate planning issues and advise clients about planning for incapacity. The attorney could help the client plan for possible long-term care needs. Locating the appropriate type of care, coordinating private and public resources to pay for care, and working to ensure the client's right to quality care are all part

of the elder law practice. A referral to an elder law attorney may be handled by a number of groups, including:

- ALZHEIMER'S ASSOCIATION
- AMERICAN ASSOCIATION OF RETIRED PERSONS
- AREA AGENCY ON AGING
- CHILDREN OF AGING PARENTS
- Health Insurance Association of America
- National Citizen's Coalition of Nursing Home Reform
- Older Women's League
- Social Security Office
- State Insurance Commissioner
- State or Local Bar Association
- Hospital or Nursing Home Social Service Department

See also NATIONAL ACADEMY OF ELDER LAW ATTORNEYS.

Elderly Nutrition Program (ENP) A government program that provides grants to support nutrition services to older people throughout the country as a way of improving nutrition among the elderly and offering participants opportunities to form new friendships and informal support networks.

The ENP provides for meals in a variety of settings, such as senior centers, schools, and in individual homes. Meals served under the program must provide at least a third of the daily recommended dietary allowances established by the Food and Nutrition Board of the National Academy of Sciences-National Research Council. In practice, the ENP's 3.1 million elderly participants are receiving an estimated 40 to 50 percent of most required nutrients. The ENP also provides a range of related services, including nutrition screening, assessment, education, and counseling. These services help older participants to identify their general and special nutrition needs, as they may relate to health concerns such as hypertension and diabetes.

The services help older participants to learn to shop for, plan, and prepare meals that are economical and healthy. The group meal programs also provide older people with contact with other seniors at the group meal sites. Volunteers who deliver meals to homebound older people are encouraged to spend some time with the elderly, and can offer an important opportunity to check on the welfare of the homebound elderly.

In addition to providing nutrition and nutrition-related services, the ENP provides an important link to other needed supportive in-home and community-based services such as homemaker-home health aide services, transportation, fitness programs, and even home repair and home modification programs.

Since American Indians, Alaskan Natives, and Native Hawaiians tend to have lower life expectancies and higher rates of illness at younger ages, tribal organizations are given the option of setting the age at which older people can participate in the program.

The program was authorized under Title III, Grants for State and Community Programs on Aging, and Title VI, Grants for Native Americans, under the Older Americans Act. Through Title III, grants are provided to the 57 state units on aging and their 655 area agencies on aging, and via Title VI, to 221 tribal organizations, representing American Indian, Alaskan Natives, and Native Hawaiians.

electroconvulsive therapy (ECT) A treatment for depression in which an electric current is passed through the brain, producing a convulsion. Before treatment, the patient is sedated; there is no memory of the shock. Several sessions may be necessary. Common side effects include headache and temporary loss of memory. Patients often report considerable relief from symptoms, but exactly why ECT works is not known.

Patients with Alzheimer's disease and behavioral disturbances, but with only mild depression, are sometimes given ECT with very poor results. They are not usually candidates for ECT unless a patient with Alzheimer's had a well-established depressive disorder before the onset of DEMENTIA.

electroencephalogram (EEG) A procedure that measures the amount and type of electrical activity in the brain. EEG measurements, which are taken from the scalp, sometimes are used to evaluate suspected cases of Alzheimer's disease. In some patients with Alzheimer's, this test reveals "slow waves." Although other diseases may evidence similar abnormalities, EEG data may help distinguish a potential Alzheimer's patient from a severely depressed person, whose brain waves are normal. However, in Alzheimer's, the EEG is usually normal, especially in the early stages.

electromagnetic fields Electromagnetic fields (EMFs) are emitted by power lines, electrical equipment, and other machinery. Most research on EMFs has concerned the relationship between ongoing exposure and cancer. However, several studies in the United States and Sweden looked at the relationship between EMFs and Alzheimer's disease.

In a study published in the *American Journal of Epidemiology* in September 1995, researchers suggested that EMFs may damage brain tissue by interfering with calcium ions inside BRAIN cells. A high level of intracellular calcium ions has been found to increase production of BETA AMYLOID, which can trigger a cascade of reactions leading to plaques in the brain. Since beta amyloid is produced in tissues outside as well as inside the brain, high EMF exposures of the hands, feet, or body also could contribute to the development of Alzheimer's disease.

Researchers found that individuals who were exposed to intense and frequent levels of EMFs in the workplace were three times more likely to suffer from DEMENTIA than those with low exposure. People in the study who once worked as seamstresses, dressmakers, and tailors (jobs in which workers are exposed to medium to high levels of EMFs) were most often affected.

Another study published in the journal *Neurology* in 1996 looked at 326 people with Alzheimer's disease over age 65 who were hospitalized at the Rancho Los Amigos Medical Center in Downey, California. They were compared to 152 others at the center who had cognitive problems but who did not have Alzheimer's. All participants were categorized based on their former occupations, and these jobs were grouped by tendency toward exposure to different levels of EMFs. Researchers found that people with higher levels of likely EMF exposure were nearly four times more likely to have Alzheimer's than those with lower exposure.

Experts agree that the research in the 1996 study needs to be repeated in larger and more diverse populations before it is clear what role EMFs play in the environment, especially with regard to Alzheimer's disease.

emergency relief programs Emergency RESPITE CARE that is available to caregivers who have an emergency and do not have a place for their family member to stay. In the case of most emergency programs, the patient stays in a care facility while the caregiver is away.

Caregivers can use this service if they are ill and cannot care for their family member, or if they need to go away for a few days. Caregivers need a break from the responsibilities of care, and it is normal for caregivers to want to get away for a few days, but this service is designed for those in desperate need of relief.

Caregivers interested in emergency relief programs can contact the local AREA AGENCY ON AGING for more information.

Emergency relief programs are often located in a long-term care facility, which provides care as if the patient was a resident of the facility.

endoplasmic-reticulum associated binding protein (ERAB) A type of protein that appears to combine with another protein called BETA AMYLOID, which accumulates in sticky plaques in the BRAINS of people with Alzheimer's disease. When ERAB combines with beta amyloid, the combination in turn attracts new beta amyloid from outside the cells. High amounts of ERAB may also enhance the nerve-destructive power of beta amyloid.

entorhinal cortex A key memory center of the brain that, according to one study, may experience changes in very early Alzheimer's disease. Researchers at the New York University School of Medicine have found shrinkages in this part of the BRAIN years before a person experiences any MEMORY loss.

The study extends previous findings that the HIPPOCAMPUS, another region of the brain associated with MEMORY and learning, gets smaller as Alzheimer's disease progresses. This progressive damage and brain cell loss is one of the hallmarks of Alzheimer's disease.

Previous studies indicated that the damage begins in the entorhinal cortex as early as age 30 and spreads to the hippocampus. In this study, researchers developed a new way to measure the size of the entorhinal cortex based on certain brain landmarks visible on MRI scans.

The technique revealed that the entorhinal cortex was 45 percent smaller among Alzheimer's patients, and 27 percent smaller in patients with very mild Alzheimer's. Scientists also found that the damage to the entorhinal cortex was more significant than to the hippocampus, and was more reliable as a disease marker.

While more research needs to be done, experts suggest that the imaging technique of specific parts of the brain may be used to diagnose Alzheimer's in patients with very mild symptoms. This would be of particular importance as new treatments are developed that may be able to stop the progression of the disease leading to brain cell death and loss of mental functioning.

environment The immediate personal surroundings can strongly affect both mood and behavior in patients with Alzheimer's disease. As the disease progresses and the patient's condition deteriorates, the environment can be frightening to people who can't remember where they are. The reason may actually lie not in the person's surroundings, but in the feelings of disorientation that are part of Alzheimer's disease. While most people can easily distinguish among many different noises, colors, or patterns in a room, a person with Alzheimer's is more likely to feel confused or overwhelmed. This kind of overstimulation can trigger feelings of hostility or worry among patients.

For these reasons, a patient with Alzheimer's disease needs a calm, quiet, familiar, enjoyable, comfortable, and organized home environment. If the person feels safe and secure, it will be easier to manage problems of wandering, anger, or agitated behavior. Something as simple as rearranging the bedroom furniture or stopping by a friend's house might be unsettling to the person with Alzheimer's.

Patients who feel secure have far less incidences of WANDERING, anger, or agitated behavior, so establishing a familiar, well-organized living area is imperative in good patient care. The more consistent and familiar the home, the better.

Caregivers can help patients retain a link to the past by displaying familiar objects such as old framed photographs, a favorite chair, cabinet, or lamp, a piece of clothing such as a hat, or a wall hanging.

Color can be used as a way to calm patients, avoiding bright primary colors such as stark white, yellow, orange, or red in favor of pastel shades such as peach, pink, beige, ivory, and light blues, greens, and lavenders. Because patients with Alzheimer's disease have trouble distinguishing between similar colors, it's a good idea to paint walls, doors, and handrails different hues.

Floor surfaces should be simple; vinyl is a good choice because it doesn't reflect light that might distract the patient from obstacles in the way. Highly patterned flooring may be perceived by the patient as cracks that need to be avoided. Carpeting is a good idea, because it can help absorb noise and prevent slipping, but wall-to-wall carpeting can be a problem with incontinent patients because it can't be easily cleaned.

Noise control is crucial if a pleasant environment for patients with Alzheimer's is to be maintained. Soft, enjoyable background music that includes favorite songs from the patients' youth is always a good choice. Lighting should be natural, and not cast a shadow that patients might find disturbing. Natural light focused directly on the area where it's needed is a good choice.

Furniture should be covered with a nonabsorbent material, and chairs used by patients should have sturdy arms that extend past the seat so the patient can get up easily.

Because patients with Alzheimer's can become confused and disoriented, caregivers should try to provide plenty of labels, pictures, and numbers that help the patient understand where he is, and what day and time it is.

Pathways should be kept clear, with no clutter or throw rugs. In addition, there should be locks on doors and cupboards, and hidden switches or controls for the stove, thermostat, and hot water heater.

Wall hangings made of various textured materials are a good choice for people with Alzheimer's, because many patients enjoy feeling textured materials such as yarn or wool and find these decorations less disorienting than those made of mirrors or glass. Small, distracting wallpaper prints should be avoided.

Pets can be a helpful, soothing part of the environment, especially if the patient has had a pet in the past. The pet should not be too energetic, and any aquarium or cage should be locked.

environmental toxins   See TOXINS.

enzyme   An organic compound that interacts with other substances to form a new chemical, either by synthesizing or degrading it. Brain function depends on chemical messages transmitted from cell to cell by neurotransmitters that depend on brain enzymes as part of their synthesis and degradation.

The enzyme choline acetyltransferase is important in the production of acetylcholine, a neurotransmitter important in memory that appears in low levels in patients with Alzheimer's disease.

episodic memory   Memory for events in a person's life ranging from the most basic to the most personally significant. Episodic memory contains both short-term and long-term memory; short-term memory involves events that have happened within the last hour, whereas long-term memory occurs more than an hour before.

At the onset of Alzheimer's disease, people don't have trouble remembering events from long ago, but may forget having set the table five minutes ago. On the other hand, distant memories may be intact, but interfere with present activities. For example, a person may speak to someone who died long ago, or act out an event which is no longer meaningful in the present.

The memory for what words mean is called SEMANTIC MEMORY, which involves definitions of a word, such as "house" or "cat." Unlike the personal characteristics of episodic memory, semantic memory is common to all those who speak the same language. Episodic and semantic memory are not located in the same part of the brain, so one type of memory may be affected by Alzheimer's disease while the other remains intact.

estrogen Hormone produced by the ovaries and testes that stimulates the development of secondary sexual characteristics and induces menstruation in women. Estrogen is also important for normal brain function and the development of nerve cells, and appears to affect brain regions relevant to memory. Some research suggests that estrogen replacement therapy may help prevent Alzheimer's disease, although the hormone hasn't been shown to affect the course of the disease once it has been diagnosed.

There is some evidence suggesting that women undergoing estrogen replacement treatment after menopause are less likely to develop Alzheimer's disease. In fact, recent studies show that estrogen replacement after menopause can reduce a woman's risk of developing Alzheimer's by 30 percent to 50 percent. In June 1997, the report of a long-term study from the National Institute on Aging (NIA) documented that estrogen replacement therapy in postmenopausal women was associated with a 50 percent reduction in the risk of developing Alzheimer's disease. In all, 472 women were studied for 16 years.

Another NIA study documented the effects of estrogen in slowing the decline of visual memory in 288 women. Other research suggests that estrogen may improve memory among postmenopausal women with Alzheimer's disease. A number of studies have reported that women taking hormone replacement therapy (in various combinations and even for brief periods) score better on verbal memory than women not on hormone replacement therapy.

A large body of data gathered over the past 25 years in animal studies supports the idea that estrogen may have some beneficial effects on memory function. Estrogen appears to have both antioxidant and anti-inflammatory effects and may enhance the growth processes from particular neu-

rons important for memory. These data have created intense scientific interest in the relationship between estrogen, memory, and cognitive function in humans.

In addition, estrogen may stimulate production of the neurotransmitters ACETYLCHOLINE and SEROTONIN, both of which are depleted in Alzheimer's patients. Estrogen also appears to smooth, relax, and open blood vessels, which may help blood flow in the brain. Estrogen is also an ANTIOXIDANT that helps clean up oxygen FREE RADICALS, the unstable particles thought to play a role in Alzheimer's. Moreover, when the level of estrogen remains above a certain threshold, it interferes with the brain's production of BETA AMYLOID, a key protein in the damaging plaques found in the brain. How estrogen controls the production of beta amyloid is not yet known.

Some experts suspect that Alzheimer's disease in older women may be related to estrogen deficiency, and that estrogen may interact with NERVE GROWTH FACTORS to delay the degeneration of neurotransmitters important in memory and learning. It could be that estrogen may be able to prevent Alzheimer's disease by protecting nerve cells in the brain that may somehow prevent nerve cell death.

While many studies indicate that estrogen may lessen the risk of Alzheimer's disease, conflicting data still exist, and larger studies are needed to conclusively establish estrogen as an effective therapy for delaying or preventing Alzheimer's disease in women. Some studies have found no beneficial effect of estrogen, and researchers point to the fact that women who take hormone replacement therapy tend to be healthier and better educated in the first place. One study of young women who had hysterectomies found no association between natural estrogen levels and mental functioning. Another found no association between different levels of natural estrogen and better or worse mental functioning in older women. An analysis of major studies reported that the largest and more rigorously conducted study found no benefits from estrogen supplements on mental functioning in healthy postmenopausal women. And a 2001 study reported no association with a lower risk for Alzheimer's disease in women taking either estrogen or estrogen-progestin combination therapies.

There are also questions about the safety of prolonged estrogen use. Because estrogen may increase the risk of breast cancer, gall bladder disease, high blood pressure, and stroke, it is often not recommended for women with a history of any of these conditions. It would also be important to develop an estrogen treatment that would not feminize men.

Although using estrogen to prevent or treat Alzheimer's disease is not generally recommended, some doctors and some women are choosing not to wait for conclusive research findings, and are trying this treatment in the hope it may work.

ethnicity and Alzheimer's disease See RACE AND ALZHEIMER'S DISEASE.

excitotoxicity Overstimulation of nerve cells by nerve impulses. Excitotoxicity often leads to cell damage or death.

executive function A broad group of behaviors that depend in particular on the frontal lobes of the brain. The behaviors include decision-making, abstract thinking, planning and carrying out plans, and so on. The frontal lobes are also involved in self-control, such as deciding what behavior is appropriate at any one time. Patients with impaired executive function (especially following damage to the frontal lobes) may be unable to perform these functions.

Exelon See RIVASTIGMINE.

exercise and Alzheimer's disease Everyone from healthy individuals to patients with Alzheimer's disease can benefit from exercise. With a physician's approval, regular exercise can help patients with Alzheimer's lead healthier lives and lessen the risk of common ailments associated with aging, including muscle shrinkage, muscle weakness, and osteoporosis.

In addition, some researchers believe that lifelong physical exercise may help protect against developing Alzheimer's disease. A 1998 study reported that people with Alzheimer's exercised less between the ages of 20 and 59 than did people who didn't develop the disease later in life.

familial Alzheimer's disease (FAD) An early onset form of Alzheimer's disease that appears to be inherited. In certain families around the world, members can point to relatives going back six or seven generations who have developed Alzheimer's before age 65. Perhaps the most famous are those who have descended from Volga Germans, a group of German families that settled in the Volga River Valley in Russia in the 1800s. Dozens of descendants have developed Alzheimer's disease in middle age.

As many as half of all cases of FAD are now known to be caused by defects in three genes located on three different chromosomes: CHROMOSOME 1, CHROMOSOME 14, or CHROMOSOME 21.

- *chromosome 1:* Mutations in a gene called presenilin 2 located on this chromosome produces an abnormal presenilin 2 protein.

- *chromosome 14:* Mutations in a gene called presenilin 1 located on this chromosome produce an abnormal presenilin 1 protein. Recently, scientists have also linked presenilin 1 to the more common, non-inherited form of Alzheimer's.

- *chromosome 21:* Mutations in the AMYLOID-PRECURSOR PROTEIN gene located on this chromosome produce an abnormal APP.

If only one of the above mutations appears in one of the two copies of a gene inherited from the parents, the person will inevitably develop early onset Alzheimer's. However, the total known number of these cases is small (between 100 and 200 worldwide).

By pinpointing gene defects related to familial Alzheimer's disease, scientists can develop tests to diagnose patients before symptoms occur, and eventually develop drugs to counteract the effects of these gene defects.

See also ALZHEIMER'S DISEASE, EARLY ONSET.

familial British dementia A disease similar to Alzheimer's disease that is characterized by progressive dementia, paralysis, and loss of balance. It usually occurs between ages 40 to 50. Just as in Alzheimer's, FBD patients have amyloid deposits associated with neurofibrillary tangles.

Recent studies have shown that a number of dementias in addition to Alzheimer's are associated with genetic defects that cause amyloid deposits in the brain. For example, in 1999 scientists in New York and London identified a defect in the gene called BRI located on chromosome 13 that is associated with the development of FBD. The mutation in the BRI gene creates abnormally long proteins that are then clipped off and deposited in the brain as amyloid plaques. An enzyme called furin is involved in the formation of fibrils in FBD.

Recently, New York University medical school researchers identified a close variant of FBD in a small Danish population characterized by severe accumulations of amyloid around blood vessels, cataracts, deafness, loss of balance, and dementia. The genetic defect is a single mutation in the same gene as FBD, which also causes abnormally long proteins that are clipped to form amyloid. Future studies of animal models that have this specific mutation may be helpful in understanding why the Danish form of the variant has abnormal amyloid deposition that is closely associated with specific blood vessels in the brain.

By studying the different amyloid types, the product of distinctly different genes and processing pathways, scientists hope to gain a better understanding of the effects of amyloid in the development of Alzheimer's.

Family and Medical Leave Act A law that entitles eligible employees to a total of 12 workweeks of leave without pay in a 12-month period to care for a family member with Alzheimer's disease (among other illnesses). The law was enacted by Congress in 1993; regulations were finalized in 1995.

Family Caregiver Alliance The first community-based nonprofit organization in the country to address the needs of families and friends providing long-term care at home.

More than 20 years ago, a small task force of families and community leaders in San Francisco joined together to create support services for those struggling to care for a loved one who didn't fit into traditional health systems. This included patients with a wide variety of conditions, including Alzheimer's disease. While the diagnoses were different, the families shared common challenges: isolation, lack of information, few community resources, and drastic changes in family roles.

FCA is now a nationally recognized information center on long-term care and the lead agency in California's system of Caregiver Resource Centers. FCA serves as a public voice for caregivers, illuminating the daily challenges they face, offering them the assistance they so desperately need and deserve, and championing their cause through education, services, research, and advocacy. For contact information, see Appendix I.

fatty acids, essential Fatty acids are the basic building blocks for all lipids, and are the nutritional components found in dietary fats and oils. Essential fatty acids (EFAs) profoundly influence the health of the human body, including brain and immune system function. Some research has suggested that people with Alzheimer's disease may have unusually low levels of EFAs in their brains, although it's not understood if this is a cause or an effect of the disease.

Although the recent trend has been toward a more fat-free diet, experts now understand that some fat is actually essential to health. The body needs essential fatty acids just as it needs other essential vitamins and minerals, to help prevent diseases and to control cellular processes. Essential fatty acids aren't produced by the body, but must be obtained through food or nutritional supplements.

There are two fatty acids that are truly essential—linoleic acid (LA) and alpha linolenic acid (ALA). A healthy body uses LA and ALA to produce other fatty acids and derivatives, including gamma linolenic acid (GLA), eicosapentaenoic acid (EPA), and DOCOSAHEXAENOIC ACID (DHA). Another derivative of linoleic acid that isn't always a "good" fat, but that is necessary in small amounts, is arachidonic acid.

The average North American typically gets too much linoleic acid from processed foods, margarine, and vegetable oils; too much sugar, alcohol, or saturated fats interfere with the body's ability to convert linoleic acid into the beneficial derivative, GLA. Insufficient quantities of zinc, magnesium, and vitamins B_6, C, and niacin also slow the process. At the same time, Americans get very little of the omega-3s (ALA, EPA, and DHA).

Eating a healthy diet and taking supplemental oils may be the best ways to ensure a healthy balance of the right fats. Americans should cut down their linoleic acid intake by eating less processed food, margarine, and vegetable oils such as corn and sunflower oils, and reduce the saturated fat intake by eating less fatty red meats, dairy products such as whole milk and butter, and deep fried foods. The EPA and DHA levels can be boosted by eating more fatty fish such as salmon, mackerel, sardines, and tuna; the ALA intake can be increased by adding milled flaxseed to salads and breads.

In addition to modifications to the diet, some experts suggest that daily supplementation with GLA, ALA, EPA, and DHA may help consumers get the health-protecting benefits of essential fatty acids. Evening primrose oil and borage oil can provide GLA; flaxseed oil can provide ALA; fish oils supply EPA and DHA. However, supplements have not been proven to work. All supplements carry the label caution that their function has not been evaluated by the U.S. Food and Drug Administration.

financial assistance There are a variety of federal, state, and local programs that can help patients with Alzheimer's disease and their families. Each program has separate eligibility requirements.

Programs that may be able to help patients include food stamps, home energy assistance programs, Internal Revenue Service reductions, meal programs, real estate tax exemptions, senior citizen rent increase exemptions, Social Security, Supplemental Security Income, and Veterans Administration benefits. Local departments of aging also may offer a variety of free or low-cost programs for older people in need of home repairs, transportation, or counseling.

Food stamps If families meet eligibility requirements, food stamps can be used in stores and toward meals served at senior centers or that are delivered to the home.

Home energy assistance programs This program pays for basic or emergency expenses for utilities for those who meet eligibility requirements.

Internal Revenue Service reductions The IRS can offer a variety of tax breaks for older people, or for families who are paying for a patient's medical care, and for some nursing home care that is not covered by MEDICARE or MEDICAID. The exact requirements change almost every year, so families should consult the IRS or an accountant.

Meal programs No matter what the income level, the Federal Older Americans Act provides for meal programs such as Home-Delivered Meals and Eating Together Congregate Meals for people over age 59. The Meals On Wheels program sends a volunteer to the patient's home once a day with a hot meal, for a nominal fee (depending on location).

Real estate tax exemptions Some homeowners may qualify for lower real estate taxes on their primary home.

Senior citizen rent increase exemptions This program allows older renters to obtain exemptions from rent increases.

Social Security In this federal program, monthly benefits are paid for retired, disabled, and blind patients who contributed to the program while they worked. Payments may also be made to the patient's nonworking spouse, widows and widowers, divorcees, dependent parents, and dependent children, in some cases.

Supplemental Security Income This federal program pays a minimum amount each month to people who are in financial need who are over age 65, or who are disabled or blind.

Veterans Administration benefits Benefits are given to any U.S. veteran, eligible dependents, or survivors of a veteran.

folic acid (B$_9$) This B vitamin can improve circulation in the BRAIN and, according to recent research, may also help prevent brain degeneration that causes Alzheimer's disease.

Folic acid has been shown to reduce the risk of disease throughout the life span, preventing birth defects, warding off coronary heart disease, stroke, peripheral vascular disease, hardening of the arteries, and possibly reducing the risk of breast and colon cancer, DEMENTIA, and DOWN SYNDROME. The B vitamins' link to MEMORY is not surprising, since the vitamins are involved in the synthesis of chemicals crucial to brain function. In addition, low levels of folic acid seem to be linked to psychiatric symptoms and depression in older individuals.

Folic acid is also a substance critical to the health of the nervous system and to a process that clears HOMOCYSTEINE from the blood. Homocysteine is a body chemical that contributes to chronic illness such as heart disease, depression, and Alzheimer's. Elevated levels of homocysteine and decreased levels of both folate and vitamin B$_{12}$ have been found in people with Alzheimer's.

In a study reported in March 2002, mouse experiments suggest that folic acid could play an essential role in protecting the brain against the ravages of Alzheimer's disease and other neurodegenerative disorders, according to scientists at the National Institute on Aging. This animal study could help researchers understand the underlying biochemical mechanisms involved in another recent finding that concluded people with high blood levels of homocysteine have nearly twice the risk of developing the disease.

In the study, investigators fed one group of mice with Alzheimer's-like plaques in their brains a diet that included normal amounts of folate, while a second group was fed a diet deficient in this vitamin. The investigators found a decreased number of neurons in the mice fed the folic acid–deficient diet. The scientists also discovered that mice with low amounts of dietary folic acid had high levels of the harmful amino acid homocysteine in the blood and brain. High levels of homocysteine in the brain has been linked to damage to nerve cells in the HIPPOCAMPUS, a part of the brain involved in memory and learning.

In mice with Alzheimer-like plaques fed an adequate amount of folate, nerve cells in this brain region were able to repair damage to their DNA. But in the mice without enough folate, nerve cells were unable to repair this DNA damage.

These new findings establish a possible cause–effect relationship between high homocysteine levels and breakdown of nerve cells involved in learning and memory in a mouse model of Alzheimer's disease.

People who have Alzheimer's disease often have low levels of folic acid in their blood, but it is not clear whether this is a result of the disease or if they are simply malnourished due to their illness. But based on emerging research, scientists suggest that consuming adequate amounts of folic acid (either in the diet or by supplementation) could help protect the aging brain against Alzheimer's and other neurodegenerative diseases.

In another study, high homocysteine levels were associated with memory loss but subjects with high folic levels appeared to be protected from memory loss even if their homocysteine levels were high. Researchers at Tufts University in Boston have been looking for a relationship between blood homocysteine levels and memory loss since earlier research had established that homocysteine levels were higher in elderly people with low intakes of B vitamins, especially folate. They had also validated reports that homocysteine—a by-product of amino acid metabolism—increases risk of stroke, which is a major player in the loss of cognitive function.

In a 1993 study of elderly Catholic nuns, low blood levels of folic acid were strongly associated with atrophy of the surface layer of the brain (CEREBRAL CORTEX) in participants with a significant amount of Alzheimer's disease lesions in the brain at death. Another study showed that low levels of folic acid boosted the risk of DEMENTIA by 300 percent.

The goal of the nun study was to determine the causes of Alzheimer's disease, other brain diseases, and the mental and physical disability associated with old age. Recent findings suggest that folic acid is important in the development of the human nervous system during pregnancy, and may also play an important role in maintaining the integrity of the brain in late life.

Folic acid occurs naturally in dark green vegetables like spinach and asparagus, and in citrus fruits and juices, peas, legumes, liver, and whole wheat bread, and dry beans. In 1998, the United States Food and Drug Administration mandated that folic acid be added to enriched grain products, such as bread, cereals, flours, corn meals, pastas, rice, and breakfast cereals, in order to increase the folate levels of the population. The current Recommended Dietary Allowance for folic acid is 400 micrograms. However, because it can take a long time for the symptoms of Alzheimer's disease to appear, researchers think it will be many years before folate supplementation in food could affect the incidence of dementia in the United States.

The nun study was completed before folic acid fortification became mandatory in the United States, so scientists don't yet know whether folic acid fortification will lower the nation's incidence of Alzheimer's disease.

food toxins   Scientists are studying the possibility of food toxins as another cause of Alzheimer's disease, since two amino acids found in the seeds of certain legumes in Africa, India, and Guam may cause brain damage, enhancing the action of a neurotransmitter implicated in Alzheimer's.

forgetfulness   Minor memory lapses that are usually completely normal. Many perfectly healthy individuals experience moments of forgetfulness. It is when serious deficits in memory occur together with distinct changes in personality and behavior that a person may be suspected to have a more serious brain disease called DEMENTIA. Alzheimer's disease is one of many types of dementia.

Forgetting the whereabouts of everyday items such as glasses or car keys is normal; forgetting that a person wears glasses or owns a car is a far more serious type of forgetting. Likewise, forgetting a pan on the stove until it boils over is normal; forgetting that dinner was prepared and starting to cook all over again is more serious.

free radicals Highly reactive forms of oxygen created in cells during normal metabolic processes, which are capable of causing damage in brain and other tissues. When free oxygen radicals interact with the lipids that compose cell membranes and vessel walls, they convert them to inactive solids that cause slow but steady cellular death.

Because free radical oxidants are so destructive, the brain and bloodstream must have an ample supply of ANTIOXIDANTS in order to survive. Antioxidants are chemicals that oxygen finds more attractive than the structural components of the cells. In a sense, antioxidants sacrifice themselves to preserve the body.

Since free radicals are the natural result of the body's metabolic reactions, the body is able to neutralize them with various antioxidant enzymes that it produces. For example, superoxide radicals are created in brain cells as a by-product of energy production in the mitochondria. These free radicals are immediately broken down by superoxide dismutase, which is one of the body's own antioxidant enzymes. Humans also depend on essential antioxidants from the daily diet.

The environment has become a perpetual source of free radical contamination, primarily from radiation and the chemical pollution in air, water, and food. Americans today are overwhelmed with more free radicals than their bodies can deal with.

Studies have shown that antioxidant levels diminish with age, which means that an aging brain is especially at risk for oxidative damage. Experts now suspect that cumulative oxidative damage to brain cells causes the poor memory, slow learning, and loss of coordination that often accompanies aging. It also has been linked to Alzheimer's disease.

Indeed, several recent studies looking at the relationship between antioxidants and Alzheimer's found that eating nuts, leafy green vegetables, and other foods rich in antioxidants (such as vitamins E and C) may reduce the risk of Alzheimer's. The findings build on growing research into the effects of antioxidants on dementia. It appears that vitamin-rich foods themselves—not vitamin supplements—have beneficial effects.

One of the studies found strong effects from vitamins E and C. In the other, results from vitamin E foods were more conclusive, but researchers said there was a suggestion vitamin C also provided benefits. Previous research suggested that vitamin E pills could slow disease progression in people already diagnosed with Alzheimer's. The new studies examined people who had not developed the condition at the start of the study.

One study funded by the NATIONAL INSTITUTE ON AGING involved 815 Chicago residents over age 65 who had no initial symptoms of mental decline. Participants answered questions about their eating habits and were studied for about four years. Alzheimer's disease eventually was diagnosed in 131 participants. In particular, it was diagnosed in 14.3 percent of those with the lowest intake of vitamin E foods, compared with 5.9 percent of those with the highest intake. When factors such as age and education were taken into account, the group with the highest intake of vitamin E foods had a 70 percent lower risk of developing Alzheimer's. Participants with the highest vitamin E intake ate amounts that could be obtained from a diet including whole-grain cereal for breakfast, a sandwich with whole-grain bread for lunch, and a dinner including a leafy green salad sprinkled with nuts.

Intake of vitamin C (in foods such as citrus fruits) also appeared to offer some protection, but those results were not statistically significant.

Vitamin E did not protect participants who carry a gene variation called APOPLIPOPROTEIN E-4 (apoE-4), which has been linked to the development of Alzheimer's.

The second study involved 5,395 people in the Netherlands over age 55 who were followed for an average of about six years. Alzheimer's developed in 146 of these participants. Those with high intakes of vitamins E and C were less likely to become afflicted, regardless of whether they had the gene variation.

freestanding dementia specific care center   A facility solely dedicated to the care of people with dementia. This building can sometimes be part of a larger campus.

fronto-temporal dementia   A range of conditions including PICK'S DISEASE, frontal lobe degeneration, and dementia that are caused by damage to the frontal lobe and/or the temporal parts of the brain, responsible for behavior, emotions, and language. These conditions may initially resemble Alzheimer's disease. Fronto-temporal dementia is rare, occurring far less frequently than Alzheimer's disease.

While many symptoms of fronto-temporal dementia are similar to Alzheimer's, there are differences. For example, in Pick's disease, damage to brain cells is more localized than in Alzheimer's, usually beginning in the front part of the brain. Personality and behavior are affected first, but in the later stages symptoms are similar to those of Alzheimer's disease. Younger people under the age of 65 are more likely to be affected.

Damage to the frontal and temporal lobe areas of the brain can cause a variety of different symptoms. Typically, the early stage of fronto-temporal dementia does not affect the memory, although personality and behavior will change. Those with fronto-temporal dementia may lack insight and lose the ability to empathize, appearing selfish and uncaring. Some patients may become outgoing when they were previously quiet, or withdrawn when they were previously extroverted. They may behave inappropriately or be rude. Some may lose inhibitions, become aggressive, or get easily distracted.

Patients with fronto-temporal dementia may also experience language problems, including problems finding the right words, or lack of speech. Patients may begin to either overeat or develop a liking for sweets.

Dementia may worsen in as little as two years or as long as 10. In later stages, brain damage is more general, and symptoms will appear more like Alzheimer's. Those affected may no longer recognize friends and family and may need nursing care.

Diagnosis

Fronto-temporal dementia is commonly misdiagnosed as Alzheimer's disease. A specialist may be able to make a diagnosis of fronto-temporal dementia by taking a detailed history of symptoms. Brain scans may be used to determine the extent of damage to the brain. An exact diagnosis may be possible only after death, when changes in the structure of the brain can be directly observed during autopsy.

Cause

There is a family history in about half of all cases of fronto-temporal dementia. In these families the course of the disease usually has a specific pattern across the generations. Some of these inherited forms have been linked to abnormalities on chromosomes 3 and 17. The causes of non-inherited fronto-temporal dementia are so far unknown.

Treatment

As yet there is no cure for fronto-temporal dementia and the progression of the condition cannot be slowed. Drugs that are designed for the treatment of Alzheimer's disease, such as Aricept and Exelon, may make symptoms worse and increase aggression.

gait   A person's style of walking. People in the later stages of Alzheimer's often have "reduced gait," meaning their ability to lift their feet as they walk has lessened.

galanin   A substance associated with learning and memory that is involved in brain function. When a nerve is cut or injured, the neuron produces extra galanin, possibly to repair or modulate the damage. A new study suggests that in patients with Alzheimer's disease, galanin may enhance the release of acetylcholine from remaining cholinergic neurons, which may delay the progression of Alzheimer's. This raises the possibility that boosting the level of galanin using NERVE GROWTH FACTOR may have a protective role against the disease.

The research findings from a Canadian study suggest that nerve growth factor, which rescues degenerating cholinergic neurons, also induces galanin gene expression in the cholinergic basal forebrain. This suggests that an increase in galanin could boost the release of acetylcholine, which would be consistent with the effects of nerve growth factor on cholinergic function.

galantamine (Reminyl)   One of four new drug treatments for Alzheimer's disease, Reminyl was approved in 2001. The drug, which is derived from daffodil bulbs, can help patients' daily function and ability to think for those people with mild to moderate disease. However, not all patients will respond to galantamine, and no patient will be cured with the drug.

Nerve cells in the brain responsible for memory and thinking communicate using a chemical called ACETYLCHOLINE. Research has shown that deterio-ration of cells that produce acetylcholine in the brains of people with Alzheimer's disease may lead to problems with memory and thought. Experts believe galantamine boosts the levels of acetyl-choline by interfering with an enzyme that breaks down acetylcholine and by stimulating the brain to release more acetylcholine.

Reminyl was developed by the Janssen Research Foundation under a codevelopment and licensing agreement with Shire Pharmaceuticals Group in the United Kingdom.

In studies ranging from 12 to 26 weeks, results showed that more patients taking Reminyl showed significant improvement in cognitive performance than those receiving a placebo. Patients taking the drug also performed better than controls using the Clinicians Interview-Based Impression of Change plus Caregiver Information Test (CIBIC-plus test).

Reminyl has been approved in 21 other countries besides the United States, including most of Europe.

Side Effects

The most common side effects are nausea, vomiting, appetite loss, diarrhea, and weight loss.

gamma secretase (gamma-secretase)   A type of enzyme that is involved in the production of plaques in the brain. Nearly one fourth of all patients with early onset Alzheimer's disease have mutations in PRESENILINS that are linked with this enzyme's activity.

Plaques begin to form in Alzheimer's when gamma-secretase and a related enzyme called beta secretase snip a larger protein into a shorter fragment called BETA AMYLOID. These fragments of beta amyloid then clump together to form the sticky plaques so characteristic of the disease.

See also GAMMA-SECRETASE INHIBITORS.

gamma-secretase inhibitors   A compound that blocks the enzyme GAMMA-SECRETASE responsible for the formation of the sticky plaques that litter the brain's neural connections in patients with Alzheimer's disease. There is evidence that these drugs may tackle the root cause rather than the symptoms of Alzheimer's disease.

Logically it would seem that compounds that block the activity of gamma-secretase should slow the progression of Alzheimer's disease, but scientists remain cautious. It may be that secretase plays a vital role in other aspects of cellular metabolism, so that interfering with it may cause serious side effects. In addition, it has still not been proven conclusively that beta amyloid is as central to Alzheimer's disease as cholesterol is to heart disease. While experimental data support that theory, scientists won't know the theory is right until there is a drug that actually prevents Alzheimer's disease.

gender and Alzheimer's disease   Women are more likely to develop Alzheimer's disease than are men, according to statistical averages. However, since the older a person gets the higher the risk for Alzheimer's, women would automatically be at greater risk because they are living longer than men.

gene   The basic unit of inheritance which is carried at a particular place on a chromosome. Located along the DNA in the nucleus of each cell, genes direct the production of all the hormones, enzymes, growth factors, and other proteins in the body. In humans, genes occur in pairs.

Genes are made up of four chemicals arranged in various patterns. Each gene has a different sequence of these chemicals, each one of which controls the production of a different protein.

Even slight changes in the DNA code of a gene can produce an abnormal protein that can lead to cell malfunction and eventually disease. Scientists have discovered evidence of a link between Alzheimer's disease and genes on four chromosomes—14, 19, and 21. The apoE-4 gene on chromosome 19 has been linked to late onset Alzheimer's disease, which is the most common form of the disease.

gene therapy   A new type of experimental surgical treatment for Alzheimer's disease in which genetically modified cells are injected into a patient's brain in order to halt or reverse brain cell loss caused by the disease. The treatment was first tried on humans on April 11, 2001, but scientists caution it may take years to discover if the therapy will work in most patients.

In the procedure, scientists harvest skin cells, isolating genes that secrete a protein called NERVE GROWTH FACTOR. The solution is injected into the patient's brain in the hope of delaying the progress of the disease and improving the patient's quality of life for several years.

The federal government approved human trials of nerve growth factor in 1999, after scientists showed the protein reversed brain deterioration in aging monkeys.

genetic theory of Alzheimer's disease   See HEREDITY.

genome   All the genes of an organism.

geriatric care manager   A professional who usually has a degree in social work, nursing, gerontology, or psychology, who specializes in helping older people and their families with long-term care arrangements. Generally fees are charged based on the service provided or time spent. A geriatric care manager may

- identify eligibility for assistance and need for services
- arrange for and monitor in-home help
- review financial, legal, or medical issues and offer referrals to geriatric specialists
- provide crisis intervention
- act as a liaison to families at a distance
- help with moving an older person to or from a retirement center or nursing home
- provide consumer education and advocacy
- counsel and support

geriatrician   A physician who specializes in the medical care and treatment of older adult patients, and who focuses on maintaining or improving the senior's ability to function in ACTIVITIES OF DAILY LIVING for the best quality of life possible. A geriatrician has additional training in disorders and conditions common in old age. In some cases, the geriatrician may act as a consultant, making recommendations and suggestions to a primary care physician but deferring overall care to the referring doctor. In other cases, the patient or even the referring physician may prefer that the geriatrician take over the comprehensive care of the older patient.

Both the American Board of Internal Medicine and the American Academy of Family Practitioners can certify a physician in geriatric medicine. To become certified in geriatrics, a physician must first hold a certification in either internal medicine or family practice. A minimum one-year fellowship in an accredited academic geriatrics program is now required, after which the physician may take the geriatrics board exam. After fulfilling the training requirements and passing the examination, the physician will be awarded a Certificate of Added Qualifications (CAQ) in geriatric medicine.

Geriatricians may work at assisted living facilities and retirement facilities, or in a Division of Geriatric Medicine at a local teaching hospital. Alternatively, faculty geriatricians may have private practices.

See also AMERICAN GERIATRICS SOCIETY, THE.

geriatric nurse practitioner A registered nurse with advanced study and expertise in the assessment and care of older adults. The nurse meets with both patients and caregivers to identify potential problems associated with cognition, function and behavior. In addition, this specialized nurse works with the family and the health care team to develop a care plan. Geriatric nurse practitioners are trained to perform physical examinations and diagnostic tests in elderly populations, and to provide patient counseling and to develop treatment programs. In most states they are authorized to prescribe medicines.

geriatric psychiatrist A physician highly trained in the diagnosis and management of emotional and behavioral problems related to aging. These disorders include DEMENTIA, DEPRESSION, ANXIETY, and late-life schizophrenia. The geriatric psychiatrist takes a comprehensive approach to diagnosis and treatment, including listening and responding to the concerns of the older adult, helping families, and when necessary, working with other health care professionals to develop effective approaches to treatment. Coexisting medical illnesses, medications, family issues, social concerns, and environmental issues are integrated into a comprehensive program of care.

The geriatric psychiatrist offers valuable help to older adults who are coping with the changes in health and function common in Alzheimer's disease. Because the geriatric psychiatrist also understands the family's role in caring for the patient, the doctor educates the family about the nature of the illness and how they can best cope, and may include referral to other appropriate services.

Geriatric psychiatrist see patients in a many settings, including office, hospital, clinic, nursing home, or an independent or assisted living facility. The family doctor can refer patients to a local geriatric psychiatrist.

The geriatric psychiatrist can help advise primary care doctors in complex situation involving both medical and mental illness, educate nurses and other health care professionals in long-term care or independent living facilities, and direct home health service providers. The geriatric psychiatrist is a good ally when it's not clear whether the patient's problem is dementia, depression, or the complications of multiple physical illnesses in addition to dementia or depression.

Gerontological Society of America, The A nonprofit professional group that was established in 1945 to promote the scientific study of aging, to encourage exchanges among researchers and practitioners from various disciplines related to gerontology, and to foster the use of gerontological research in forming public policy.

While the society has grown in numbers and scope along with the field, the founding mission remains the same. GSA members have succeeded in exploding the myths of the frail and dependent aged, demonstrated their potential, and attacked the scientific, medical, and political barriers for a healthier and more productive old age. From biology to medicine, from social work to psychology, from architecture to law, GSA members in the past 50 years have contributed to the body of gerontological knowledge and science.

The research areas now addressed by members extend well beyond the society's initial biomedical boundaries. More than 30 disciplines are now represented among GSA's membership; nurses are the fastest-growing segment. For contact information, see Appendix I.

gerontologist A specialist with advanced knowledge and training in a broad range of aging issues. The gerontologist can help identify problems, assist with referrals, and serve as an information resource for questions that arise. Gerontologists may have a degree in gerontology or may be trained in nursing, sociology, psychology, or other human service-related professions. A gerontologist may work within existing professions or in new, emerging nontraditional fields.

Gerontologists often work with other professionals, such as occupational and physical therapists, dietitians, or lawyers, to improve the quality of life of elderly persons. Nursing homes, senior citizens centers, and other community facilities also rely on gerontologists, who may conduct research on aging and the living environments of older persons. Many gerontologists also are involved in education, and may teach at a junior college, provide education to the elderly, produce educational materials, offer counseling for the elderly and their families, or serve as a consultant for business, industry, and labor interests.

Gerontology is a multidisciplinary career that draws from a variety of fields, and the length of training requirements vary. Many colleges and universities offer associate, bachelor's, and master's programs in gerontology; some schools offer research programs at the doctoral and postdoctoral levels. Currently, no accreditation or registration is required.

gila monster saliva See GILATIDE.

Gilatide An experimental drug derived from the saliva of the venomous Gila monster aimed at improving memory and learning that may be a treatment for Alzheimer's disease. Although the bite of the Gila monster (a lizard native to the southwestern United States and Mexico) can be deadly, its saliva also contains a chemical that affects a previously unknown pathway in the brain that affects memory.

New York-based biotechnology company Axonyx Inc., which is developing the drug, hopes to study its effects in patients with Alzheimer's disease by 2003. In rat studies, researchers found that Gilatide had a potent and long-acting ability to improve memory with no observable side effects. Gilatide produces impressive benefits in helping rats to remember how to run a maze after just one dose of the drug.

Research shows that various peptides released in the stomach interact with memory receptors in the brain, which is probably an evolutionary adaptation to help animals remember where they caught food. Scientists believe they have discovered a new gene-signaling pathway in the brain that controls memory. Gilatide stimulates specific receptors, which in turn activate a series of genes involved in this new pathway for memory.

If Gilatide is also effective in humans, it could provide a novel treatment that can boost memory and thinking skills in healthy people, in addition to improving learning and memory in age-related memory loss, attention deficit disorder, and various dementias.

ginkgo biloba A tree whose extract has been used in traditional Chinese medicine for thousands of years as a memory tonic, and is still widely used today in Europe and in the United States. Some studies suggest that the herb may stabilize or improve the quality of life for patients with mild to moderate Alzheimer's disease. However, most experts agree that the treatment does not result in big improvements among patients with severe Alzheimer's.

Ginkgo biloba is the oldest living tree species in the world, whose extracts are made up of flavone glycosides, several terpene molecules unique to the tree, and organic acids. Scientists believe the special terpenes improve circulation in the brain, and extracts are thought to have both anti-inflammatory and antioxidant properties. Some experts believe ginkgo biloba may have both antioxidant and anti-inflammatory properties that protect cell membranes and regulate neurotransmitter function. It may be that ginkgo improves memory by directly stimulating nerve cell activity and protecting cells from the toxic effects of beta amyloid protein, which makes up the plaques littering the brains of patients with Alzheimer's disease.

Researchers at McGill University in Canada showed that a standardized extract of ginkgo biloba could protect cells in the HIPPOCAMPUS (involved in memory) from the deadly effects of beta amyloid. In this study, researchers grew hippocampal cells in a dish, and then exposed them to beta amyloid. Without any protection, the cells died, but when the researchers added a standardized extract of ginkgo biloba developed in 1964 by a German pharmaceutical company, the hippocampal cells were able to survive the exposure to beta amyloid.

The ginkgo extract used in the study is known as EGb 761 and has been standardized to contain specific percentages of its chemical components: 24 percent flavonoids, 6 percent terpenoids, 5 percent to 10 percent organic acids, and more than 0.5 percent proanthocyanidins. This extract and its components have been used in hundreds of research studies. In this study, both EGb 761 and its flavonoid component protected brain cells; the flavonoid component was slightly less protective than the whole extract. However, the terpenoid components tested in the study did not protect against beta amyloid toxicity.

Although scientists don't fully understand how beta amyloid works, they suggest that it may trigger the production of free radicals. Since flavonoids have been shown to act as an antioxidant, these results indicate that the beneficial effects of the ginkgo biloba extract may be due in part to its antioxidant properties. Since the terpenoids—which act as an anti-inflammatory—did not protect the cells against beta amyloid, the protective effects of ginkgo are probably not attributable to anti-inflammatory action.

In a study published in the October 22, 1997, issue of the *Journal of the American Medical Association,* researchers found ginkgo biloba may slightly help some individuals with Alzheimer's disease. This 52-week study initially involved 309 patients suffering from mild to moderately severe dementia caused by either Alzheimer's disease or multi-infarct dementia. Researchers found those who took ginkgo had modest improvements in cognition, ACTIVITIES OF DAILY LIVING (such as eating and dressing), and social behavior, but no measurable difference in overall impairment.

According to a 1992 article published in the British medical journal *Lancet,* more than 40 double-blind controlled trials have evaluated the benefits of ginkgo in treating age-related mental decline. Of these, eight were rated of good quality, involving a total of about 1,000 people and producing positive results in all but one study.

Ginkgo appears to be very safe, since very high doses have been safely given to animals for long periods of time. In clinical trials of ginkgo with more than 10,000 people, only 21 cases of stomach distress were reported, and even fewer cases of headaches, dizziness, and allergic skin reactions.

However, because ginkgo may reduce the ability of the blood to clot; it should not be used with drugs that also thin the blood, such as Coumadin (warfarin), heparin, or even aspirin. Ginkgo also should be used with caution, if at all, by those with bleeding disorders, before or after surgery, and before labor and delivery. Safety for pregnant or nursing women and those with severe liver or kidney disease has not been established.

Most American experts believe it is premature to recommend ginkgo as a specific treatment for Alzheimer's disease without more rigorous research. People with Alzheimer's should consult their doctors before taking any drug because of potential side effects when drugs are combined. Because ginkgo is an herb, it is not regulated by the U.S. Food and Drug Administration; therefore, commercially available ginkgo products may not contain uniform amounts of active ingredients.

global deterioration scale of primary degenerative dementia A test that can provide caregivers with an overview of the stages of cognitive function for those suffering from Alzheimer's disease.

The scale is divided into seven different stages, with the first four describing pre-dementia. Stages five through seven describe the stages of dementia, in which an individual can no longer survive without help.

Within the scale, each stage is numbered from one to seven, given a short title (such as "forgetfulness" or "early confusional") followed by a brief listing of the characteristics for that stage. This helps caregivers understand in general terms how advanced a patient's condition has become by noting the person's' behavior and comparing it to the scale.

glucocorticoids   Hormones that normally enhance the manufacture of glucose and reduce inflammation in the body. Studies in older animals showed that exposure to glucocorticoids contributed to neuron death and dysfunction in the HIPPOCAMPUS, a part of the brain important in learning and memory.

Several studies are currently exploring how glucocorticoids might be linked to Alzheimer's disease by contributing to neuron death through their effect on glucose metabolism.

glucose   The primary substance that the brain uses for energy. The brain uses glucose as its primary energy source for thought processes, and is dependent on receiving an adequate supply of glucose from the body. Disruption of glucose metabolism may contribute to cognitive changes in Alzheimer's disease. Indeed, some studies have shown that adults with Alzheimer's disease show a reduced sensitivity to insulin, the main peptide that promotes glucose utilization. Further studies have shown that temporarily overriding insulin insensitivity by infusing insulin and glucose results in improved memory function in patients with Alzheimer's disease.

glutamate   A neurotransmitter normally involved in learning and memory that under certain circumstances may cause nerve cell death in Alzheimer's disease. Scientists suspect that in certain situations, high levels of glutamate can disrupt the metabolism of brain cells, leading to their eventual death. Glutamate triggers action in a neuron, stimulating the flow of calcium into the cell. If it is produced in higher-than-normal lev-

els, it can overexcite a neuron, bringing in too much calcium.

Even in normal levels, glutamate can be dangerous to a neuron if glucose levels are low. Therefore, if a problem with metabolism leads to low levels of glucose, this could allow glutamate to overexcite the cell, leading to its death.

green tea   A Japanese study suggests green tea, a form of tea popular in Japan, may help people with Alzheimer's disease and vascular DEMENTIA. The 2000 study followed 485 people over age 80 for two years, and found that 96 percent of those who drank 10 cups of green tea a day did not show any cognitive impairment. In contrast, 12 percent of those people who drank less than three cups of green tea a day showed a cognitive decline. Previous research has shown green tea to be effective in preventing vascular diseases such as stroke.

grief   A common feeling of loss and despair upon receiving a diagnosis of Alzheimer's disease. It is common for both the impaired person and the caregiver to experience these feelings. As the patient begins to experience feelings of loss when realizing the gradual changes in abilities, and the caregiver experiences feelings of personal loss, many people progress through the phases of grieving: denial, anger, guilt, and acceptance.

Although the patient is not dying, as function decreases many caregivers experience true grief reactions as the changes in memory, thinking, and personality progress.

At first, many caregivers go through a period of denial in which they can't believe the person is really sick. This may be followed by physical symptoms such as helplessness, weeping, loss of appetite, exhaustion, and insomnia. As the situation continues, caregivers may feel frustrated with the endless tasks of caring for the patient, together with guilt, despair, or depression. Caregivers may begin to withdraw from friends and even from an emotional interaction with the patient. Eventually, as the caregivers work through the grieving process, they reach a point where they accept the disease and the reality of caring for a terminally ill patient.

grooming In the early stages of Alzheimer's disease, a decline in good grooming habits may be one of the first signs that something is wrong. A previously well-groomed person with Alzheimer's may gradually become untidy, unbathed, or have uncombed hair. Although eventually patients will completely lose interest in their appearance, in the earlier stages the lack of good grooming may be caused by forgetting how to take care of themselves.

A patient with Alzheimer's disease should have hair brushed at least once a day and washed twice a week, with hands washed daily, nails trimmed, lotion applied to dry skin, and deodorant applied after bathing. Men may need to shave and women may need to shave their legs. If a woman wore makeup in the past, she should be helped to apply it.

growth factors Naturally occurring substances that affect the nervous system and that may contribute to the dysfunction or death of brain cells in Alzheimer's disease. Some scientists believe that the reason brain cells die in Alzheimer's disease is that there is a decline in growth factors that maintain the functioning of brain cells or a spontaneous increase in factors that are toxic to brain cells.

Experiments in aged rats indicate that specific NERVE GROWTH FACTORS (NGFs) can stimulate the growth of new connections between nerve cells in the HIPPOCAMPUS, the part of the brain crucial to learning and memory. This could help restore some memory loss. Although there could be neurotoxic as well as growth-enhancing effects in the use of NGF, scientists are looking at way to safely use NGF in humans, perhaps through the transplant of genetically engineered cells.

guardian An individual appointed by the courts who is authorized to make legal and financial decisions for another individual.

guilt Most caregivers feel guilt at some point during the care of a patient with Alzheimer's disease and for many, the feelings may be overwhelming. When guilt occurs, and how long it may last, varies with the severity and length of the disease.

There are many common sources of guilt among caregivers charged with the responsibility of a patient with Alzheimer's. Some caregivers may feel that they may have contributed to in the past to the person's condition. Others worry that they should have done something differently after the person was diagnosed with the condition. An extremely common cause of guilt is the uncomfortable feeling that the caregiver is still able to enjoy life while the patient can no longer do so.

Many caregivers also experience profound guilt and feelings of failure when a patient must be placed in a nursing home. Because the responsibility and stress of caring for a patient with Alzheimer's can be extreme, it is quite common to have negative thoughts about the patient, even wishing that the person would die. While quite common, these feelings can cause significant guilt in caregivers who understand the patient is truly ill.

Quite often the burden of patient care falls to one family member who lives nearby; other family members may feel guilty for not "doing their share," and the caregiver may feel angry at family members who either criticize the care or who remain uninvolved.

In many cases, feelings of guilt are linked with unrealistic expectations or thoughts such as "I should have done . . . ," "I must always feel love for the person," and "I must do everything for the person." Some caregivers and family members who are forced to place the patient in a nursing home believe they should visit the person every day, and feel guilty when they cannot. Often caregivers who did not have an ideal relationship with the patient before the diagnosis are consumed with guilt about this, and the realization that now it may be too late to repair the relationship.

Caregivers should understand that guilt is a normal part of loss and grief, and that all that can be expected is that they made the best decision possible with the information available at the time. Feeling guilty is really only a waste of emotional energy; it will not improve the reality of the disease, nor will it help the patient.

Some caregivers find it helpful to share feelings with a sympathetic friend, or to join a support group for relatives of patients with Alzheimer's. Talking to others about feelings and experiences will provide emotional support. Joining a support group offered by a local chapter of the ALZHEIMER'S ASSOCIATION may help ease the feelings of isolation and loneliness. A therapist who has had professional training in grief and mourning may help caregivers work through the overwhelming issues they may confront.

Those who feel they had problems in a relationship with a patient may want to work through those issues by writing a letter asking for forgiveness that is never mailed.

While it may be difficult, caregivers should try to accept that they deserve good things that still occur in their lives, getting involved in new activities, or resuming previous hobbies begun before the diagnosis. Many caregivers find it difficult to spend time caring for themselves, but renewing the spirit can actually help the patient as well.

Haldol   See HALOPERIDOL.

hallucinations   Perceptions of things such as smells, sounds, physical sensations, tastes, or visual objects that do not really exist. Hallucinations are common symptoms of Alzheimer's disease. Hallucinations can be frightening, and can make patients become agitated or afraid to go to sleep.

Often there are physical factors that will contribute to the hallucinations, such as bladder or kidney infections, dehydration, side effects of medications, cataracts, glaucoma, eye surgery, or intense pain. The most common hallucinations are those which involve sight or hearing.

The reaction of the person with DEMENTIA to the hallucinations may vary. Some patients may realize the hallucination is not real, whereas others may not be able to decide if it is real or not. Patients may require reassurance that what they are seeing, hearing, or experiencing is not reality. As the dementia becomes more severe, the person may become convinced that the hallucination is real, which can be very frightening. However, not all hallucinations are upsetting.

Hallucinations are less likely to occur when a patient is occupied or involved. If the hallucinations persist or the person with dementia becomes distressed, antipsychotic medication may help.

Hallucinations are caused by changes within the brain that result from Alzheimer's disease. Visual hallucinations are the most common type experienced by people with dementia. The person may see people, animals, or objects that may involve complicated scenes or bizarre situations. Such hallucinations can be the result of the person's brain misinterpreting everyday objects. The patient may see faces in fabrics, or believe that pictures are real people or animals, or that a reflection in the mirror is another person. Many people with dementia only experience visual hallucinations occasionally, but sometimes they are more persistent and troublesome.

Hallucinations can be caused by a physical illness, such as an infection, or by side effects of some medications. A doctor should be able to help rule out these possibilities. Visual hallucinations may be due to poor eyesight.

People with LEWY BODY DEMENTIA often have a mixture of the symptoms found in Alzheimer's disease and Parkinson's disease. People with this form of dementia are more likely to have persistent visual hallucinations together with stiffness and slowing of movement and marked fluctuations in their abilities. In these cases, some antipsychotic medication, which are sometimes prescribed for hallucinations, can make the stiffness worse. It should, therefore, only be prescribed in small doses, if at all, and reviewed regularly.

Auditory hallucinations occur when a person hears voices or noises although nothing is there. As with visual hallucinations it is important to rule out physical causes such as physical illness and the side effects of medication. It is also worth checking the person's hearing and make sure that their hearing aid is working properly if they wear one. One indication that the person may be experiencing auditory hallucinations is when they talk to themselves and pause, as though waiting for someone else to finish speaking before continuing. However, talking to oneself is very common—not everyone who does this is having an hallucination.

Shouting at people who are not there also suggests the possibility of hallucinations. People are less likely to hear voices when they are talking to someone real, so company can help prevent this type of hallucination.

haloperidol (Haldol) An older drug commonly used to treat AGITATION in patients with Alzheimer's disease. However, the first large controlled study of these drug treatments found that they are only marginally effective at best. The Alzheimer Disease Cooperative Study (ADCS) reports that only 34 percent of patients improved; agitation worsened in 46 percent of patients, and did not change in 20 percent. Haldol use has lessened with the introduction of atypical antipsychotics such as Risperdal and Zyprexa.

head injury and Alzheimer's disease People who suffer a moderate or severe head injury may have more than double the risk of developing Alzheimer's disease and other forms of DEMENTIA later in life. Moreover, the more severe the head injury, the higher the risk.

Moderate head injury (in which a person has a brief loss of consciousness or amnesia) increases the risk of Alzheimer's by 2.3 times and nearly triples the risk of dementia. A severe head injury involving unconsciousness or amnesia for more than 24 hours more than quadruples the risk of both types of dementia. In the first study of its kind, researchers from Duke University Medical Center looked for an association between head injury and Alzheimer's disease and other dementias in more than 7,000 World War II veterans. Researchers also tested for apoE, an important gene in cases of hereditary Alzheimer's disease. Men who had the apoE-4 form of the gene were 14 times more likely to get Alzheimer's, and 10 times more likely to have dementia, but there did not seem to be any link between head injury and the type of apoE gene predicting the risk of dementia.

In another study, researchers discovered that mice who had been repeatedly knocked on the head (similar in severity to injuries sustained by professional boxers or football players) developed deposits of a plaquelike protein faster than mice who did not suffer head trauma. The protein, called BETA AMYLOID, seemed to appear in response to the injuries. These are the same protein-riddled plaques that are found in brains of Alzheimer patients. Even without head trauma, the mice eventually developed the harmful plaques later in life, but those with head injuries produced symptoms of Alzheimer's disease much more quickly. The mice used in the study contain the human gene that produces the protein.

Although the findings could be a promising development in Alzheimer's research, using mice as a research model has limitations. In human brain diseases in which the primary concern is behavior, it is not easy to form a link between brain changes and behavior. While in some ways mice are very much like humans, in other ways they are quite different.

head size and Alzheimer's disease The risk of developing Alzheimer's disease may be higher for people with small head sizes who also carry an Alzheimer's-related gene variant APOLIPOPROTEIN E-4 (APOE-4), some research suggests.

People with both these risk factors may be 14 times more likely to develop Alzheimer's disease than people without that combination. Having a small head size without the gene does not appear to significantly increase the risk of developing Alzheimer's.

This finding supports the idea that having a large brain reserve protects against Alzheimer's. The theory is that the symptoms appear when the loss of brain cells goes below a critical threshold of brain reserve. People with the apoE-4 gene variant are at risk for more rapid brain cell damage, but those with large brain reserves may not show symptoms until much later because they have more brain cells to lose.

The head size study involved 1,869 healthy Japanese Americans over age 65 in King County, Washington. Study participants were divided into three groups, based on head circumference. Only the group with the smallest head circumference (less than 21.4 inches), and apoE-4, had a significantly greater risk of Alzheimer's. The study participants were followed for an average of 3.8 years. During that time, 59 people developed Alzheimer's disease. Those who developed Alzheimer's were also older, less educated, shorter, lighter, and had lower estimated verbal IQ scores than those who did not develop Alzheimer's during the study period.

While brain growth is controlled in part by genetics, it may also be influenced by factors during the first 10 years of life, such as malnutrition, poverty, infection, parental occupation and educational status, family size, and birth order. Later in life, factors such as higher education and income, and mental and physical exercise may play a role in delaying the onset of Alzheimer's disease.

Scientists wonder if this means it might be possible to prevent this disease if brain reserves were systematically boosted throughout life. In the study, 18 percent of the risk of Alzheimer's was attributable solely to small head size. Therefore, if it were possible to increase brain reserve by preventing brain damage over the years, it might be possible to say that nearly 20 percent of the disease among these individuals might be preventable.

Several other studies with other groups have also shown a relationship between head circumference and cognition, and rates of developing Alzheimer's.

health care proxy   A legal document (also called a health care power of attorney or a medical power of attorney) that permits individuals to convey their wishes regarding medical treatment. The designated agent will then be allowed to make health care decisions in accordance with the person's wishes. The person writing the health care proxy has the right to place specific limitations on the agent's authority. Specific desires to limit the agent's authority should be explained in the proxy.

Without a formally appointed person, many health care providers and institutions will make critical decisions for the incapacitated patient, not necessarily based on what the person would want. In some situations, a court-appointed guardian may become necessary unless the person has a proxy, especially where the health care decision requires that money be spent for care.

heart disease and Alzheimer's disease   Growing evidence suggests that all the risk factors for heart disease (high blood pressure, excess weight, high cholesterol, lack of exercise, and diabetes) also may play a role in the development of Alzheimer's disease.

Over the past few years scientists have begun to understand the important links between lifestyle and Alzheimer's. Aging is the primary risk for Alzheimer's—the risk of incidences of disease doubles every five years after age 65—but today scientists realize that healthy aging can actually lower the chance of Alzheimer's.

Scientists do not know what causes the sticky brain deposits that inevitably kill off neural cells until memory disintegrates and ultimately the patient dies, but research first presented in the summer of 2002 suggests people may be able to reduce their chances of developing Alzheimer's by treating high blood pressure.

One 21-year study by Finnish researchers found that among 1,449 people, high cholesterol and high blood pressure seemed to be more strongly linked to the risk of developing Alzheimer's than a gene variation previously linked to the condition.

Taking cholesterol-lowering drugs also can reduce the chances of developing Alzheimer's, according to researchers at Boston University medical school, who found that patients taking CHOLESTEROL-LOWERING DRUGS called statins reduced the risk of developing Alzheimer's by 79 percent. With 2,378 patients, it is the largest study to investigate the connection and the first to include large numbers of black Americans, who are disproportionately more likely to develop Alzheimer's. The study also found that types of cholesterol-lowering drugs other than statins were not linked with a reduced risk of Alzheimer's.

Scientists know that high cholesterol can narrow the arteries and raise the risk of heart disease; today, scientists suspect that high cholesterol also may affect brain arteries and boost the clumping of BETA AMYLOID protein, which is thought to damage the brain in Alzheimer's. Beta amyloid occurs normally in the body, but in people with Alzheimer's, it builds up between brain cells, clumping into sticky plaques. Clogged with plaque, brain cells eventually die, which leads to a gradual loss of memory and control of body function. By the time a patient has noticeable symptoms of Alzheimer's, significant amounts of amyloid have already built up in the brain.

Still another study by British scientists found that statins dramatically reduced the production of beta amyloid. The small amounts of beta amyloid normally found in the blood of healthy people are quickly cleared from the brain. In the general population, people taking statins to reduce their blood cholesterol also have a 70 percent lower chance of Alzheimer's.

heredity and Alzheimer's disease   It's quite clear that genes are involved in at least a few types of Alzheimer's disease; some experts suspect that genes may be involved in more than half of all cases of Alzheimer's. While scientists know that in some families, Alzheimer's disease is an inherited condition, the full extent of its hereditary nature remains unclear.

Many people are affected with this disease who don't have a strong family history, and the genetic factors associated with the disease vary from family to family. There may be a number of subtypes of Alzheimer's disease, with differing risk factors and causes for each. This is why the National Institute on Aging cautions that while a genetic test is available and may be useful in diagnosing someone with symptoms, it shouldn't be used for those without symptoms because the limits of the test are not known.

Researchers are working to discover not only what gene mutations cause the disease and how they initiate the disease process, but also what risk factor genes might work together to make individuals more susceptible to late onset disease.

Two types of Alzheimer's disease exist: familial Alzheimer's disease (FAD), which follows a certain inheritance pattern, and sporadic Alzheimer's, in which there is no obvious genetic cause. Alzheimer's is further described as either "early onset" (occurring before age 65) or "late onset" (occurring after age 65). Early onset Alzheimer's is rare, occurring in between 5 percent and 10 percent of all cases, and generally affects people between ages 30 and 60.

As many as half of all cases of FAD are now known to be caused by defects in three genes located on three different chromosomes: CHROMO-SOME 1, CHROMOSOME 14, or CHROMOSOME 21.

- *chromosome 1:* Mutations in a gene called presenilin 2 located on this chromosome produce an abnormal presenilin 2 protein.

- *chromosome 14:* Mutations in a gene called presenilin 1 located on this chromosome produce an abnormal presenilin 1 protein. Recently scientists have also linked presenilin 1 to the more common, non-inherited form of Alzheimer's.

- *chromosome 21:* Mutations in the applipoprotein gene located on this chromosome produce an abnormal APP.

If only one of the above mutations appears in one of the two copies of a gene inherited from the parents, the person will inevitably develop early onset Alzheimer's. However, the total known number of these cases is small (between 100 and 200 worldwide), and there is as yet no evidence that any of these mutations plays a major role in the more common, sporadic (non-genetic) form of late onset Alzheimer's.

Since the genes were first discovered in 1995, scientists have found that the mutated forms of the genes may cause Alzheimer's by boosting production of BETA AMYLOID, a protein that creates the plaques found in the brain of Alzheimer's patients. Scientists believe that a buildup of beta amyloid damages cells, and that the presenilins also participate in cellular suicide, sending precise chemical messages to cells urging them to die. This mechanism of cell death begins in healthy people at around age 45. People with the mutated form of the presenilin gene are far more sensitive to these proteins.

Apolipoprotein E-4

Although there is no evidence that inheriting mutated genes causes late onset Alzheimer's, genetics does appear to play an indirect role in the development of this more common form of the disease. In the early 1990s, researchers discovered that one form of the apolipoprotein (apoE) gene on chromosome 19 is much more common among patients with Alzheimer's disease. Therefore, a person with this one form is at higher risk of developing the disease.

The genes that produce apoE come in several forms—apoE-2, apoE-3, and apoE-4. ApoE-3 is most commonly found in the general population, but apoE-4 appears in 40 percent of people with Alzheimer's. Interestingly, even people who don't have a family history of Alzheimer's but who develop the disease are also more likely to have the apoE-4 version of the gene.

The finding that people who inherit the apoE-4 form of the gene are at higher risk for developing Alzheimer's has helped explain some of the variations in age of onset of the disease, based on whether a person has inherited none, one, or two copies of the apoE-4 form from their parents. The more apoE-4 forms inherited, the sooner the disease will develop. People who inherit two apoE-4 genes (one from the mother and one from the father) are at least eight times more likely to develop Alzheimer's disease than those who have two of the more common E-3 version. People with one E-2 and one E-3 gene have only one-fourth the risk of developing Alzheimer's as people with two E-3 genes.

The relatively rare apoE-2 form may protect some people against the disease, since it seems to be associated with a lower risk for Alzheimer's and a later age of onset if the disease does develop.

Inheriting one or two apoE-4 forms does not mean a person will definitely develop Alzheimer's. Unlike early onset FAD, which is caused by specific genetic mutations, a person can have one or two apoE-4 genes and still not get the disease, and a person who develops Alzheimer's may not have any apoE-4 genes at all. ApoE-4 genes simply increase the *risk* of developing Alzheimer's; they do not cause the disease.

Exactly how apoE-4 increases the chances of developing Alzheimer's is not known, but scientists suspect that apoE-4 may help beta amyloid build up in plaques, which causes the person to develop Alzheimer's earlier. Other scientists think the gene may interact with cholesterol levels or cause nerve cell death.

Scientists also have noticed that patients with Alzheimer's who have the apoE-4 gene also have neurons with shorter dendrites (the branchlike extensions that receive messages from other neurons). It appears as if these smaller dendrites have been somehow cut back, which limits the neuron's ability to communicate with other neurons. Although this pruning can also occur in people without the apoE-4 gene form, it happens 20 or 30 years earlier in people who do have the apoE-4.

Unfortunately, apoE-4 is not a consistent marker for Alzheimer's; this means that some people with the gene don't develop Alzheimer's, and others who don't have the gene do develop the disease. For this reason, a test identifying apoE-4 is not reliable to predict disease.

The apoE-4 gene contributes to the development of more than 60 percent of all late onset Alzheimer's cases, but that means 40 percent of cases are caused by something else. For this reason, scientists assume there must be other Alzheimer' susceptibility genes.

Interleukin-1

In late spring 2000, another mutant gene (this one causing inflammation) was discovered to be associated with Alzheimer's disease. Scientists know that some genes produce an inflammation-promoting protein called interleukin-1 (IL-1). This protein is produced in the brains of Alzheimer's patients, and researchers have found that several variations of the protein-producing gene can significantly boost the risk of developing Alzheimer's disease. One variation of the gene, called A2, triples the risk if a person receives a copy from each parent. Furthermore, if a person has two copies of this A2 gene and has another variation of that gene called B2, they have 10 times the risk of developing the disease. Some evidence suggests that anti-inflammatory drugs play a role in preventing Alzheimer's disease.

hippocampus A part of the brain important in learning and memory that lies under the medial temporal lobe, one on each side of the brain. The hippocampus is critical for the formation of new autobiographical and fact memories, and may function as the entrance through which new memories must pass before becoming stored in long-term memory. Damage to this area can cause a loss of ability to form new memories, although older memories are not disturbed. The hippocampus is one of the first brain areas to show damage in Alzheimer's disease. Among patients with Alzheimer's, nerve cells in the hippocampus stop working properly, triggering failure of short-term memory. As this part of the brain becomes damaged, the person's ability to do familiar tasks begins to decline.

The paired structures found on each side of the brain link nerve fibers involved in touch, vision, sound, and smell with the limbic system.

The hippocampus receives nerve cell input from the cortex and appears to consolidate information for storage as permanent memory in another brain region. The hippocampus appears to be particularly important in learning and remembering spatial information.

The hippocampus is related to memory because of its response to repetitive stimulation; its synapses change according to previous experience, which may form the structural basis of memory itself. But because research shows that a person with a damaged hippocampus can still retain long-term memory, it is not likely that this part of the brain is the primary storehouse for this type of memory.

A damaged hippocampus interferes with the ability to form new memory, but only the conscious memory or recall of facts and events is lost. The hippocampus does not play a vital role in storing older memories but is profoundly important in the short-term memory of contextual information (such as the series of clues a person would recall when trying to find a parked car in a crowded lot). This is one area that causes particular difficulty in patients with Alzheimer's.

Both the neurotransmitter GLUTAMATE and the inhibitor neurotransmitter gaba are important in the proper function of the hippocampus; an imbalance in either of these transmitters will cause memory disorders.

Hispanics and Alzheimer's disease   Recent studies suggest the risk of Alzheimer's disease may be higher for Hispanics than for Caucasians. The study underscores the critical need for more research to find the unknown factors that are responsible for the differences in risk. In one study of more than 1,000 people in New York City who did not carry a copy of the gene for Alzheimer's, the risk of the disease was two times higher for Hispanics than for Caucasians.

See also RACE AND ALZHEIMER'S DISEASE.

hoarding   Collecting and hiding things or animals in a guarded manner until they interfere with day-to-day functions such as home, health, family, work, and social life. Severe hoarding causes safety and health hazards. Hoarding is a common behavioral problem among patients with Alzheimer's disease, who may collect items or save food or dirty clothes and hide them in strange locations. Many patients hoard because objects represent security to patients who, by the nature of their disease, are profoundly insecure. In addition, throwing something away requires making a decision to throw it away. Many patients with Alzheimer's have lost the ability to distinguish between something of value and something that is worthless, and become afraid to discard anything.

The same insecurity that leads to hoarding behavior can also reveal itself in the form of painful anxiety about money matters, or in an apprehensive reaction whenever any money must be spent.

The most obvious reason the patient hoards things is because of decreasing brain function. The patient doesn't realize that taking things that are not theirs is wrong, so if they see something they want, they take it and hoard it. Common hiding places are under cushions, in drawers, under beds, or in closets. Hoarders often will use the same spot.

hobbies and Alzheimer's disease   Adults with hobbies that exercise their brains, such as reading, jigsaw puzzles or chess, may be much less likely to have Alzheimer's disease.

A recent survey of people in their 70s showed that those who regularly participated in hobbies that were intellectually challenging during their younger adult years were two and a half times less likely to develop Alzheimer's disease. The finding supports other studies showing that brain power is linked to cognitive strength.

Scientists studied the leisure activities in young and middle adulthood of 193 patients with Alzheimer's and of 358 healthy subjects. All the participants were in their 70s when the survey was conducted. The information about the Alzheimer's patients was gathered from family and friends, while the healthy subjects were interviewed directly. The researchers gathered information on how the subjects spent their leisure time during their early adulthood, age 20 to 39, and during their middle adulthood, age 40 to 60. The survey centered on passive activities like watching TV or talking on the phone; intellectual pursuits such as reading, jigsaw or crossword puzzles, playing musical instruments, chess or other board games, knitting or woodwork, and physical activity like sports, bike riding, swimming, walking, or skating. The Alzheimer's patients were less active in all these activities except for television watching.

Intellectual activities seemed particularly protective, no matter what the profession or the amount of education. Of course, intellectual stimulation in early and middle adulthood is not a guarantee that Alzheimer's won't develop later in life, but the activities could delay the disease for years.

Scientists believe that healthier brain cells are better able to control or slow the Alzheimer's process. It appears that brain-challenging activities build up a reserve of brain cell connections, so that it takes longer for the Alzheimer's process to destroy enough cells for symptoms to appear. Intellectual stimulation may delay the onset, but there is no evidence that it will actually alter the disease course. Of course, delaying the disease onset would give many more years of healthy life before people would eventually develop the disease.

holidays Holidays can be opportunities for togetherness, laughter, and memories, but they also can be wrought with stress, disappointment, and sadness for patients with Alzheimer's disease and their families.

Patients with Alzheimer's may feel a special sense of loss during the holiday season, and caregivers may feel overwhelmed by the effort to maintain holiday traditions while juggling caregiving responsibilities. Caregivers also may hesitate to invite family and friends into the home to share the holiday because of the patient's changed personality. It's perfectly normal for caregivers to feel overwhelmed with guilt, anger, or frustration during the holidays.

Before the holiday, discuss upcoming celebrations with relatives and close friends to ensure that everyone understands the situation and has realistic expectations. Some caregivers write a letter to potential guests explaining the patient's cur-

rent status, as well as what can be expected, and perhaps enclosing a photo. It's also helpful to make a few suggestions of what visitors could do or how they might interact with the patient in meaningful ways.

Caregivers should not worry about not being able to re-create past celebrations; caring for a patient with Alzheimer's is a full-time job. There may not be much time left over to maintain every holiday tradition.

Patients with Alzheimer's can still be involved in holiday preparations as long as they are well supervised for safety reasons. Patients may be able to help prepare simple foods, wrap packages, hang decorations, or set the table. The patient's schedule should remain the same as much as possible so that the preparations don't become confusing or upsetting. While the patient's memory may be faltering, old memories, holiday songs, and traditions may still bring a great deal of pleasure to patients.

Even patients with Alzheimer's can still enjoy receiving gifts. Practical, useful gifts for people with this condition include identification bracelets, comfortable, easy-to-remove clothing, music tapes or CDs, family videos, photo albums, subscriptions to magazines, cable television gift certificates, or long distance phone cards. People should avoid giving patients dangerous tools or instruments, utensils, challenging board games, complicated electronic equipment, or pets.

Good gifts for caregivers include gift certificates to restaurants or a therapeutic massage; maid, laundry, or dry cleaning services; videotapes; a gift certificate for "respite care"; and so on.

The patient may enjoy helping with gift-giving by helping to bake cookies and packing them in boxes, or wrapping a gift bought by a caregiver.

Instead of hosting an elaborate evening meal, some caregivers prefer to celebrate with a lunch or brunch, so as to avoid the risk of SUNDOWNING behavior. The number of visitors at one time also should be limited.

home health care The delivery of clinical, social, and supportive services at home or in the community to help patients maintain or regain the highest possible level of health, functioning, and comfort. An essential element of home health care's success has been the emphasis on patient and family education.

Home health care services can help prevent hospitalizations or institutionalization. While home health care services aren't appropriate for every situation, many patients with Alzheimer's can receive care at home, at least in the early stages of their disease.

Home health care professionals offer comprehensive, advanced care in the community along with solid clinical, educational, and supportive services. Services are usually provided by home care organizations or from registries and independent providers. Home care organizations include home health agencies, hospices, homemaker and home care aide (HCA) agencies, staffing and private-duty agencies, and companies specializing in medical equipment and supplies, pharmaceuticals, and drug infusion therapy. Several types of home care organizations may merge to provide a wide variety of services through an integrated system.

Home care services are usually available 24 hours a day, seven days a week. Depending on the patient's needs, services may be provided by one person or a team of specialists.

See also HOME HEALTH CARE AGENCY.

home health care agency   A home care provider that is usually certified by Medicare to have met federal minimum requirements for patient care and management; this means the agency can provide Medicare and Medicaid home health services. Patients who need skilled home care services usually get their care from a home health agency. Because of legal requirements, services provided by these agencies are highly supervised and well controlled.

Some agencies deliver a variety of home care services through physicians, nurses, therapists, social workers, homemakers and home care aides, and volunteers. Other agencies focus on delivering nursing and one or two other specialties. If a patient needs care from more than one specialist, home health agencies can put together a caregiving team to administer comprehensive services.

See also HOME HEALTH CARE.

home modifications   When a person is diagnosed with Alzheimer's disease, family members may want to consider modifying the home to accommodate the special needs of someone with this condition.

Areas of the house that will need to be considered off-limits to someone with Alzheimer's are the garage, basement, and closets where breakable, dangerous, or valuable items have been stored. Doors leading to these restricted areas and to the outside should be locked, alarmed, or controlled by wander-prevention devices.

It is also important to set aside an area dedicated to the caregiver where the person can retreat to recover from the stress of caring for an Alzheimer's patient. While the caregiver is in this respite zone, the patient should be cared for by someone else.

The patient with Alzheimer's should be able to roam around the rest of the home. Caregivers should provide tamper-proof plug outlets and remove medicines, dangerous tools, appliances, and chemicals, as well as important documents, bills, and valuable or breakable objects. Safety-proofing the home is critical for the safety of a patient. Eventually, a person with Alzheimer's loses the ability to think clearly. The caregiver should approach safety-proofing as if there were a young, curious toddler living in the home.

Windows and balcony doors on upper floors must be secured, since patients may not remember they live aboveground. Hardware can prevent a window or sliding door from opening wide enough to allow a person to walk through.

Both poisonous and harmless products that are toxic if eaten in excess should be removed. Sharp utensils and electrical appliances must be kept out of the patient's reach. Because the garbage disposal is often an attractive spot for patients to hide things, it should be disconnected.

All electrical appliances should be removed from counters, as well as the control knobs from the stove, oven, and inside the refrigerator.

The home's electrical lighting should be maintained to help the person with Alzheimer's see, especially in dark hallways. A patient with Alzheimer's may not remember how to turn around and come back down a darkened hallway.

The thermostat on the hot water heater should be reset to the lowest setting (no higher than 120 degrees) to prevent accidental burns. Inexpensive anti-scalding devices can be installed on faucets of the sinks, showers, and bathtubs. A seat and a hand-held showerhead in the bath or shower is a good idea to help with the sometimes-difficult bathing activities. Grab bars and nonslip bath and shower mats are a good idea.

If the patient begins to fall, furniture should be moved so as to provide support when the person moves through a room. Flimsy furniture that rolls or falls over easily should be removed, together with throw rugs and low furniture that can cause falls. Furniture that is hazardous or hard to see, such as glass tables, should be removed. Extension cords and telephone lines that may be tripped over should be rerouted or taped into place.

Locks should be removed from any doors that lock from the inside. An extra front door key should be well hidden or given to a trusted neighbor for emergencies.

The yard is also a dangerous place for a patient with Alzheimer's disease. All poisonous or thorny plants should be removed. The yard should be enclosed with a fence that cannot be easily climbed, and gates should be locked.

Because WANDERING is a serious problem for patients with Alzheimer's, a simple door alarm on the knob of the bedroom door should be installed. If the knob is turned, the alarm will sound and alert the caregiver that the patient is trying to leave.

In addition to safety proofing, caregivers should remove clutter from the home and simplify choices whenever possible, such as putting out one kind of facial soap instead of three or four. The home should be a calm, safe environment that encourages decisions and tasks that can be completed successfully. Large, simple signs or pictures cut out of magazines can be placed on cabinets and drawers to illustrate the contents.

As the disease progresses, modifications may need to be changed or eliminated completely. For example, a large mirror may encourage the patient at first to remember grooming, but may only confuse and frighten the patient later in the disease process. As the disease continues, it is likely the patient will spend most of the time in fewer rooms. Supplies should be moved as the person's world shrinks.

homocysteine An amino acid (the building block of protein) that circulates in the blood that at high levels may contribute to memory problems and Alzheimer's disease, in addition to other chronic illnesses such as heart disease, stroke, and depression. According to one study, patients with high levels of homocysteine in their blood had nearly double the risk of developing Alzheimer's. In an Australian study, healthy seniors with high homocysteine levels were twice as likely as those with normal levels to show loss of brain cells.

As a group, Alzheimer's patients tend to have elevated homocysteine levels, together with low levels of folate and vitamin B_6. High homocysteine levels typically are found in about 5 percent to 7 percent of the general population as well.

The relationship between Alzheimer's and homocysteine is of particular interest to scientists because blood levels of homocysteine can be easily lowered by getting more folic acid (or folate) and vitamins B_6 and B_{12}, although no one knows whether lowering the homocysteine level can postpone Alzheimer's. The federal Alzheimer's Disease Cooperative Study, a nationwide consortium of research centers, is already working on a clinical trial to see whether boosting folate and vitamins B_6 and B_{12} can slow the rate of cognitive decline in people diagnosed with Alzheimer's.

In a recent Boston study, researchers analyzed the homocysteine levels of participants in the well-known Framingham Heart Study who had no memory problems—well before any evidence of dementia. It provided the clearest demonstration yet of the relationship between elevated homocysteine levels and dementia, because those who had high levels were more likely to develop Alzheimer's later in life.

The analysis showed further that people with consistently high levels of homocysteine throughout the period of the study were at highest risk for dementia and Alzheimer's. The researchers also found that early high levels of homocysteine—at least eight years before a diagnosis of Alzheimer's—was strongly linked to the development of

Alzheimer's, regardless of other known risk factors such as age, gender, or apoE genotype.

Other studies have found that folic acid is critically important in clearing homocysteine from the blood. In one recent study, high levels of homocysteine were associated with memory loss but subjects with high folic levels appeared to be protected from memory loss even if their homocysteine levels were also high. Researchers at Tufts University in Boston have been looking for a relationship between blood homocysteine levels and memory loss since earlier research had established that homocysteine levels were higher in elderly people who didn't get enough B vitamins (especially folate). They had also validated reports that homocysteine increases risk of stroke, which is a major factor in the loss of the ability to think clearly.

In a 1993 study of elderly Catholic nuns, low blood levels of folic acid was strongly associated with atrophy of the surface layer of the brain in participants with a significant amount of Alzheimer's lesions in the brain at death. Another study showed that low levels of folic acid boosted the risk of DEMENTIA by 300 percent.

Scientists speculate that consuming B vitamins by diet or supplementation might help reduce levels of homocysteine in some individuals. Findings from the DASH (Dietary Approaches to Stop Hypertension) study suggest that a diet rich in leafy green vegetables, low-fat dairy products, citrus fruits and juices, whole wheat bread, and dry beans can significantly lower levels of homocysteine. The Food and Drug Administration (FDA) now requires the addition of folic acid to enriched breads, cereals, flours, cornmeals, pastas, rice, and other grain products. Good sources of folic acid include citrus fruits and juices, tomatoes, vegetables, and grain products such as bread, cereal, and pasta. Vitamin B_6 is found in meat, poultry, fish, fruits, vegetables, and grain products, and vitamin B_{12} is plentiful in meat, poultry, fish, and dairy products. Americans can get a sufficient amount of all three nutrients if they eat a varied, well-balanced diet.

hospice   A concept rather than a place of care that focuses on a holistic model of services designed to neither hasten nor postpone death, but rather to make a patient's final days as positive and symptom-free as possible.

Although many people assume that late-stage Alzheimer's patients can't benefit from the services that hospice provides, there are many ways to reach dying people suffering from Alzheimer's, such as massage and music therapy. Hospice workers are expert in managing specific symptoms of late-stage Alzheimer's, including problems with skin, mouth, eating, bowel and bladder, safety, restlessness, and sleep.

Hospice is a medical benefit covered by most insurance plans, enabling patients to stay home at the end of their lives. They receive care from an integrated hospice team of nurses, medical social workers, physical and occupational therapists, nutritionists, home aid workers, pastoral counselors, and trained volunteers. Patients can continue to be treated by their own physician or by the hospice physician. Smaller hospices may require that a family member or friend be in the patient's home to act as a primary caregiver.

While patients are at home, all necessary symptom-relieving medications are provided by hospice workers, along with any necessary special medical equipment. Assistance is available 24 hours a day, seven days a week. In emergencies, hospice workers take patients to a hospital or hospice inpatient unit designed to be as homelike as possible. Inpatient respite care is also available to provide a break for families.

Besides medical aid, hospice workers help patients with practical support (such as shopping) and emotional support, including life-closure, grief and spiritual counseling. Depending on the hospice's resources, it may also provide other services such as art, touch, and music therapy.

Medicare law states that to qualify for hospice care, a patient must have "a medical prognosis that life expectancy is six months or less if the illness runs its normal course." However, it's difficult to predict how much time is left to a patient with Alzheimer's disease. It is therefore important to remember that hospice beneficiaries are not restricted to six months of coverage.

Hospice Foundation of America   A nonprofit organization that promotes HOSPICE care and educates professionals and those they serve about caregiving, terminal illness, loss, and bereavement. The foundation provides leadership in the development and application of hospice and its philosophy of care. Hospice Foundation, Inc. was chartered in 1982 as a way to help raise money for hospices operating in south Florida, prior to passage of the Medicare hospice benefit. In 1990, the foundation expanded its scope to a national level in order to provide leadership in the entire spectrum of end-of-life issues.

To more accurately reflect its national scope, in 1992 the foundation opened a Washington, D.C., office and in 1994 changed the name of Hospice Foundation, Inc. to Hospice Foundation of America. For contact information, see Appendix I.

hospitalization   Spending time in a hospital can be a frightening and uncomfortable experience for anyone, but it is even more so for someone with Alzheimer's disease. Moving a person with Alzheimer's from the quiet familiar home setting to the noisy, strange world of a hospital may emphasize memory loss and trigger difficult behavior. Other challenges involve the stress of the illness, the potential of surgery and anesthesia, and possible drug interactions.

It is always best to avoid hospitalization by using day surgery or having procedures completed in a doctor's office. If hospitalization is unavoidable, caregivers should involve patients in discussions and decision making as much as possible. Caregivers should try to find out if any tests can be completed before admission that might shorten the hospital stay.

If financially possible, patients should be placed in a private room. Shortly before leaving for the hospital, caregivers should explain that the patient needs to spend a short time in the hospital. Caregivers may want to bring some familiar objects along, including photographs, familiar objects, or a familiar blanket or bedspread from home.

Caregivers should try to stay with the patient as much as possible, appearing in the room when patients wake up in the morning, when medications are given, when IVs or catheters are inserted, or when the doctor makes morning rounds. All hospital workers should understand that the patient has Alzheimer's, what they may expect, and how the patient may need to be helped. For example, it may be important to explain that the patient can still use the bathroom, but must be taken there every few hours if incontinence is to be averted. Hospital staffers should also be informed if the patient tends to wander so they can be sure to protect the person's safety. A typed list of suggestions for hospital staffers may help.

Because general anesthesia can sometimes depress a patient's central nervous system, some doctors prefer to use local or spinal anesthesia.

Caregivers should keep complete records during the hospitalization, including which drugs are ordered each day, and when they can be stopped. Caregivers should pinpoint the expected length of hospitalization and how long it will take to recover. Caregivers should also know what to expect, such as whether the patient will experience fatigue, exercise limitations, whether there will be pain, and so on. Once the illness or condition has improved, it's a good idea to discharge the patient as quickly as possible.

huperzine A (Cerebra)   An extract of club moss (Huperzia serrata) that has been used in traditional Chinese medicine for centuries as a memory enhancer. Because it can boost levels of ACETYL-CHOLINE, a chemical linked to memory deficits in people with Alzheimer's disease, it is now being considered as a potential treatment for the memory problems of Alzheimer's. Research suggests it may be just as potent as DONEPEZIL, RIVASTIGMINE, and TACRINE. However, as an herb, huperzine A is unregulated and manufactured with no uniform standards.

Huperzine A works very much like standard Alzheimer's drugs that inhibit the enzyme that breaks down acetylcholine, which raises acetylcholine levels in the brain.

Although it comes from a plant, this substance is highly purified in the laboratory and is sold as a single chemical, not an herb that contains hundreds or thousands of chemicals. Huperzine A much more closely resembles drugs such as digoxin or codeine, which are also highly purified chemicals derived from plants. Huperzine A is a highly potent compound with a recommended dose of only .05 mg twice a day for age-related memory loss.

Although it appears to have few side effects, children, pregnant or nursing women, or people with high blood pressure or severe liver or kidney disease should not take huperzine A except on a doctor's recommendation. Patients who use this chemical need to understand there could be dangers associated with its use. Using huperzine with donepezil, rivastigmine, galantamine, or tacrine can lead to overdose of these drugs.

The Alzheimer's Disease Cooperative Study has begun a trial to evaluate huperzine A.

Hydergine (ergoloid mesylates) A medication made from an extract of ergot (a fungus that grows on rye), once used as a popular treatment for all forms of DEMENTIA in the United States. Hydergine has been approved by the U.S. Food and Drug Administration (FDA) as a treatment for Alzheimer's disease, but today it has been superseded by more effective medications.

Hydergine may be effective in improving symptoms of senility by interfering with dangerous forms of oxygen called FREE RADICALS, enhancing brain cell metabolism and increasing blood supply and oxygen to the brain. Some scientists believe it may boost memory by mimicking the effect of NERVE GROWTH FACTOR, a substance that stimulates dendrite growth in the brain.

Originally produced and distributed by Sandoz Pharmaceuticals, the original patent has expired, which means that many generic versions are now available by prescription in various strengths. According to FDA guidelines, prescription is permitted for anti-senility treatment only, but many healthy adults also take the drug to improve memory. In Europe, Hydergine is prescribed in higher doses than those usually approved in the U.S.

Studies have found that more than 1,000 patients with senile disorders at a number of U.S. labs who took Hydergine had consistently higher scores in mental alertness, clarity and mood.

Side Effects

Hydergine is nontoxic; its potential side effects include mild nausea and stomach problems. The drug should not be taken by people who have low blood pressure, an abnormally slow heartbeat, or who are psychotic.

Hydrocephalus Association, The A nonprofit organization founded in 1983 dedicated to providing support, education, and advocacy for individuals, families, and professionals. The group offers personal support, comprehensive educational materials, and ongoing quality health care. For contact information, see Appendix I.

hyperbaric oxygen treatments A treatment in which patients in a specialized chamber inhale pure pressurized oxygen in order to reduce air bubbles that can form in blood vessels during medical procedures, reverse carbon monoxide poisoning, spur regrowth of crushed or irradiated blood vessels, cure chronic wounds and bone infections, help heal burns, and offset "the bends" that could otherwise kill deep-sea divers. It has been suggested as a possible treatment for Alzheimer's disease, but no study has ever found any benefits for this treatment.

Oxidation is a chemical reaction during which one molecule donates electrons to another. The molecule getting the electrons is said to be oxidized (and the one losing electrons is said to be reduced). Often the electrons come from an oxygen molecule (O_2)—hence the term oxidation. A certain amount of oxidation has to happen for the body to function. Oxidation therapy is based on the theory that repeated environmental stress cuts down on the ideal amount of oxidation. Restoring it with extra doses of oxygen—in one of several forms—is supposed to boost these reactions and heal the patient.

Some people take antioxidants such as vitamins C and E to prevent a chemical process called oxidation that may be involved in cell destruction in Alzheimer's. The theory behind using oxygen to help Alzheimer's disease is based on the idea that oxygen—the main agent that does the oxidizing—is beneficial. Hyperbaric oxygen therapy is helpful in a range of medical conditions, but using this therapy to treat or relieve symptoms of senility is much more speculative and too uncertain to justify using this costly therapy. In addition, highly pressurized oxygen can cause serious damage (including ruptured membranes, collapsed lungs, and cataracts).

ibuprofen   See NONSTEROIDAL ANTI-INFLAMMATORY DRUGS.

incontinence   The loss of bladder or bowel control and bedwetting. Incontinence is a common problem in later stages of Alzheimer's disease that is usually devastating for a caregiver. Incontinence is one of the main reasons a caregiver seeks nursing home care for a patient.

When a patient first shows signs of incontinence, the doctor should make sure the problem is not caused by an infection. There may be several reasons incontinence occurs in a person with Alzheimer's disease. Some patients forget some of their body signals, such as the urge to urinate or defecate. Others forget where the bathroom is or what it is used for. Emotional stress or an infection can sometimes cause incontinence, as can some medications such as diuretics, tranquilizers, or sedatives. Beverages such as hot coffee or tea, or caffeinated sodas, also can have a diuretic effect.

Urinary incontinence may be controlled for some time by monitoring frequency of liquid intake, feeding, and urinating. Once a schedule has been established, the caregiver may be able to anticipate incontinent episodes and get the patient to the toilet before they occur. Caregivers can sometimes improve incontinence by making sure the patient goes to the bathroom at regular intervals, especially after meals, before bedtime, after getting up from bed, and every two hours while awake. A sign or picture on the bathroom door will help patients find the room and help them remember what it is for. Beverages should be limited in the evening, as long as the patient is drinking enough during the day.

Patients who are incontinent should be kept very clean, since urine and feces can cause infections, pressure sores, and odors.

independent living   A type of housing option for older people often referred to as a retirement community, congregate living, or senior apartments. They are designed specifically for independent senior adults who want to enjoy a lifestyle filled with recreational, educational, and social activities with other seniors. These communities are designed for older people who are able to live on their own, but desire the security and conveniences of community living. Some communities offer an enriched lifestyle with organized social and recreational programs as a part of everyday activities, while others provide housing with only a minimal amount of amenities or services, such as senior apartments.

Some independent living communities offer a wide range of recreational activities that may include swimming pools, spas, exercise clubs, lounge, and reading room or library. Communities may also provide laundry facilities, linen service, meals, local transportation, and planned social activities.

An age inclusive community attracts retirees, but does not have age requirements; an age exclusive community requires that residents be of a certain age (usually over age 55). Most require that prospective residents be reasonably healthy and free from Alzheimer's disease or other dementias.

Although normal fees don't include health care, many communities will allow residents to pay for a home health aide or nurse to come into the apartment or cottage to help with medicines and personal care.

Prices vary according to locale, although there are some subsidized senior apartments that cater to seniors with limited incomes. Residences are usually paid for privately, although some senior apartments are subsidized and accept Section 8 vouchers. Medicare and Medicaid do not cover payment since no health care is provided.

Regulation

These communities are not licensed by local, state, or federal agencies. In those communities that provide services and activities, the rules are established by the management company providing the services. In other communities, an on-site or off-site manager can handle any problems.

independent providers   Nurses, therapists, aides, homemakers, geriatric care workers, and companions who are privately hired by individuals who need such services. Aides, homemakers, chore workers, and companions are not required to be licensed or to meet government standards except in cases where they receive state funding.

The responsibility for recruiting, hiring, and supervising the independent provider rests with the client. This also means that finding back-up care in the event that the provider fails to report to work or fulfill job requirements is the client's responsibility. Clients also pay the provider directly and must comply with all applicable state and federal labor, health, and safety requirements.

Indocin (indomethacin)   See NONSTEROIDAL ANTI-INFLAMMATORY DRUGS.

indomethacin (Indocin)   See NONSTEROIDAL ANTI-INFLAMMATORY DRUGS.

inflammation   Many scientists believe that inflammation may be an important component of the Alzheimer's disease process, triggering the sticky BETA AMYLOID protein plaques that stud the brains of many patients with Alzheimer's.

As beta amyloid breaks down, it releases unstable chemicals called oxygen FREE RADICALS. Once released, these oxygen free radicals bind to other molecules through a process called oxidation. The immune system responds to oxidation by triggering an inflammatory response, which is designed to fight harmful agents or manage injuries. When the inflammatory response becomes pronounced, however, inflammatory factors can actually begin to damage the body's own cells.

Inflammatory factors of specific interest in Alzheimer's research are the enzyme cyclooxygenase (COX) and its products, called prostaglandins. High levels of these factors may boost levels of GLUTAMATE, an amino acid that excites nerves and, when overproduced, can kill nerve cells.

Recent studies have found that NONSTEROIDAL ANTI-INFLAMMATORY DRUGS (NSAIDs) may reduce the inflammation of Alzheimer's, in some cases reducing the overall risk of Alzheimer's by 50 percent. Researchers believe that NSAIDs may influence inflammation by interfering with the actions of some proteins, thus lessening their harmful effects. A long-term study of nearly 7,000 Dutch volunteers found that people who regularly take aspirin-like drugs for at least two years are 80 percent less likely to develop Alzheimer's disease.

However, this doesn't mean everyone should start taking NSAIDs to prevent Alzheimer's. Some NSAIDs seem to have no effect on the risk of Alzheimer's, and people who begin taking the drugs run a higher risk of gastrointestinal hemorrhage, one of the more common causes of death in the United States.

Researchers found that dose size didn't seem to be important. Lower doses, similar to those available as over-the-counter medicines in the United States, seemed to work as well as some of the higher doses prescribed for arthritis.

Doctors have long suspected a link between Alzheimer's and inflammation. But earlier research examining whether NSAIDs might help have produced inconclusive results. The newer findings suggested that the earlier studies did not last long enough. The Dutch team followed patients over age 55 for an average of seven years, and discovered that the longer people had been taking NSAIDs, the lower their chances of getting Alzheimer's. It is not known whether anti-inflammatory drugs prevent the disease, but it seems clear that they do nothing to treat the disease.

inhibition, lack of A behavioral characteristic of people with Alzheimer's disease that other people find embarrassing. Uninhibited behavior may occur as a result of the patient's failing memory and confusion, or it may be due to specific damage to the brain. The patient may undress or appear without clothes in public, lift a skirt, or touch the genitals in public. Other uninhibited behavior may involve rude or insulting behavior, swearing, or spitting in public.

Caregivers should react calmly in the face of a patient's uninhibited behavior, and try to distract the patient or discourage the behavior whenever possible. A patient who is rude or insulting should not be corrected or disagreed with, but should be distracted.

insomnia Nighttime wakefulness is very common among patients with Alzheimer's disease. Although many patients can still correctly interpret a clock, many lose a real sense of time, so that when they wake up, they get up. Unfortunately, most sleep medications cause side effects that can worsen the confusion and agitation common in Alzheimer's disease.

instrumental activities of daily living Secondary level of activities important to daily living, such as cooking, writing, and driving. They are less basic than ACTIVITIES OF DAILY LIVING such as eating, dressing, and bathing.

insulin-degrading enzyme (IDE) An enzyme that breaks down both insulin and BETA AMYLOID protein, which has been implicated in the development of Alzheimer's disease. Some scientists suspect that a malfunction of this enzyme could be responsible for Alzheimer's in some families.

Patients with Alzheimer's have excessive levels of a protein called beta amyloid, which accumulates in their brains and forms sticky plaques. In a few cases, it seems that genetic mutations speed up the production of beta amyloid. Some scientists wondered if the beta amyloid buildup also could be caused by sluggish enzymes responsible for breaking down beta amyloid that aren't working fast enough.

In 1997, researchers found that insulin-degrading enzyme (IDE) breaks down beta amyloid in a test tube. Several years later, Harvard Medical School scientists discovered that IDE seemed to dispose of most naturally secreted beta amyloid. Blocking IDE activity stopped about 70 percent of beta amyloid breakdown in brain cell membranes, while overproducing IDE boosted beta amyloid breakdown.

Together with scientists at Massachusetts General Hospital, researchers found that mutations in the gene for IDE might contribute to Alzheimer's in people with a family history of the disease. In this study, seven families had Alzheimer's that seemed to be linked to the region of chromosome 10 that holds IDE. Members from one family had significantly less beta amyloid breakdown than normal, suggesting that a broken IDE can contribute to the disease.

intellectual stimulation Mental exercise may help delay the onset of Alzheimer's disease. Scientists have discovered that people whose leisure activities provide some type of intellectual stimulation are less likely to develop Alzheimer's than those who spend more time on passive activities. In one study, those who spent most of their leisure time on intellectual activities between the ages of 20 and 60 were 2.5 times less likely to have Alzheimer's.

Passive activities involve watching television, talking on the phone, or listening to music. Intellectual activities include things such as reading, playing chess, doing puzzles, knitting, woodworking, and playing musical instruments.

Studies don't show that intellectual stimulation can prevent the disease—just that it may delay onset. Scientists suspect this may be because intellectual stimulation increases the number of brain cell connections, so that it would then take longer for Alzheimer's disease to destroy enough brain cells to cause symptoms.

Another study of older nuns also suggests that intellectual ability plays a role in the risk of developing Alzheimer's. When researchers reviewed autobiographies the nuns in Wisconsin had written nearly 60 years earlier, they found that those women whose writing contained less complex ideas and simpler grammar were more likely to develop Alzheimer's disease than those whose autobiographies suggested greater intellect.

Earlier studies have shown that the onset of Alzheimer's disease is also delayed among people with more education and who have intellectually demanding jobs.

interleukins   Proteins that trigger inflammation and are linked with the development of Alzheimer's disease. Scientists know that some genes produce an inflammation-promoting protein called interleukin-1 (IL-1). There are two different versions of IL-1: interleukin-1 alpha (IL-1A) and interleukin 1-beta (IL-1B). These variations of the gene can significantly boost the risk of developing Alzheimer's disease.

Those people who have two copies of a specific variation in the gene for IL-1A (called IL-1A2)—one from each parent—have three times the risk of Alzheimer's than those with other versions of the gene. Those who have two copies of IL-1A2 in addition to a second variation in IL-1B (IL-1B2) are more than 10 times as likely to have Alzheimer's disease. A variation in IL-1A also appears to be linked to the development of Alzheimer's disease at an earlier age.

A separate Italian study found that people who had an IL-1A variation were almost five times as likely as others to develop Alzheimer's before the age of 65 years. Those with an IL-1B variation had nearly double the risk of developing the early onset version of the disease. Overall, people with the IL-1A variation developed Alzheimer's nine years earlier than people with other forms of the gene.

These results clearly demonstrate an association of certain IL-1 genes with Alzheimer's disease, and help to explain why many studies show that NON-STEROIDAL ANTI-INFLAMMATORY DRUGS delay the onset of Alzheimer's disease in some patients.

international statistics   DEMENTIA is a global problem, and two out of three people with dementia live in developing countries, according to the World Health Organization. Currently, there are about 29 million people worldwide with dementia, and two-thirds of these live in developing countries. By 2025 in Africa, Asia, and Latin America, this figure will nearly triple, to 55 million. Much of this increase will be in rapidly developing and heavily populated regions such as China, India, and Latin America.

Dementia primarily affects older people; before age 65, it develops in only about one person in 1,000. The chance of having the condition rises sharply with age, so that one person out of every 10 over the age of 65 has dementia. Over the age of 80, this figure increases to one person in two.

Of the approximately 580 million elderly people over age 60 in the world today, about 355 million live in developing countries. Over the last 50 years, mortality rates in developing countries have declined dramatically, raising the average life expectancy at birth from about 41 years in the early 1950s to almost 62 years in 1990. By 2020, it is projected to reach 70 years. At that point, the number of elderly people worldwide will reach more than 1 billion with more than 700 million of them in developing countries.

Over the next 25 years, Europe is projected to retain its title of "oldest" region in the world. The "oldest" nation by 2020 will be Japan (31 percent) followed by Italy, Greece, and Switzerland (above 28 percent). Currently, the countries with the highest proportion of elderly people are Greece and Italy (both 23 percent in 1998). By 2020, the proportion of population over age 60 is projected to reach 23 percent in North America, 17 percent in East Asia, 12 percent in Latin America, and 10 percent in South Asia.

In 2020, the proportion of the oldest old (over age 80) in the above-60 group is projected to be 22 percent in Greece and Italy, 21 percent in Japan, France, and Spain, and 20 percent in Germany. In several developing countries, including Uruguay, Cuba, and Argentina, this proportion will be between 15 percent and 20 percent.

jogging   Recent studies suggest that daily jogging might prevent the deterioration of brain cells that can lead to Alzheimer's disease, according to researchers at UC Irvine's College of Medicine. The researchers' work indicates that regular exercise controls the expression of genes in an area of the brain important for memory and maintaining healthy cells in the brain; this maintenance breaks down in cases of Alzheimer's.

Rats who ran in wheels for three weeks had increased expression of some genes and decreased expression of others. Many of these genes are responsible for helping the brain respond to stress, learning, and a wide range of other outside influences.

Studies have indicated the benefits of exercise in preventing Alzheimer's disease, but this recent study shows why exercise might help the brain prevent the cell degradation that can lead to the disease. There is a connection between the genes that control growth hormones and other important molecules and the genes' ability to be stimulated by exercise.

Researchers found that after three weeks of running, rats had changed the activity of genes in the HIPPOCAMPUS, a brain structure associated with higher cognitive functions such as memory, thinking, and learning. These changes in gene activity could make the hippocampus more able to adapt to changing circumstances. Even walking at least 20 minutes, three times a week can slow the onset of Alzheimer's disease.

John Douglas French Alzheimer's Foundation   A nonprofit charitable organization dedicated to generating money for research into the cure for Alzheimer's disease within the next decade. Funding is targeted to areas of research typically not supported by government agencies.

The group was founded by Dorothy Kirsten French and Richard K. Eamer in August 1984 to honor Dorothy's husband, Dr. John Douglas French, who suffered with Alzheimer's disease from 1977 until his death in 1989. The group provides money for fellowships and grants for talented young scientists in the early stages of their research careers, encouraging them to use new technological skills of study, including the exploration of less traditional avenues of research. The group also provides money for projects investigating new frontiers of research.

In the past 15 years, the foundation has raised more than $18 million for 110 special grants for research scholars and 67 scientific symposiums and conferences. For contact information, see Appendix I.

language areas of the brain The areas of the brain associated with language reception, comprehension, processing, and production are still not fully understood, but functional brain scans have helped explain how the brain interacts with language. In late-state Alzheimer's disease, language ability begins to fail because of damage to these parts of the brain.

Different parts of the brain control different language processes; for example, the motor portion of speech production versus the cognitive task of sentence planning. While the original data on locations of functional areas in the brain were based on persons with language defects, studying their problems and then looking at their brains after death, functional imaging technology has allowed assignments of function to be based on data from normal individuals without damage to their brains. Being able to base data on healthy brains is much more exact, since damage to one area of the brain could have multiple effects on a vast number of functions.

Broca's Area

Most studies agree that this area of the frontal lobe in the dominant hemisphere is primarily related to speech production. Broca's area is usually associated with maintenance of a list of words and parts of words used in producing speech, and their associated meanings. It has been linked to articulation of speech and to semantic processing, or assigning meanings to words.

The original area described in 1861 by Pierre Paul Broca to be the "seat of articulate language" has now been further studied and subdivided by functional imaging studies (fMRI and PET) into smaller subsections, each of which participate differently in language tasks. Semantic processing has been linked to the upper portion of the area, while

articulation falls within the center of Broca's original region of importance.

Broca's area is not simply a speech area, but is associated with the process of articulation of language in general. It controls not only spoken, but also written and signed language production.

M1-Mouth Area

This area of the brain is responsible for controlling the physical movements of the mouth and articulators used to produce speech. It is part of the motor cortex, and controls the muscles of the face and mouth just as the rest of the motor cortex controls various other parts of the body's movement. It is not involved with the cognitive aspects of speech production, though it is located near Broca's area and is activated in speech tasks along with Broca's area.

Wernicke's Area

This semantic processing area is associated with some memory functions, especially the short-term memory involved in speech recognition and production, as well as some hearing function and object identification. Wernicke's area is most often associated with language comprehension, or processing of incoming written or spoken language.

This distinction between speech and language is key to understanding the role of Wernicke's area in language. It does not simply affect spoken language, but also written and signed language. Wernicke's area works with Broca's area, Wernicke's handling incoming speech and Broca's handling outgoing speech.

Auditory Cortex

The areas of the brain responsible for recognizing and receiving sound are closely linked with language processing. In spoken language tasks, without correct auditory input, language comprehension can't happen. As people speak or read words aloud, there is also evidence that they listen to themselves as they are speaking in order to make sure they are speaking correctly. Areas around the auditory cortex near Wernicke's area have also been suggested to be involved in short-term memory, specifically a loop in which language heard is continuously repeated in the brain in order to maintain that language in the memory.

Visual Cortex

The area responsible for vision, also known as the striate cortex, is important in reading words and recognizing objects as an initial step in naming objects. The visual areas of the brain are usually among the first parts of the brain activated in reading and object-naming activities for speech tests in fMRI and PET scans. Other than this primary visual area located in the occipital lobe, another set of areas associated with vision are located in the parietal lobe, above the visual cortex. This region is associated with object naming and word reading, and is thought of as supplementary to the primary visual cortex. The visual cortex, along with the auditory cortex, is one possible first step on the path to language comprehension.

lecithin   A substance used to treat high cholesterol for many years that has more recently been proposed as a remedy for Alzheimer's disease. Lecithin contains a substance called phosphatidylcholine (PC), which plays a role in proper nerve function. It is broken down by the body into CHOLINE, which is used to make ACETYLCHOLINE, a nerve chemical essential for proper brain function.

Patients with Alzheimer's disease lack the enzyme responsible for converting choline into acetylcholine in the brain. Because lecithin is a major dietary source of choline, some people suspect that consuming more lecithin might reduce the progression of dementia.

However, evidence from randomized trials does not support the use of lecithin in the treatment of patients with dementia. Although a moderate effect cannot be ruled out, results from the small trials to date do not suggest lecithin has a major impact on the disease.

In the past, lecithin/phosphatidylcholine was one of the most commonly recommended natural treatments for high cholesterol. But this treatment appears to rest entirely on preliminary studies that lacked control groups. A more recent small, double-blind study of 23 men with high blood cholesterol levels found that lecithin had no significant effects on blood levels of total cholesterol, HDL ("good") cholesterol, LDL ("bad") cholesterol, or triglycerides (harmful fats found in the blood).

Because phosphatidylcholine plays a role in nerve function, it has been suggested as a treatment for various psychological and neurological disorders, such as Alzheimer's disease. However, the evidence that it works is limited to small studies with somewhat conflicting results.

Dosage

Lecithin is believed to be generally safe. However, some people taking high dosages (several grams daily) experience minor but annoying side effects, such as abdominal discomfort, diarrhea, and nausea. Maximum safe dosages for young children, pregnant or nursing women, or those with severe liver or kidney disease have not been determined.

Neither lecithin nor its ingredient phosphatidylcholine is an essential nutrient. For use as a supplement or a food additive, lecithin is often manufactured from soy. While ordinary lecithin contains about 10 to 20 percent phosphatidylcholine, European research was based on products concentrated to contain 90 percent phosphatidylcholine in lecithin. For Alzheimer's disease, studies have used doses as high as 5 to 10 grams three times a day.

leisure activity   Participating in everyday activities seems to protect healthy individuals against cognitive decline in later life. Leisure activities such as reading a book or magazine, going for a walk, watching a movie, or visiting a friend or relative can reduce the risk of developing Alzheimer's disease, according to one recent study at Columbia University. Reading and engaging in other leisure activities may reduce the risk or delay onset of clinical manifestations of dementia.

Earlier studies have found that education and successful jobs are also associated with reduced risk of Alzheimer's, but now researchers have found that leisure activities all by themselves can help reduce the risk of dementia among people of any education or job level.

In the study, 1,772 people over age 65 who were not demented at the beginning of the study were evaluated over a seven-year period to discover their participation in 13 common leisure activities categorized as intellectual, physical, and social pursuits. No matter what ethnic group, education, or job, subjects with high leisure activity had 38 percent less risk of developing dementia. The study also showed that the more leisure activities a person participates in, the better—there was an additional 8 percent risk reduction associated with each leisure activity.

All three activity categories were helpful in preventing Alzheimer's, although the intellectual activities were associated with highest risk reduction.

The study suggests that aspects of life experience provide a set of skills that allows a person to cope with Alzheimer's symptoms for a longer time before the disease becomes obvious.

Lewy body dementia A common condition (also called dementia with Lewy bodies) similar to Alzheimer's disease that describes several common disorders causing dementia. Its name comes from the presence of "Lewy bodies"—abnormal lumps of protein which develop inside deteriorating nerve cells.

When Lewy bodies disperse throughout the brain, it causes a dementia with symptoms much like Alzheimer's disease, with progressive loss of memory, language, calculation, and reasoning, as well as other higher mental functions. However, the condition progresses differently from Alzheimer's, involving hallucinations and fluctuations in impaired thinking.

Lewy body dementia was first described in 1961 and has been more often diagnosed over the past five to 10 years. Sometimes it occurs alone as the presenting illness, but more often it appears simultaneously with Alzheimer's or Parkinson's disease. Autopsies of the brains of people who had dementia suggest that Lewy body is relatively common, but the exact prevalence is not known. It appears to affect men and women alike.

Cause

Several key areas of the brain undergo degeneration in this form of disease, beginning with an area in the brain stem called the substantia nigra. Normally, the substantia nigra contains nerve cells responsible for making the neurotransmitter dopamine. In both Parkinson's disease and Lewy body dementia, these cells die. Remaining nerve cells contain abnormal structures called Lewy bodies, which are a hallmark of the disease. Shrinkage of the brain is particularly seen in the temporal lobe, parietal lobe, and the cingulate gyrus.

Doctors aren't sure what triggers these brain changes, although there appears to be a genetic component in some people. Genetic studies are beginning to show a group of different genes which may contribute to the development of DLB. In the genetic cases of Lewy body disease, families inherited the condition as an autosomal dominant disease, which means that anyone who carries the gene will develop the disease. The children of such a person have a 50 percent chance of inheriting the illness.

Symptoms

People with Lewy body dementia may have problems with short-term memory, finding the right words, sustaining a line of thought, and locating objects in space. They also may be anxious or depressed, with acute episodes of confusion that vary from hour to hour. Because the person is not always confused, however, it may seem as if the person is only pretending to be confused.

Hallucinations are another early characteristic of this condition, and may occur at any time, but are often worse during the times of acute confusion. The most common hallucinations are visual and often involve people, colored patterns, or shapes. These hallucinations often are not distressing and many people learn to distinguish between real and unreal images; in fact, some people come to enjoy the hallucinations.

On the other hand, patients may experience visual hallucinations together with unpleasant persecution delusions. Some develop the features of Parkinson's disease (rigidity, tremor, stooped posture, slow shuffling movements), followed later by the typical fluctuating cognitive performance, visual hallucinations, memory loss and progressive dementia. Others experience the cognitive symptoms first and go on to develop Parkinsonian features later in the disease.

DLB v. Alzheimer's

An important feature that can help to distinguish DLB from Alzheimer's disease is the presence of striking fluctuations in cognitive performance during the early stages of the disease. For example, one day a DLB patient may be able to hold a sustained conversation when next day he may be drowsy, inattentive or mute. The basis of these fluctuations is not clear.

Diagnosis

There are no specific diagnostic tests for the disease, although detailed psychological exams may help confirm the pattern of dementia, and brain scans may show generalized brain atrophy. It is important to be able to diagnose DLB, because the condition improves when Alzheimer's drugs (such as DONEPEZIL, GALANTAMINE, or RIVASTIGMINE) are given.

Treatment

While there is no cure for Lewy body disease, it is possible to treat some of the symptoms. For example, the depression that often accompanies the disease usually responds to antidepressants. Occasional unpleasant hallucinations may respond to medication.

Alzheimer's drugs such as rivastigmine may help ease some symptoms. In one study, rivastigmine improved apathy, indifference, anxiety, delusions, hallucinations, and abnormal movements. Subjects taking rivastigmine were significantly faster in their reactions, particularly in tasks focusing on attention. At the end of a three-week drug holiday, study participants taking rivastigmine had scores that showed the beneficial effects of the drug were wearing off.

On the other hand, patients with DLB react badly to neuroleptic drugs such as thioridazine or haloperidol, and their parkinsonism gets worse.

Outlook

In almost all patients, the disease is relentless and progressive; eventually, patients become profoundly demented and immobile, and usually die from pneumonia or another illness after an average of seven years. The overall course of the disease seems to be quicker than Alzheimer's or Parkinson's disease alone.

limbic system   A network of ring-shaped structures in the center of the brain's neocortex on top of the brain stem, associated with emotion and behavior (especially motivation, gratification, memory, and thought). It is also responsible for controlling body temperature, blood pressure, and blood sugar. Damage to certain structures that are part of the limbic system, such as the HIPPOCAMPUS and AMYGDALA, are common in patients with Alzheimer's disease.

It is the complexity of emotions as mediated by the limbic system, together with a sophistication of sensory and motor systems, that lead to the profoundly complex behavior that is uniquely human. While much is still to be learned, scientists do know that the limbic system and the hypothalamus are interconnected with emotional feelings and with certain types of basic primitive behaviors such as eating, drinking, and sexual activity.

The limbic system developed early in evolution, which is not surprising considering that this area governs such basic survival necessities as fear, aggression, hunger, and sexual desire. The neural function and connectedness of the limbic system are fundamentally similar in all mammals. This extensive system includes a range of substructures such as the hippocampus, cingulate gyrus, and amygdala. Because it contains the mechanisms that make an organism warm-blooded, it is known as the mammalian brain.

The structures of the limbic system receive input from all the senses, but in most animals (and to some degree, humans) the sense of smell plays an especially important part in the system. Other parts of the brain that connect closely with the limbic system include the association areas of the cerebral cortex involved in higher thought processes, and midbrain structures such as the reticular formation governing awareness and attention.

The effects of the limbic system are widespread, including the formation of tears, sweating, heart rate regulation, hormone release, and motor activity (such as facial expressions). Most of the messages sent by the limbic system end up in the hypothalamus. Connected directly to the pituitary gland below, it controls the body's hormones and regulates instinctive behavior and the autonomic nervous system.

Patients in late-stage Alzheimer's experience severe problems due to the damage in the limbic system. Patients begin to live in an eternal present, not able to remember what has happened in the past or what is happening around them. At this stage, patients start to forget the events that occurred even five minutes before, and are not able to relate to what is happening around them. Patients will experience very frequent emotional changes due to the damage in the limbic system as well as the deterioration of the neocortex.

linguistic skills There is a strong relationship between poor linguistic skills in early life and Alzheimer's disease in later life, according to a 1996 study of nuns. Understanding the link between linguistic skills and Alzheimer's may help doctors detect the disease at an earlier age, boosting the chance of early intervention and treatment.

In the study, scientists found that people with poor linguistic abilities were much more likely to experience cognitive decline and Alzheimer's disease than were those with better skills, even though the writing samples had been done nearly 60 years before. Moreover, women who scored poorly on measures of cognitive ability as young adults were found to be at higher risk for Alzheimer's disease and poor cognitive function in late life.

The groundbreaking study of nearly 100 nuns revealed that the complexity of the sisters' writing when they were young was strongly linked with how well they maintained thinking skills later in life. Scientists found that 90 percent of the sisters with Alzheimer's disease confirmed at autopsy had low linguistic ability in early life, compared with only 13 percent in those without evidence of the disease.

A decade ago, Kentucky researchers began the NUN STUDY, working with 678 School Sisters of Notre Dame aged 75 to 102 years who agreed to undergo physical and psychological tests and to have their brains studied after death. For the study of linguistic ability, researchers concentrated on those nuns who joined the Milwaukee convent from 1931 through 1939 and who had written autobiographies at an average age of 22.

The autobiographies were examined for linguistic ability as a test of cognitive function in early life. One component of linguistic ability, idea density, defined as the average number of ideas for each 10 written words, is associated with educational level, vocabulary, and general knowledge; while a second measure (grammatical complexity) is linked with working memory, performance on timed tests, and writing skills.

About 58 years after they had written their autobiographies, the women took part in tests of cognitive abilities. For the 25 nuns who died, brain tissue was examined at autopsy.

The study found that low idea density shown in the writings of the young women was strongly linked with low cognitive test scores and the presence of Alzheimer's disease in late life. For example, the nuns with low idea density scores were 30 times more likely to do poorly on a standard measure of cognitive function, the MINI-MENTAL STATUS EXAMINATION, than those with more complex writings. An even more dramatic difference was observed when cognitive ability and characteristics of brain tissue were compared in the nuns who died. Neurofibrillary tangles of Alzheimer's disease appeared in about 90 percent of those nuns who had low linguistic ability in early life.

David A. Snowdon, Ph.D., of the University of Kentucky's Sanders-Brown Center on Aging and lead author of the report, says the findings show that written linguistic performance—the study's measure of cognitive ability in early life—may be a potent marker for cognitive problems, Alzheimer's disease, and brain lesions in late life.

Why there should be a relationship between the two is not clear. Snowdon and his colleagues have suspected that developing the brain and thinking abilities early in life might offer some type of reserve that protects people from Alzheimer's disease and cognitive problems later.

Educational differences, however, did not explain the relationship between low linguistic ability in early life and poor cognitive function later on. Combining that with the study's findings on the nature of lesions in the brain, the scientists concluded that poor linguistic ability in early life could actually already be a subtle symptom of very early changes in the brain that ultimately lead to Alzheimer's disease.

Scientists note that the nun study is one of the first long-term studies in a well-controlled population to suggest that the process of Alzheimer's disease may begin earlier in life than previously thought. But linguistic ability in early life, while possibly a marker for Alzheimer's disease, needs to be examined further.

Researchers note that other factors could explain the link between early cognitive differences and disease in old age. The link might be related to inherited differences in cognitive ability, so that those with stronger linguistic ability early in life may be more resistant to later influences which lead to the disease, while those with poorer ability as young adults may be more at risk.

living trust　A notarized legal document in which a person states that his or her property be held in trust by a trustee, simplifying the eventual disposition of the estate and, in some cases, avoiding probate of the estate after the person's death. One of its advantages is that the patient's assets move to heirs without having to go through probate—the process by which the state examines a will and declares it valid. That's a plus in states like California and Florida, where probate can drag on for months. And if you own property in several states, multiple probate proceedings may be required.

A revocable living trust can be useful if a patient with Alzheimer's disease becomes incapable of taking care of personal financial affairs. In this case, the successor trustee—the person who would have distributed trust property after the patient's death—can also, in most cases, take over manage-ment of the trust property if the patient becomes incapacitated.

A living trust is also private, while probate is a public process. But living trusts aren't for everyone. At $2,000 to $3,000 each, they cost more than wills to prepare, and to make them effective, all the person's assets must be transferred into the trust.

living will　A legal document that allows a patient with Alzheimer's disease to outline what is to be done about specific health care decisions and whether life-sustaining treatment is to be carried out. Most states recognize living wills.

For a sample of a living will, see Appendix V.

long-term planning　A type of financial and social planning that may span several decades. When a diagnosis of Alzheimer's disease is given, long-term planning becomes very important. Caregivers should work with a knowledgeable attorney who specializes in geriatric issues to discuss durable POWER OF ATTORNEY, LIVING WILL, health care preferences, or guardianship.

The health care team should include a doctor who specializes in geriatrics, a nurse (especially one who makes house calls), and a social worker. In addition, caregivers might want to become familiar with nursing homes in the area, whether or not institutionalization is planned. Some nursing homes offer specialized care for patients with Alzheimer's, but they often have long waiting lists.

RESPITE CARE can be identified by contacting the local AREA AGENCY ON AGING; ADULT DAY CARE CENTERS; local hospitals; family, friends, and neighbors; church and community groups; private agencies; the ALZHEIMER'S ASSOCIATION.

Other helpful services to investigate include low-cost van services, half-price taxi fares for seniors, meal and chore services, doctors with staff who make house calls, mobile X-ray services, and handyman services.

magnetic resonance imaging A brain scan technique that allows scientists to look at changes in structure and function in the living brain, and that can be used to measure the size of various brain structures. Many studies have shown that Alzheimer's disease causes some shrinkage in brain structures (particularly the HIPPOCAMPUS) early on in the disease. Several teams of scientists have established the usefulness of MRI as a research tool to help determine which people with memory problems are in the earliest stages of Alzheimer's, to identify people who later will be diagnosed with the condition, to distinguish between people with MILD COGNITIVE IMPAIRMENT and those with no memory or learning problems, and between people without Alzheimer's and those with very mild Alzheimer's.

During the procedure, the patient lies back on a narrow table, and transmitters are positioned on the body. The cushioned table that the patient is lying on moves into a long tube containing the magnet. Once the area to be examined has been properly positioned, a radio pulse is applied, and a two-dimensional image corresponding to one slice through the area is made. The table then moves a fraction of an inch and the next image is made. Each image exposure takes several seconds; the entire exam lasts from 30 to 90 minutes. Depending on the area to be imaged, the radio-wave transmitters will be positioned in different locations.

magnetic resonance spectroscopy imaging (MRSI) A non-invasive analytical technique that has been used to study metabolic changes in the brain in order to diagnose Alzheimer's disease, as well as tumors, strokes, seizure disorders, depression, and other diseases affecting the brain. It has also been used to study the metabolism of other organs.

Magnetic resonance spectroscopy is similar to MAGNETIC RESONANCE IMAGING (MRI), but it depends on the behavior of other chemical elements, such as phosphorus and calcium, to identify the chemical composition of diseased tissue and produce color images of brain function. MRSI uses a continuous band of radio-wave frequencies to excite hydrogen atoms in a variety of chemical compounds other than water. These compounds absorb and emit radio energy at characteristic frequencies that can be used to identify them. Generally, a color image is created by assigning a color to each distinctive spectral emission. This makes up the "spectroscopy" part of MRSI.

MRSI, which is still experimental and is available in only a few research centers, can be done as part of a routine MRI, but MRSI and MRI use different software to acquire and mathematically manipulate the signal. Whereas MRI creates an image, MRSI creates a graph arraying the types and quantity of chemicals in the brain.

Medicaid A state program that may provide payment for nursing home care, adult day care, or at-home nursing care for patients with Alzheimer's if the person meets the financial need requirements. Medicaid also covers hospitalization, some medications, physical exams, and more. Patients usually become eligible for Medicaid only when their own money has been depleted to the point where they are below the federal poverty level. Eligibility is calculated not just on the patient's income, but also on the spouse's situation.

In order to prepare for accessing Medicaid, it is possible to transfer assets from a patient's name to another person (such as an adult child); however, this transfer must take place at least 30 months before the patient applies for Medicaid coverage.

Each state has different Medicaid rules and regulations. In some states, adult children and spouses are not legally required to spend their own money to support family members in nursing homes, but in other states, relative responsibility laws require a family to financially support the patient.

Medicare   A federal social security program that provides money for health care for patients age 65 or older, or who are disabled at any age. In 2000, Medicare spending for Alzheimer's disease was $31.9 billion; by 2010, that could increase to $49.3 billion.

If a patient with Alzheimer's disease gets sick, Medicare should cover the temporary illness, although maximum coverage is just 150 days and involves a co-payment. Medicare does not cover the two greatest expenses incurred by Medicare beneficiaries with Alzheimer's: long-term care and prescription drugs. Congress is now debating ways of adding a prescription drug benefit, but funding for long-term care is provided only through Medicaid once patients spend their remaining assets.

Recent rulings now require Medicare to pay doctors and other health care professionals for neurodiagnostic testing, medication management, and psychological therapy for patients with Alzheimer's disease. Previously, about 40 percent of Medicare carriers had been rejecting claims for treatment of patients with Alzheimer's and other types of DEMENTIA under the assumption that treatment would be futile. However, the legislation did not authorize any additional services exclusively for Alzheimer's patients. In addition, the person with Alzheimer's must still be able to derive benefit from the service in order to qualify for Medicare coverage. For example, if a patient with Alzheimer's breaks a leg and needs physical therapy, the person would have to be able to follow the therapist's instructions in order to qualify for Medicare coverage.

Many claims for patients with Alzheimer's disease are denied simply because they are coded improperly. For example, if a patient needs physical therapy to recover from the broken leg, the leg injury should be the primary diagnosis, not the Alzheimer's disease.

Medicare will cover "reasonable and necessary" evaluation and management visits by doctors or other health care providers; physical, occupational, and speech therapy; psychotherapy or other behavior management therapy provided by a mental health provider. Medicare will also cover HOME HEALTH CARE if the patient is homebound and requires a skilled service, such as nursing services, or physical, occupational, or speech therapy, even if the patient attends adult day care. It also covers medically necessary services, such as physical, occupational, and speech therapy or hospice care.

Medicare will not cover prescription drugs for Alzheimer's disease, adult day care, room and board in an assisted living facility, custodial care in a nursing home, or 24-hour personal care in the home.

The federal Centers for Medicare and Medicaid Services has instructed its claims payers to continue to scrutinize claims, since people with dementia can still be denied coverage for some Medicare services. Also, different states claims payers have leeway to decide whether to cover specific services.

Caregivers can find more information about Medicare coverage in Alzheimer's disease by contacting the federal government's Centers for Medicare and Medicaid Services, (1-800-MED-ICARE, or through the website, http://www.medicare.gov).

Families who believe that the patient is being denied service due to the Alzheimer's diagnosis, and who believe that the patient is cognitively able to benefit from that service, can call the ALZHEIMER'S ASSOCIATION for advice. If improper coding is not the problem, the patient's physician may be able to help with an appeal to the provider for review of the denial. The Health Insurance Counseling Advocacy Program can help caregivers review insurance coverage and file a claim if appropriate, and there is no charge for their services. The program offers Medicare information and support, assistance with coverage and regulatory issues, and help with preparation and filing of appeals to Medicare or an HMO. The program maintains a website with several fact sheets on the appeals process for both Medicare and Medicare HMOs at http://www.cahealthadvocates.org/facts.cfm.

The Centers for Medicare and Medicaid Services (CMS) at (415) 744-2986 also may be able to help caregivers Staffer specialists can advise caregivers how to file an appeal to Medicare, and whether they think a claim fits with the regulations. This process can take as little as three weeks, or up to a year if it is denied, and goes before an Administrative Law Judge. Information on filing an appeal can also be found at the CMS website at http://www.hcfa.gov, or the Medicare website: www.medicare.gov.

Mellaril   See THIORIDAZINE.

memantine (Akatinol)   A drug that acts on a key central nervous system receptor that may help slow the progression of moderately severe to severe Alzheimer's disease. Memantine is used in Germany to treat memory loss, and is being considered for approval in the United States.

Current drug treatments for Alzheimer's, called acetylcholinesterase inhibitors, have been approved by the U.S. Food and Drug Administration (FDA) for people with mild to moderate Alzheimer's disease. These drugs are designed to increase the amount of ACETYLCHOLINE, a substance that transmits nerve impulses in the brain.

Memantine is not an acetylcholinesterase inhibitor. Instead, it involves a different chemical and structural system called the NMDA receptor that is involved in the memory process.

In one study, researchers found that after six months, both the placebo group and the treatment group declined, but researchers found that the group who had taken memantine performed significantly better than the placebo group in thinking skills and daily life activities.

Researchers could not reverse the disease process with memantine, but they were able to slow the clinical decline over a six-month period. Memantine was safe and well tolerated by the patients with advanced Alzheimer's disease.

See also DRUG TREATMENTS.

memory   A biological phenomenon rooted in the senses that begins with perception. Memory is a complex construction that actively utilizes many areas of the brain to reassemble a thought into a coherent whole. When a person rides a bike, for example, the memory of how to ride the bike comes from one set of brain cells; the memory of how to get from here to the end of the block comes from another; the memory of biking safety rules from another. Yet people are never aware of these separate mental experiences, nor that they're coming from all different parts of the brain, because they all work together so well. In fact, experts say there is no firm distinction between how a person *remembers* and how they *think.*

This doesn't mean that scientists have figured out exactly how the system works. They still don't fully understand exactly how a person remembers, or what occurs during recall. The search for how the brain organizes memories and where those memories are acquired and stored has been a never-ending quest among brain researchers.

Still, there is enough information to make some educated guesses. The process of memory begins with encoding, and then proceeds to storing and then retrieval.

Encoding

Encoding is the first step to creating memory. Each sensation travels to the part of the brain called the HIPPOCAMPUS, which integrates these perceptions as they occur into one single experience. The hippocampus, experts believe, consolidates information for storage as permanent memory in another part of the brain (probably the cortex).

A memory begins with perception, yet it is encoded and stored using the language of electricity and chemicals. Nerve cells communicate with other cells at a point called a SYNAPSE, where all the action in the brain occurs as electrical pulses carrying messages leap across gaps between cells. The electrical firing of a pulse across the gap triggers the release of chemical messengers called neurotransmitters. These neurotransmitters diffuse across the spaces between cells, attaching themselves to neighboring cells. Each brain cell can form thousands of links like this, giving a typical brain about 100 trillion synapses. The parts of the brain cells that receive these electric impulses are called dendrites, feathery tips of brain cells that are near the neighboring cell.

The connections between brain cells can change all the time. Brain cells work together in a network, organizing themselves into groups that specialize in different kinds of information processing. As one brain cell sends signals to another, the synapse between the two gets stronger. The more active the two brain cells are, the stronger the connection between them grows. Thus with each new experience, the brain slightly rewires its physical structure. In fact, how people use their brain helps determine how the brain is organized. It is this flexibility, which scientists call plasticity, that can help a brain rewire itself if it is ever damaged.

As a person learns and experiences the world, changes occur at the synapses and dendrites as more connections in the brain are created. The brain organizes and reorganizes itself in response to experiences, forming memories triggered by the effects of outside input prompted by experience, education, or training. These changes are reinforced with use, so that as a person learns and practices new information, intricate circuits of knowledge and memory are created in the brain. If a musician plays a piece of music over and over, for example, the repeated firing of certain cells in a certain order in the brain makes it easier to repeat this firing later on. The result: The person gets better at playing the music, able to play it faster with fewer mistakes. Practice it long enough and the musician can play it perfectly. Yet if practicing stops for several weeks, the person will probably notice that the result is no longer perfect. The brain has already begun to forget what it once knew so well.

There are four types of remembering:

- *Recall:* the active, unaided remembering of something from the past.
- *Recollection:* the reconstruction of events or facts on the basis of partial cues which serve as reminders.
- *Recognition:* the ability to correctly identify previously encountered stimuli—such as when someone sees an old girlfriend's face across the room and recognizes who she is.
- *Relearning:* the evidence of the effects of memory—material that's familiar is often easier to learn a second time.

To properly encode a memory, a person must first be paying attention, which is why most of what occurs every day is simply filtered out, so that only a few stimuli pass into conscious awareness. If a person remembered every single thing, memory would soon become bogged down and overloaded. What scientists aren't sure about, however, is whether stimuli are screened out during sensory input or after the brain processes its significance. Scientists do know that how someone pays attention to information may be the most important factor in how much is remembered.

Once a memory is created, it must be stored. Many experts think that memories can be stored in three ways: as sensory input, in short-term memory, and ultimately, long-term memory. Because there is no need to maintain everything in the brain, the different stages of human memory function as a sort of filter that helps to protect people from the flood of daily information.

The creation of a memory begins with its perception—the registration of this information during perception occurs in the brief sensory storage that usually lasts only a fraction of a second. It's a person's sensory memory that allows a perception such as a visual pattern, a sound or a touch to linger for a brief moment after the stimulation is over.

After that first flicker, the sensation is stored in short-term memory, a fairly limited cache that lasts for just 20 or 30 seconds before being replaced with other material (unless it is constantly repeated). Most people find it impossible to remember a phone number or word after using it the first time because it is only stored in the ultra-short-term memory. However, after using or thinking about something more frequently, the information will then become part of short term and later part of the long-term memory. Important information is eventually transferred from short-term memory into long-term memory (this is called retaining). Long-term memory has an unlimited capacity store; unlike sensory and short-term memory, which decay rapidly, long-term memory can store information indefinitely.

People tend to store material on subjects they already know something about, since the information has more meaning to them. This is why someone with a normal memory may be able to remember in depth more information about one particular subject.

Most people think of long-term memory when they think of memory itself but most experts believe information must first pass through sensory and short-term memory before it can be stored as a long-term memory. When a person wants to remember something, it is first retrieved on an unconscious level, and then brought into the conscious mind at will.

While most people think they either have a "bad" or a "good" memory, in fact most people are fairly good at remembering some things, and not so good at others. If someone has trouble remembering something (assuming the person is healthy) it is usually not the fault of the entire memory system, but an inefficient component of one part of the memory system.

That assembly process of memory first begins with the onset of sexual maturity, and tends to get worse as people reach middle age. This age-dependent loss of function appears in many animals.

As a person learns and remembers, the connections between new cells are reinforced and made stronger, but with age, these synapses begin to falter. This begins to affect how easily a person can retrieve memories.

Aging

What may be lost

- attention span—gets shorter
- thinking—slows down
- learning—takes longer

What will probably be maintained

- short-term memory
- retention of well-known information
- searching techniques

Researchers have several theories behind this deterioration, but most suspect that aging causes major cell loss in a tiny region in the front of the brain that leads to a drop in the production of a vital neurotransmitter called ACETYLCHOLINE. Acetylcholine is vital to learning and memory.

In addition, some parts of the brain itself vital to memory are highly vulnerable to aging. One area, called the HIPPOCAMPUS, loses 5 percent of its nerve cells with each passing decade or a total loss of 20 percent by the time people reach their 80s. In addition, the brain itself shrinks and becomes less efficient as the brain ages.

Of course, other things can happen to the brain to speed up this decline—a person may have inherited some unhealthy genes, might have been exposed to poisons, or perhaps smoked or drank too much. All these things speed up memory decline.

This is why as a person gets older, some physical changes in the brain can make it more difficult to remember efficiently. This does not mean that memory loss and dementia is inevitable, however. While some specific abilities do decline with age, overall memory remains strong for most people throughout the 70s. In fact, research shows that the average 70-year-old performs as well on certain cognitive tests as do many 20-year-olds, and many people in their 60s and 70s score significantly better in verbal intelligence than do younger people.

Studies also have shown that many of the memory problems experienced by older people can be improved or even reversed. Studies of nursing home populations show that patients were able to make significant improvements in memory when given rewards and challenges. Physical exercise and mental stimulation also can really improve mental function.

Evidence from animal studies suggests that stimulating the brain can stop cells from shrinking and can even increase brain size in some cases. For example, studies show that rats living in enriched environments with lots of toys and challenges have larger outer brains with larger, healthier brain cells. And animals given lots of mental exercise have more dendrites, which allow their cells to communicate with each other. With age, research has shown that a stimulating environment encourages the growth of these dendrites and a dull environment impedes that growth.

As the brain ages, a person may not learn or remember as well as in youth, but that individual will likely learn and remember nearly as well. In many cases, an older person's brain may be less effective not because of a structural problem, but simply through lack of use.

memory, active working   A type of short-term memory that enables a person to hold information in mind while manipulating or using it. For example, when adding several numbers together, a person might hold the amount "carried" in active working memory while adding a new row of numbers.

Research suggests that remembering gets easier with age because using these processes becomes more automatic after extended use and practice. Active working memory also allows a person to return to earlier steps in a problem-solving sequence so the process can be integrated. Because it has a limited capacity, this kind of memory is linked to attention.

Active working memory is critical to success at home, on the job, and in personal relationships, and it's a fundamental component in the process of reading and writing. It enables reflection on past events and helps monitor the passing of time. Individuals who are experiencing severe Alzheimer's disease find it difficult to use active working memory effectively.

See also MEMORY.

Memory Impairment Study   A nationwide research study to determine whether medical intervention in people with MILD COGNITIVE IMPAIRMENT (MCI), characterized primarily by memory problems, can help delay the onset of Alzheimer's disease. The study is sponsored by the NATIONAL INSTITUTE ON AGING (NIA), the first step in the Alzheimer's disease prevention initiative made possible by increased funding for Alzheimer's disease research provided by Congress.

Older adults with MCI appear to be at increased risk of developing Alzheimer's disease at a rate of 12 to 15 percent per year, whereas people over age 65 with normal memory develop Alzheimer's at a rate of perhaps 1 to 2 percent per year.

The Memory Impairment Study includes about 720 men and women aged 55 to 90 with an obvious memory problem but no other cognitive impairment. This study is not for people diagnosed with Alzheimer's disease or for those who, through testing, show a level of impairment equal to Alzheimer's disease. Between 65 and 80 centers across the United States and Canada are participating in the study, which will test vitamin E and DONEPEZIL (Aricept) in the treatment of memory loss and possible delay of the onset of Alzheimer's disease.

It is important to find ways to intervene early in the disease process before significant brain cell damage has occurred, and to stop the disease from occurring.

The study is as much a trial of the research methodology as it is of the particular drugs being used, because scientists aren't yet certain if it is possible to conduct a trial on Alzheimer's disease prevention. A key factor is whether it is possible to effectively identify and recruit people who do not yet have Alzheimer's but are at higher risk for the disease.

The study is being implemented through the Alzheimer's Disease Cooperative Study (ADCS) at the University of California, San Diego, the NIA's consortium of Alzheimer's disease clinical centers.

memory loss vs. Alzheimer's   There is a great deal of difference between normal, everyday forgetting and Alzheimer's disease. Many memory changes are only temporary, such as those that occur during any stressful situation that makes it hard to concentrate. The differences between normal behavior and Alzheimer's symptoms include

- *Daily life:* Alzheimer's often affects daily life and job skills. It's normal to occasionally forget a task or a person's name, but frequent FORGETFULNESS or unexplainable confusion at home or in the workplace may signal that something is wrong. It's normal for someone to misplace a pair of glasses, but not to forget that the person *wears* glasses.

- *Familiar tasks:* It is normal to forget a pan on the stove, but patients with Alzheimer's might forget to serve an entire meal—or even that they cooked it.

- *Language problems:* It's normal to forget a word sometimes, but a person with Alzheimer's disease forgets many words and also substitutes inappropriate words so that sentences become hard to understand.

- **Disorientation:** It is normal to momentarily forget what day of the week it is, but people with Alzheimer's disease not only forget the day, they get lost on their own street.
- **Poor judgment:** A person with Alzheimer's often exhibits bad judgment; for example, DRESSING inappropriately by wearing pajamas to the workplace.
- **Abstract thinking problems:** Most everyone occasionally forgets a multiplication fact now and then, but people with Alzheimer's forget how to recognize numbers, and can no longer add or subtract.
- **Misplacing things:** Everyone forgets things like where the car keys are, but people with Alzheimer's forget they have a car.
- **Personality changes:** Occasionally crankiness or depression is normal, but a person with Alzheimer's can change dramatically and become suspicious or fearful.

Alzheimer's disease begins slowly with mild forgetfulness that leads to problems finding the right word. Ever so gradually, it progresses to an inability to recognize objects, and ultimately, to an inability to use even the simplest things, such as a hairbrush. This gradual degeneration often lasts more than 10 years.

A person with mild DEMENTIA can usually live independently with only minor problems in work or social activities, but as the dementia continues, although the patient may seem capable, independent living becomes increasingly dangerous. The person may begin to dress carelessly and neglect work and family responsibilities. He may leave the stove or iron turned on and become lost while away from home. As short-term memory falters, the patient can no longer perform everyday tasks such as zipping a zipper. Behavioral symptoms are also quite common, since the damage to the brain can cause a person to act in different or unpredictable ways.

Some people become anxious or aggressive, while others engage in repetitive behavior. Other behavioral symptoms may include AGITATION, COMBATIVENESS, DELUSIONS, DEPRESSION, HALLUCINATIONS, SLEEP PROBLEMS, and WANDERING.

As the dementia becomes severe, the person must be constantly supervised; by now, he may string together unrelated words into meaningless sentences. Eventually the failing nervous system affects the entire body and he becomes completely incapacitated—even unable to eat. Death usually follows as the result of pneumonia or an infection.

menopause and Alzheimer's disease Several studies have suggested that the lower levels of estrogen that occur after menopause may be linked to an increased risk of developing Alzheimer's disease. The results of several studies suggest that estrogen may reduce the risk of Alzheimer's by as much as 50 percent. Other studies have suggested that estrogen or hormone supplementation helps to slow the progression of Alzheimer's.

For example, one 1996 study showed that patients with Alzheimer's were significantly less likely to have taken estrogen after menopause (7 percent versus 18 percent). In addition, the study found that four of seven Alzheimer's patients taking daily estrogen improved on mental test scores. However, further work still needs to be done in this controversial area.

Estrogen facilitates networking between nerve cells, promoting their ability to communicate and influencing memory, language skills, mood, attention, and a number of other functions. Estrogen receptors are present in several regions of the brain, including those involved in memory, and when estrogen activates these receptors, it triggers processes that are beneficial to the brain. In addition, estrogen may boost levels of certain neurotransmitters, including ACETYLCHOLINE (implicated in memory), SEROTONIN and noradrenaline (mood), and dopamine (motor coordination).

Researchers at the NATIONAL INSTITUTE ON AGING discovered that by maintaining optimal levels of estrogen, postmenopausal women may be able to protect themselves from memory decline associated with aging. Adequate levels of estrogen appear to protect parts of the brain that are most vulnerable to neuron loss.

mental exercise and Alzheimer's disease Some studies seem to suggest that mentally exercising the brain may postpone the development of Alzheimer's. Scientists suspect this may be because an intellectually stimulated brain produces more connections between brain cells. People with more connections to lose would therefore not experience the symptoms of Alzheimer's as quickly as someone with fewer neural connections. Research suggests that the more connections (synapses) people have between brain cells, the more resistant they are to the effects of Alzheimer's.

One Columbia University study published in 1995 showed that people with less than an eighth-grade education had twice as much risk of developing Alzheimer's as those with more education. When those with less education also worked at mentally unstimulating occupations, their risk was three times higher. Similarly, the Kentucky NUN STUDY found that nuns with poor linguistic skills in their early 20s were far more likely to develop Alzheimer's when they grew old. And a large Massachusetts General Hospital study of more than 1,000 people ages 70 to 80 found that both physical and mental factors seem to determine which elders hold on to their intellects. Key elements revealed in this study were education, which seems to increase the number and strength of synaptic connections; strenuous physical exercise, which improves blood flow to the brain; and good lung function, which provides a lot of oxygen for the blood.

mental status testing A diagnostic tool used by a doctor to help determine the extent of behavioral and thinking problems. In such an exam, the patient is asked questions such as "What is today's date?" and "Who is the president of the United States?" Patients might be asked to draw a clock face in an empty circle, count backward by sevens from 100, or put a stamp on an envelope in the correct place. A numerical score is given at the end of the test that can be compared to average scores of people at different levels of impairment.

There is a range of other tests that have been designed to assess the degree of impairment in patients with Alzheimer's, including behavior problems, thinking problems, and functional impairment. Some of these tests include the MINI-MENTAL STATUS EXAMINATION, the Blessed Dementia Rating Scale or the Mattis Dementia Rating Scale. The Hamilton Rating Scale for Depression can help determine how depressed a patient may be. The Present State Examination can assess DEPRESSION, ANXIETY, DELUSIONS, and HALLUCINATIONS.

mercury A metal used in dental fillings that had in the past erroneously been linked to the development of Alzheimer's disease. According to recent studies at the University of Kentucky, although very small amounts of mercury are released from dental amalgam when eroded from brushing or eating, they are not taken up by the brain.

Dental amalgam has been used since the early 1830s because of its strength and durability, but because it is composed of 50 percent mercury—a neurotoxin—its use has caused controversy over a possible public health risk. Some dentists have encouraged patients to have their amalgam fillings removed and replaced by other restoration materials, but up to 76 percent of dentists still use it as their primary restoration material.

At the same time, trace levels of many metal elements—including mercury—have been reported to be imbalanced in patients with Alzheimer's disease. Some experts have speculated that the imbalance may play a role in the development of Alzheimer's disease.

The Kentucky researchers began their study in 1991, funded by a grant from the National Institutes of Health. They examined the brains of 68 people with Alzheimer's and a control group of 33 who were not affected, and determined the number and location of existing teeth, and amalgam restorations. Dental histories of each subject's 32 teeth were completed and information was obtained on non-dental exposure to mercury. The authors then measured mercury levels in multiple brain regions and performed full nervous system disease evaluations to confirm the normal status of the brain or the presence of Alzheimer's disease.

Researchers found no association between brain mercury levels and dental amalgam, and no significant difference in brain mercury levels between subjects with Alzheimer's and the control subjects without the disease. The definitive study was published in the February 1999 issue of *The Journal of The American Dental Association.*

metabolism All of the physical and chemical processes that take place in the body. Some experts believe that metabolic problems may be implicated in the development of Alzheimer's disease in some patients.

Some researchers are studying whether changes or an imbalance in the metabolism of certain elements (such as CALCIUM) in brain cells may be part of the process by which the cells degenerate and die in Alzheimer's. Brain cells use calcium to help transmit signals in the brain, but too much calcium can kill a cell. Some scientists think that cell death in Alzheimer's patients may be caused by high levels of calcium. This excess calcium level could be caused by a number of problems, such as a defect in the structures that store calcium in the cell, or those that pump it out of the cell.

Other experts suspect the hormone GLUCOCORTICOID, which normally enhances the manufacture of sugar in the body and lessens inflammation. Animal studies have suggested that long exposure to glucocorticoids contribute to cell death and dysfunction in the HIPPOCAMPUS.

metacognition The awareness and knowledge of an individual's own mental processes; the ability to think about thinking. Metacognition refers to a person's understanding of what strategies are available for learning and what strategies are best used in which situations. Metacognition skills are directly related to reading, writing, problem solving, and any process that requires error monitoring.

metrifonate (ProMed) A drug that had been studied as a potential treatment for Alzheimer's disease whose application for approval from the U.S. Food and Drug Administration (FDA) was suspended by its manufacturer because studies reported some cases of respiratory paralysis and problems in neuromuscular transmission. Metrifonate has joined a list of drugs that are no longer in development, which is not uncommon in the drug development process.

Earlier studies had shown positive results in metrifonate's ability to improve cognition and behavioral symptoms in mild and moderate Alzheimer's disease, with only "weak indications" of adverse effects.

The FDA originally had approved metrifonate (ProMed), which would have been the fifth medication for the treatment of some of the symptoms of Alzheimer's disease. Like the other four, metrifonate is a CHOLINESTERASE enzyme inhibitor. Medications already approved to treat loss of memory and decline in abilities such as thinking and reasoning include TACRINE (Cognex), available by prescription since 1993; DONEPEZIL (Aricept), available since 1996; RIVASTIGMINE (Exelon), approved in 2000; and GALANTAMINE (Reminyl), approved in 2001. All these drugs work by increasing the brain's supply of ACETYLCHOLINE. (Galantamine also affects some of the brain's receptors that respond to acetylcholine). By slowing down the metabolic breakdown of acetylcholine, more of the brain chemical is available for communication between cells. Although these drugs help slow the progression of Alzheimer's, they don't cure the disease. All of these drugs are most effective if taken early in the disease when there are more functioning brain cells to produce acetylcholine. After too many cells die, the drug no longer works.

microglia (microglial cells) A type of scavenger immune cell found in the brain that engulfs dead cells and other debris. In Alzheimer's disease, microglia are associated with dying nerve cells and BETA AMYLOID plaques.

mild cognitive impairment A condition characterized by mild recent memory loss without DEMENTIA or significant impairment of other thought functions to an extent that is beyond what would be expected for age or educational background. This condition is more serious than simple forgetfulness, but not as severe as Alzheimer's disease. Because 80 percent of people with MCI go on to develop Alzheimer's within 10 years at a rate of 10 percent to 15 percent of patients per year, many experts consider MCI not a distinct condition, but simply an early stage of Alzheimer's. Only 1 percent of healthy people over age 65 develop Alzheimer's each year. Still, some individuals with MCI never develop Alzheimer's disease.

The idea that MCI might be an early form of Alzheimer's is also based on physiological similarities between the two conditions. Many MCI patients present with significant atrophy of the brain in the temporal lobe area, while others have abnormal concentrations of a protein that is associated with the plaques common to Alzheimer's.

There are also genetic similarities between the conditions. The strongest predictor of inherited Alzheimer's, for example, may be the presence of the APOLIPOPROTEIN E GENE (ApoE), which is present in both Alzheimer's and MCI patients. These characteristics, together with the fact that the onset of Alzheimer's is gradual and progressive, suggest that brain problems exist many years before any symptoms occur. From this scientists deduce that in many cases MCI is an early sign of Alzheimer's.

Symptoms

Patients with MCI perform worse on memory tests than do healthy people, but they are normal in other thinking areas. They aren't generally confused or disoriented, and they can perform ACTIVITIES OF DAILY LIVING that would be impossible for a patient with Alzheimer's. However, as time passes, people with MCI experience a decline in mental and functional abilities more quickly than do normal healthy aging people. For example, people with MCI have a much harder time remembering a fact after a relatively short time. In cognitive testing, people with MCI remember significantly less of a paragraph they have read or details of simple drawings they have seen compared to people with normal memory changes associated with aging.

A person with MCI is likely to forget important events repeatedly, while significant information is retained in normal aging. Other memory lapses in MCI might include repeatedly missing appointments, telling the same joke over and over again, or forgetting the names of close colleagues. In other words, a diagnosis of MCI is made when a person's memory impairment begins to interfere with the activities of daily living.

As its name indicates, MCI is a condition of mild impairment, specifically in the area of memory, while dementia is characterized by additional and severe problems in other areas of cognition, such as orientation, language, and attention. Alzheimer's disease is the most common form of dementia among people age 65 and older.

A diagnosis of MCI can be made on the basis of five symptoms:

- memory complaints
- abnormal memory for age
- ability to carry out normal activities of daily living
- normal general cognitive function
- no dementia

Diagnosis

MCI can't be diagnosed by one test alone; a doctor must check both physical and neurological assessments in order to uncover the memory problems that may be abnormal for the person's age and educational level. Normal memory loss generally associated with aging is characterized by misplacing an item, forgetting someone's name, or forgetting to pick something up at the store. Memory loss associated with MCI is more severe and involves continuing problems in delayed recall of information. Abnormal memory loss associated with Alzheimer's or dementia is characterized by even more severe problems, such as disorientation and general confusion.

Tests such as the SHORT PORTABLE MENTAL STATUS QUESTIONNAIRE (SPMSQ), the MINI-MENTAL STATUS EXAMINATION (MMSE), or the CLINICAL DEMENTIA RATING SCALE (CDR) usually identify cognitive impairment.

Treatment

There is currently no approved treatment for MCI. Those who believe that MCI is really early Alzheimer's may start treatment with cholinesterase inhibitors even at this early stage.

Mini-Mental Status Examination (MMSE) A test of orientation and simple thinking ability that is often used for a quick clinical assessment of patients with Alzheimer's disease. The MMSE includes assessments of orientation, memory, attention and calculation, language, ability to follow commands, reading comprehension, the ability to write a sentence, and the ability to copy a drawing. The MMSE is often used in clinical settings because it tends to take less time to administer than some of the longer, more involved assessments.

However, a patient's education, job, and cultural and background factors can strongly influence MMSE scores. The test may falsely indicate DEMENTIA in normal but poorly educated patients, or may indicate that a mildly demented person is normal. This is why the dividing line between "normal" and "demented" should be used only in context with the person's history and overall condition. This is especially the case in people with Alzheimer's, which may cause a wide variety of different symptoms in behavior and thinking skills. Cultural, educational, and social factors must also be considered when attempting a diagnosis.

In the beginning of the test, the doctor will assess how well a patient is oriented in place and time by asking for the date, and then specifically asking for any omitted information.

Next, the doctor will ask patients to name three unrelated objects clearly and slowly, about a second apart. After all three objects have been named, the patient is asked to repeat them. The first repetition determines the score.

Next, the patient is asked to begin with 100 and count backward by sevens. After five subtractions, the doctor will score the response (one point for each correct subtraction). Alternatively, the doctor may ask patients to spell a five-letter word backward (the score is the number of letters in correct order.)

Patients are then asked to recall the three objects they were previously asked to remember. To test skills in naming objects, patients are shown two objects and asked to name each item. Then patients are asked to repeat a sentence.

To assess reading ability, the doctor will print clearly on a piece of paper in large letters the command: "Close your eyes," and then ask patients to read and perform the command. To assess complex three-stage commands, patients are then given a piece of paper and asked to repeat the command.

Next, patients are given a blank piece of paper and asked to write any sentence of their own; it must contain a subject and a verb to score 1 point. Punctuation does not matter.

On another clean piece of paper with a picture of intersecting pentagons, each side measuring 1 inch, patients are asked to copy the figure. The patient's drawing must include all 10 angles and the two figures must intersect to score one point. Any rotation of the figures or tremor does not matter.

A score of less than 24 suggests the presence of delirium, dementia, or another problem affecting the patient's mental status, and it may indicate the need for further evaluation

See also CLINICAL DEMENTIA RATING SCALE; MENTAL STATUS TESTING; SHORT PORTABLE MENTAL STATUS QUESTIONNAIRE (SPMSQ).

money Mishandling money is fairly common among patients with Alzheimer's disease, who may accuse caregivers or family members of stealing their money.

Having and handling money is one of the symbols of a person's independence and competence. Patients with Alzheimer's may blame others for money mistakes because they are trying to protect their self-esteem and maintain independence. Early problems with memory and reasoning abilities that are the hallmark of Alzheimer's can make it hard to handle more complex financial matters. Trying to perform calculations becomes frustrating.

The spouse or adult child should assume the responsibility for financial matters, monitoring monthly bills and contacting creditors about unusual charges. Legal arrangements such as a POWER OF ATTORNEY or GUARDIAN can help protect the person's financial security.

music Music can have a calming effect on patients with Alzheimer's disease, lessening WANDERING, improving mood, behavior, and attention—as long as it is music that holds significance for the patient.

A number of studies have found music has enhanced physical and mental functioning in neurologically impaired patients. Meaningful music can help patients organize and make incoming stimuli comprehensible. People with Alzheimer's disease have not lost their memories or their former personalities—they simply have lost access to them. For many people, the key to opening the locked door to long-term memories is the therapeutic use of the right music.

While the music is playing, patients have been able to recall and reaccess speech, perceptual and thinking skills, and past memories, for a brief period.

A study on the impact of music therapy on DEMENTIA patients, conducted by Eastern Michigan University, determined that patients consumed 20 percent more calories when music was played during lunchtime. The Alzheimer's Association notes that music can stir memories and encourage group activity through singing and clapping. Other studies have shown improvements in loneliness, DEPRESSION, and brain chemistry in people with Alzheimer's.

Music therapy appears to have healing and relaxing effects by triggering the release of neurotransmitters and hormones in the brain. Scientists have noted changes in the level of melatonin, norepinephrine, epinephrine, serotonin, and prolactin following music therapy. The melatonin increase lasted as long as six weeks after the therapy, which may have contributed to patients' calmer moods. Norepinephrine and epinephrine levels increased significantly after four weeks of music therapy, but returned to pretreatment levels at a six weeks' follow-up. Serotonin levels remained unchanged after four weeks of music therapy and at six weeks' follow-up.

multi-infarct dementia   A form of dementia (also known as vascular dementia) caused by a number of strokes in the brain, that may resemble Alzheimer's disease. MID affects about four out of 10,000 people; it is estimated that up to 20 percent of all dementia is caused by multi-infarct dementia.

MID leads to the deterioration of mental function and memory, impaired motor and walking skills, and hallucinations, delusions, or depression. The strokes typically begin between the ages of 60 and 75, affecting men more often than women.

Causes

As multiple blood clots throughout the brain block small blood vessels, a steady oxygen supply is cut off, leading to the brain damage and dementia seen in MID. The disorder is associated with atherosclerosis, a condition where fatty deposits build up in the inner lining of the arteries. MID is not caused directly by deposits of atherosclerotic plaque in the blood vessels of the brain, but by a series of strokes that leave areas of dead brain cells. This occurs when plaques cause multiple, scattered blood clots that block off the small blood vessels and prevent the brain from receiving blood and oxygen.

Symptoms

Symptoms include confusion, problems with recent memory, wandering or getting lost in familiar places, incontinence, inappropriate laughing or crying, and problems following instructions or handling money.

At first, the damage is so slight that changes are barely noticeable, but as time goes on, more small vessels become blocked, which leads to a stepwise mental decline.

Memory impairment is often an early symptom of the disorder, followed by impaired judgment. This often progresses slowly to delirium, hallucinations, and impaired thinking. Personality and mood changes accompany the deteriorating mental condition. Apathy and lack of motivation are common. Catastrophic reaction, where a person reacts to tasks by withdrawal or extreme agitation, is common. Confusion that occurs or is worsened at night is also common.

Risk

Risk factors for the development of MID include a personal or family history of MID, stroke, high blood pressure, smoking, and atherosclerosis.

Diagnosis

The disorder is diagnosed based on history, symptoms, signs, and tests, and by ruling out other causes of dementia, including dementia due to metabolic causes. Characteristics that suggest multi-infarct dementia include abrupt onset, physical complaints, emotional changes, and localized neurologic symptoms.

A neurologic examination shows variable deficits depending on the extent and location of damage. There may be multiple localized areas with a specific loss of function. Weakness or loss of a function may occur on one side or only in one area, with abnormal reflexes or loss of coordination.

A brain CT or MRI scan may reveal changes that indicate multi-infarct dementia.

Treatment

Recent research shows that GALANTAMINE can improve cognitive and behavioral symptoms in these patients.

It is important to provide a safe environment with control of aggressive or agitated behavior; this may require home health care or adult day care, or nursing home care. The patient should be surrounded by familiar objects and people, with a simple schedule of activities.

The prognosis for patients with MID is generally poor. Individuals with the disease may improve for short periods of time, then decline again. Death may occur from stroke, heart disease, pneumonia, or other infection.

multi-photon microscope A new imaging device that provides images of the protein deposits in the brains of living creatures. Before the invention of this device, the only way to confirm the presence of these deposits and to diagnose Alzheimer's disease with 100 percent accuracy was at death with direct examination of the brain during autopsy.

mutant proteins For nearly a century scientists have wondered which of the brain lesions associated with Alzheimer's disease is the cause: the plaques that clutter up the empty spaces between nerve cells, or the stringy tangles that erupt from within those cells.

In the mid-1980s, researchers discovered a class of sticky proteins called BETA AMYLOID in the plaques of patients with Alzheimer's. A short time later, four research teams found the gene that makes the protein. They realized that beta amyloid is a fragment of a much larger protein called AMYLOID-PRECURSOR PROTEIN (APP), which is involved in cell membrane function and is found in the brain, heart, kidneys, lungs, spleen, and intestines. Scien-

tists discovered that the plaques typical of Alzheimer's are created when an enzyme snips APP apart at a specific place and then leaves the beta amyloid fragments behind, where they clump together in abnormal deposits in the brain.

Beta amyloid protein is produced by cells throughout the body, but it is found in large amounts in the brain. Its normal function remains mysterious, although scientists know it occurs in two lengths, and that in the brain the slightly longer version is more likely to clump into plaques. For some reason, in Alzheimer's disease the brain identifies the tiny broken bits of beta amyloid as foreign, and immune cells try to clear them away. The result is a state of chronic inflammation that progressively injures nearby nerve cells.

Among the powerful weapons the brain's immune system uses to fight off the beta amyloid bits are FREE RADICALS of oxygen, which is one reason many think that substances that fight free radicals—like vitamin E and the drug Eldepryl—may be helpful against Alzheimer's.

What is even more intriguing is that beta amyloid plaques occur early in the disease, before there is any damage to surrounding brain cells—as early as 10 to 20 years before symptoms develop.

Tau Protein

While plaques are made of beta amyloid clumps, the tangles are made of another kind of protein called TAU. Scientists know that normally, tau protein plays a critical role in the brain. The internal support structure for nerve cells depends on the normal functioning of tau, which acts like the rungs of a ladder, holding the two parallel branches of axons apart. In cells of Alzheimer's patients, however, this parallel structure of axons collapses as the tau protein "crosspieces" twist the paired filaments so they collapse and tangle together and they can no longer shuttle substances throughout the cell. The axons then shrivel and die.

Beta Amyloid v. Tau

Together, beta amyloid and tau form the plaques and tangles that have been the hallmarks of the disease since it was first described in 1907 by Alois Alzheimer. Scientists disagree about whether it is the sticky plaques of beta amyloid in the brain, or the tangles of tau protein inside brain nerve fibers, that play a more central role in the destruction of brain cells.

Although tangles of tau have been found in the brains of people with Alzheimer's, many scientists believe that the tangles are probably a secondary part of the disease. Instead, most Alzheimer's researchers have focused attention on beta amyloid as the substance that kills brain cells.

Others think the plaques and tangles are really a marker left by nerve cells that were killed by some other cause.

The key question scientists need to resolve is the relationship between beta amyloid and tau, and whether these substances trigger the disease, or are merely the by-product of some other brain process gone terribly awry.

What scientists do know is that the more beta amyloid in brain tissue, the more severe the mental decline; the highest levels of beta amyloid are found in the brains of patients with the most dementia.

myths about Alzheimer's disease   There are a number of myths about Alzheimer's disease that are widely believed but which actually are not true. They include

"Memory loss is a natural part of aging":   In fact, everyone occasionally forgets where the car is parked or the name of a colleague, and many people who are perfectly healthy are less able to remember certain kinds of information as they get older. However, the symptoms of Alzheimer's are much more severe and consistent, and affect communication, learning, thinking, and reasoning.

"Alzheimer's disease is always hereditary":   Alzheimer's disease occurs as either early onset or late onset. The early onset form of the disease is very rare and mainly begins between age 30 and age 50. This form of the disease has been linked to three different genes and has been observed in only 120 families around the world. People who

carry one of the early onset genes will probably develop Alzheimer's disease.

The late onset form, which occurs after age 65, accounts for more than 90 percent of all cases of Alzheimer's. It is unclear whether a genetic abnormality, environmental factors or a combination of both causes this form of the disease.

What scientists do know is that a person's risk of developing Alzheimer's at any given age appears to increase if an immediate relative (parent or sibling) has the disease.

"Alzheimer's disease is not fatal":   Alzheimer's disease is a fatal, progressive, degenerative disease that attacks the brain and impairs memory, thinking, and behavior. It is the most common form of DEMENTIA and is the fourth leading cause of death in people over age 65.

"Aluminum in cans or pots can lead to Alzheimer's disease":   Based on current research, getting rid of aluminum cans, pots, and pans will not prevent Alzheimer's. Aluminum is one of 90 naturally occurring elements—the third most common element in the earth's crust. The exact role (if any) of aluminum in Alzheimer's disease is still unclear, but most researchers believe that not enough evidence exists to consider aluminum a risk factor for Alzheimer's or a cause of dementia.

"Aspartame causes memory loss":   Several studies have found no link between aspartame and memory loss in humans or animals. Aspartame (marketed as Nutrasweet and Equal) was approved by the U.S. Food and Drug Administration (FDA) in 1996 for use in all foods and beverages.

"There are treatments that can stop the progression of Alzheimer's":   At this time, there is no medical treatment that can either cure, prevent, or stop the progression of Alzheimer's. Four FDA-approved drugs—TACRINE (Cognex), DONEPEZIL (Aricept), RIVASTIGMINE (Exelon), and GALANTAMINE (Reminyl)—may temporarily relieve some symptoms of the disease in people with mild to moderate Alzheimer's.

naloxone hydrochloride (Narcan) A narcotic antagonist that combines competitively with opiate receptors currently being studied as a possible treatment for the DEMENTIA of Alzheimer's disease.

naproxen See NONSTEROIDAL ANTI-INFLAMMATORY DRUGS.

naps Many Alzheimer's disease patients develop a pattern of disrupted nighttime sleep and daytime naps. Experts suggest that CAREGIVERS should discourage daytime napping in order to limit evening WANDERING.

National Academy of Elder Law Attorneys A nonprofit association which helps lawyers, bar organizations, and others who work with older clients and their families. Established in 1988, the academy acts as a resource for information, education, networking, and assistance for those who must deal with the many specialized issues involved with legal services to the elderly and disabled. Some of the issues NAELA members handle include public benefits, probate and estate planning, guardianship/conservatorship, and health and long-term care planning.

NAELA members are attorneys who deal with legal issues affecting the elderly and disabled. Members also include judges, professors of law, and students. The primary focus of the academy is education; the group sponsors continuing legal education programs on elder law for attorneys throughout the year, and provides publications and educational materials to its members on a wide range of elder law topics.

The academy also tries to help other organizations serving the elderly, although it does not provide direct legal services.

For contact information, see Appendix I.

National Adult Day Services Association The only organization that provides a focal point for adult day services at the national level. The association, formerly known as the National Institute on Adult Daycare (NIAD), tries to promote the concept of adult day services as a workable community-based option for disabled older persons.

The group provides information on all aspects of adult day services, provides help to adult day service programs, works closely with national, state, and local organizations and governmental agencies, and supports research projects. The group is also interested in stimulating action on legislative, public policy, and service delivery issues.

For contact information, see Appendix I.

National Alzheimer's Coordinating Center (NACC) A national coordinating center designed to facilitate research on Alzheimer's disease by providing a place to analyze combined data from all Alzheimer's Disease Centers. Until the NATIONAL INSTITUTE ON AGING (NIA) established the NACC in 1999, each Alzheimer's center collected its own information separately. Now there is a central data coordinating center where data from all Alzheimer's disease centers are being analyzed.

The NACC assembles, maintains, analyzes, and disseminates data, catalogs brain tissue and other samples, and coordinates meetings to discuss progress.

National Association of Area Agencies on Aging The umbrella organization for the 655 area agencies on aging and more than 230 Native American aging programs in the United States. Through its presence in Washington, D.C., the association advocates on behalf of the local aging agencies to ensure that needed resources and support services are available to older Americans. The fundamental mission is to provide services which make it possible for older individuals to remain in their homes, thereby preserving their independence and dignity. These agencies coordinate and support a wide range of home- and community-based services, including information and referral, home-delivered and congregate meals, transportation, employment services, senior centers, adult day care, and a long-term care ombudsman program.

The association's primary mission is to build the capacity of its members to help older persons and persons with disabilities live with dignity and choices in their homes and communities for as long as possible.

National Association of Professional Geriatric Care Managers

A nonprofit professional organization of practitioners interested in providing dignified care for the elderly and their families. With more than 1,500 members, GCM is committed to helping elders remain independent while striving to ensure that the highest quality and most cost-effective health and human services are used.

The association has developed a *Geriatric Care Managers Resource Guide and Directory* to help consumers find qualified GERIATRIC CARE MANAGERS.

For contact information, see Appendix I.

National Council on the Aging

The nation's first association of organizations and professionals dedicated to promoting the dignity, self-determination, well-being, and contributions of older persons. Founded in 1950, the group's members include senior centers, area agencies on aging, ADULT DAY SERVICES, congregations, senior housing, health centers, employment services, and consumer organizations. The council helps community organizations enhance the lives of older adults, turning creative ideas into programs and services that help older people in hundreds of communities. The council advocates for public policies, societal attitudes, and business practices that promote vital aging.

For contact information, see Appendix I.

National Family Caregivers Association

A grassroots organization created to educate, support, empower, and speak for the millions of Americans who care for chronically ill, aged, or disabled loved ones. NFCA focuses on reaching across the boundaries of different diagnoses, different relationships, and different life stages to address the common needs and concerns of all family caregivers. The association provides information, education, support, public awareness, and advocacy.

For contact information see Appendix I.

National Indian Council on Aging, Inc.

The nation's foremost nonprofit advocate for the nation's 296,000 American Indian and Alaska Native elders. The council was established by a group of tribal chairmen in 1976 to better the lives of the nation's indigenous seniors through advocacy, employment training, dissemination of information, and data support.

For contact information, see Appendix I.

National Institute on Aging (NIA)

One of the 25 institutes and centers of the National Institutes of Health (NIH) that leads a broad scientific effort to understand the nature of aging. NIA also provides specific information about Alzheimer's disease through the Alzheimer's Disease Education and Referral Center (ADEAR), which provides publications about symptoms, diagnosis, and treatment of Alzheimer's. ADEAR information specialists can provide referrals to supportive services as well as referrals to research facilities or the nationwide network of NIA-funded Alzheimer's Disease Centers.

The NIA was established by Congress in 1974 to provide leadership in aging research, training, health information dissemination, and other programs relevant to aging and older people. Subsequent amendments to this legislation designated the NIA as the primary federal agency on Alzheimer's disease research.

The NIA's mission is to improve the health and well-being of older Americans through research, and to support research, train research scientists, and provide information to the public.

NIA sponsors research on aging at universities, hospitals, medical centers, and other public and private organizations nationwide. The intramural program conducts basic and clinical research in

Baltimore, Maryland, and on the NIH campus in Bethesda, Maryland.

For contact information, see Appendix I.

National Institute of Environmental Health Sciences A federal health institute that supports scientists examining the ways in which metals and other compounds found in the environment may affect brain tissues and possibly contribute to the development of Alzheimer's disease.

For contact information, see Appendix I.

National Institute of Mental Health Federal institute that supports research on the causes of Alzheimer's disease, its treatment, and services for patients. Researchers supported by NIMH have made advances in a number of areas, including the use of advanced imaging techniques, improvements in understanding mental illnesses in both caregivers and patients, and some of the basic underlying molecular and genetic causes of the disease.

For contact information, see Appendix I.

National Institute of Nursing Research National institute that supports research on biobehavioral aspects of Alzheimer's disease and related dementias. The primary focus of current studies is on behavioral, physical, and functional problems of these patients, such as WANDERING, AGITATION, and AGGRESSION, and maintaining ACTIVITIES OF DAILY LIVING.

For contact information, see Appendix I.

National Institute on Adult Care The original name for the NATIONAL ADULT DAY SERVICES ASSOCIATION.

National Institute on Neurological Disorders and Stroke Federal institute and part of the National Institutes of Health that supports scientists studying the brain processes responsible for a variety of neurodegenerative disorders, including Alzheimer's disease and Parkinson's disease.

For contact information, see Appendix I.

National Senior Citizens Law Center Nonprofit national support center that promotes the independence and well-being of low-income elderly individuals, as well as people with disabilities, with particular emphasis on women and racial and ethnic minorities. NSCLC advocates through litigation, legislative and agency representation, and provides help to attorneys and paralegals.

For contact information, see Appendix I.

nerve cell Also known as a neuron, this is the basic working unit of the nervous system. In the brain, nerve cells are responsible for information processing, converting chemical signals to electrical signals and back again. Nerve cells are composed of a cell body containing the nucleus, several short branches (dendrites), and one long arm (the axon). Each nerve cell receives electrical impulses through dendrites, which lie adjacent to each other in a gigantic web whose tiny branches direct signals toward the body of the nerve cell. If enough arriving signals stimulate the nerve cell, it fires, sending this electrical pulse down its axon, which connects through synapses into the dendrites of other nerve cells.

Information is carried inside a nerve cell by electrical pulses, but once the signal reaches the end of the axon it must be carried across the synaptic gap by chemicals called NEUROTRANSMITTERS. On the other side of the synapse is another dendrite, containing receptors that recognize these transmitting chemicals.

A single nerve cell can receive signals from thousands of other nerve cells, and its axon can branch repeatedly, sending signals to thousands more. Most researchers agree that when a person experiences a new event, a unique pattern of nerve cells is activated in some way, and within the entire configuration of brain cells, certain cells light up. As knowledge is acquired, circuits break apart and re-form, constantly rewriting themselves and influencing a person's representations of the world. Thus, the more a person repeats the experience, the stronger the connection between the nerve cells.

There are about 50 million nerve cells in the cerebral cortex, 40 billion more in the cerebellum, and another 10 billion in the rest of the brain and spinal cord—about the same as there are stars in the galaxy. The average number of nerve cells varies dramatically from one person to the next, but seems to have nothing to do with general intelligence (some animals have more nerve cells than humans). Apparently, quantity is less important than the quality of the connections between the nerve cells.

nerve growth factors (NGF)   One of several naturally occurring nourishing proteins in the brain that promotes nerve cell growth and survival. Some scientists believe that low levels of NGF might contribute to Alzheimer's disease.

In Alzheimer's, brain cells die in areas responsible for memory and rational thought. In particular, cells that supply ACETYLCHOLINE, a vital chemical messenger to key areas of the brain, begin to die. These cells are located fairly deep in the brain, in a structure called the BASAL FOREBRAIN. Their job is to provide acetylcholine to the HIPPOCAMPUS, which is involved in memory and emotion, and the CEREBRAL CORTEX, where higher thought processes take place.

While nerve cells in the brain do not divide in large enough numbers to vanquish Alzheimer's, they can repair themselves after injury, and NEUROTROPHIC FACTORS promote this regeneration. Scientists hope that by protecting these crucial cells, they can fend off Alzheimer's disease.

Growth factors (there are at least eight different varieties currently being studied) each have a different target cell in the body, and each has a possible role in protecting the body's nerve cells against damage from disease.

Working with rats and monkeys, several research teams have taken cells genetically engineered to produce NGF and transplanted them into parts of the brain where cells are dying. The transplants not only keep the nearby damaged cells alive, but they also act as a bridge across which the cells can grow back again. The grafts also appear to improve memory in aging rats, who often have trouble navigating mazes as they get older. These studies have not been done in humans, and much more research is needed before they become potential treatments, but experiments on rats also show that NGF promotes growth of new connections between synapses in the brain, which could help restore memory loss.

In a 1988 study, a team of researchers showed that grafts of modified skin cells containing an NGF gene could prevent acetylcholine-producing neurons from dying and help the damaged ones regrow. Because they were working with rats, which do not get Alzheimer's disease, they used a surgical incision to mimic the nerve degeneration. The study was the first to confirm the usefulness of gene transfer in a model of a nervous system disorder.

Another scientist went on to try similar experiments in monkeys, with equal success, finding that transplanting NGF-producing cells is safe and effective, and it appears to last for a long time—at least one year in rats and eight months in monkeys. In addition to protecting the dying cells, the grafts also help the surviving cells produce higher levels of acetylcholine. In primates, scientists have also successfully used cells taken from the skin of the same animal, modified them to produce NGF, and transplanted them back into the host.

In another study, scientists took a group of older rats and tested them in mazes to find out which ones were memory-impaired. These rats received transplants of NGF-secreting cells and were then able to run the same maze test they had failed before—in effect, the transplants reversed the age-related memory loss.

Scientists at the University of Lund in Sweden took a group of middle-aged rats who were not yet showing any signs of age-related decline, giving half the NGF grafts. During the next nine months, the control rats began to have trouble with the maze tests, but the NGF-treated rats kept up a level of performance comparable to rats in their prime. This suggested to the scientists that treatment with NGF can actually prevent cognitive impairments.

In a variety of learning and memory tests, California researchers have shown that infusions of nerve growth factor into the brain could improve learning capacity and increase the size of brain cells that had previously shrunk. In a study in the mid-1980s, scientists took several rats with memory impairment and gave them nerve growth factor. The rats' ability to negotiate the maze improved, coming close to the ability seen in older rats with no impairment.

In 1999, scientists at the University of California at San Diego showed that brain cells in aging monkeys were restored to near-normal size and quantity after surgical implants of cells genetically altered to produce NGF. The researchers took skins cells from older monkeys, inserted a gene that makes human nerve growth factor, and then injected the modified cells into the brains of four monkeys. Once in the monkeys' brains, the modified cells began making nerve growth factor and appeared to revive brain cells.

The federal government approved human trials for nerve growth factor in 1999 after a team of researchers showed the protein reversed deterioration in the brains of aging monkeys. Because of this study and several similar ones, NGF intrigues neuroscientists as a possible treatment for Alzheimer's disease.

Working with these factors is not easy, however; most of these protein molecules are large and hard to handle; they must be pumped directly into the brain, because they will not cross the blood-brain barrier.

It is not so easy to test NGF in humans. A few years ago NGF was tested in humans by directly infusing the substance into the spinal fluid surrounding the brain, but the study was discontinued when the drip became painful to the subjects. Scientists now believe this was an effect of NGF on the nervous system that is sensitive to pain; cellular transplants would avoid this problem by being directly inserted only into the basal forebrain area itself.

NGFs were first discovered in the 1950s by developmental biologist Rita Levi-Montalcini, who won a Nobel Prize in 1986 for that work.

neural graft An experimental procedure in which brain cells are implanted into a brain and allowed to grow together into the existing brain tissue. In rat studies, implanted neurons seem to substitute for original neurons by reconnecting to neurons whose connections had been lost. It appears that the brain may be able to allow surviving, healthy neurons to establish new connections with surviving or implanted neurons. This means that one day it may be possible to repair neurons in brains damaged by Alzheimer's.

neural transplant See NEURAL GRAFT.

neuritic plaque See BETA AMYLOID.

neurofibrillary tangles A type of abnormal brain lesion typically found in Alzheimer's disease that is made up of a kind of protein called TAU. Tau protein plays a critical role in the brain. In healthy neurons, the internal support structure for nerve cells (called microtubules) is shaped like two train rails; these long parallel tracks are joined together by crosspieces that function like rungs of a ladder to hold the tracks apart. These crosspieces are made of tau protein. Microtubules are essential to healthy cells, since they carry nutrients from the body of the cells down to the ends of axons.

In cells affected by Alzheimer's, the tau that normally forms the crosspieces between the microtubules begins to twist, like two threads wound around each other, until the entire microtubule collapses and becomes hopelessly entangled. Eventually, the entangled axons shrivel and die. When scientists look at the brain of a person who has died from Alzheimer's disease, neurofibrillary tangles typically appear throughout the brain.

There is also a close correlation between the degree of memory problems in people with Alzheimer's, and the number of these neurofibrillary tangles, according to researchers from the University of Kentucky's Sanders-Brown Center on Aging in Lexington. In the now-famous NUN STUDY of 678 School Sisters of Notre Dame, aged 75 to 102 years, researchers compared the levels and distribution of neurofibrillary tangles in the nuns' brains with the results of cognitive tests taken within months before their deaths. From the subjects in the earliest stages of neurofibrillary tangle deposition, to those in the latest stages, which are characterized by heavy and widespread tangles, the degree of neurofibrillary tangles was matched by increasingly poor performance on cognitive tests. The data also indicate that subjects with memory impairments in addition to other cognitive deficits had more of the tangles than subjects with non-memory cognitive deficits alone, and were more likely to be diagnosed with Alzheimer's disease over a four-year period.

Another study has found that these tangles appear to be more dense in people with Alzheimer's who develop hallucinations and delusions (psychosis), which occur in about half of all Alzheimer's patients. In addition to memory loss, depression, and personality changes, psychosis is commonly associated with the disease. In a study of 109 Alzheimer's disease patients, researchers found that neurofibrillary tangles in one region of the brain were more than twice as dense in patients with psychotic symptoms compared with those without such symptoms. These differences were particularly notable in patients with mild Alzheimer's disease.

Tangles also tended to be denser in patients with more severe dementia. The study found no relationship between psychotic symptoms and tangles found in other parts of the brain, or with plaques that also have been linked to Alzheimer's disease. Scientists believe that some process that causes psychosis may worsen tangles.

The tangles were first described by German neuropathologist Alois Alzheimer in 1906.

neurologist A specialist in the diagnosis and treatment of diseases and disorders of the brain and nervous system. Neurologists conduct examinations of patients' nerves, reflexes, motor and sensory functions, and muscles to determine the cause of a particular problem. In patients with suspected Alzheimer's disease, detailed questions regarding memory, speech and language, and other cognitive abilities will be part of the examination. Patients with Alzheimer's may use a neurologist as a primary care physician. Neurologists also may serve as consultants to other physicians treating Alzheimer's patients.

A neurologist can perform detailed examinations of all the neurological structures in the body, including the nerves of the head and neck, muscular strength and movement, sensation, balance, and reflex testing. In some cases, detailed questions about memory, speech and language, and other cognitive functions are part of the examination.

Neurologists also use other common tests, including CT (computerized axial tomography) and MAGNETIC RESONANCE IMAGING (MRI) scans to provide detailed pictures of the brain, spinal structures, and blood vessels. A neurologist can also perform a lumbar puncture (spinal tap) to obtain a patient's cerebrospinal fluid for analysis. A neurologist does not perform surgery.

A neurologist must complete a four-year premedical university degree and four years of medical school, followed by at least three years of specialty training in an accredited neurology residency program. After residency training, neurologists may choose to enroll in a one- or two-year fellowship program, which offers the opportunity to focus on a subspecialty of neurology such as stroke, dementia, or movement disorders.

After completing the educational requirements, neurologists may seek certification from the American Board of Psychiatry and Neurology (ABPN). To be eligible for certification, an applicant must be a licensed physician with the required years of residency who has passed both a written and oral exam administered by the ABPN.

The AMERICAN ACADEMY OF NEUROLOGY offers a "Find a Neurologist" option for patients with Alzheimer's at http://www.aan.com/fan.

neuropsychiatry The branch of medicine that deals with the relationship between psychiatric symptoms and neurological disorders, such as Alzheimer's disease. Neuropsychiatry is also concerned with subtle forms of brain damage that may underlie psychotic illness. This could include conditions such as traumatic brain injury, cerebral vascular disease, seizure disorders, neurodegenerative diseases (such as Alzheimer's or Parkinson's disease), brain tumors, infectious and inflammatory diseases of the central nervous system (CNS), alcohol-induced mental disorders, and developmental disorders involving the brain.

Generally, neuropsychiatrists use medication to treat neuropsychiatric disorders and use very specialized equipment to determine the degree of physical defects in the brain. To a greater degree than most psychiatrists, neuropsychiatrists are able to determine specifically what medications should be used and what their effects might be, as opposed to trying various medications on an experimental basis.

Technically speaking, all psychiatrists can present themselves as neuropsychiatrists because board certification for psychiatrists includes a joint certification in both psychiatry and neurology. However, The American Board of Psychiatry and Neurology issues certificates based on different tests. Most practicing psychiatrists pass tests that ask two-thirds of their questions on psychiatry and one-third on neurology. A neuropsychiatrist has passed the test that devotes half of its questions to neurology and half to psychiatry.

neuropsychological tests Assessments that can evaluate the extent of memory loss, brain damage, and the probable presence of Alzheimer's disease. This kind of testing was first used as a way to distinguish between those whose abnormal behavior was caused by brain dysfunction and those whose problems were caused by psychological factors.

In recent findings, researchers report that it may be possible to predict the onset of Alzheimer's disease with paper-and-pencil neuropsychological tests administered to healthy subjects averaging 75 years of age, because studies revealed early signs of cognitive decline in tests of those subjects who later developed Alzheimer's disease.

In an analysis of cognitive performance test data from 40 participants enrolled in a long-term study at the UCSD Alzheimer's Disease Research Center, a research team from the Veterans Affairs San Diego Healthcare System and the University of California/San Diego medical school noted subtle evidence of changes that might signal the onset of cognitive decline. All participants were symptom-free when they took the test, but 20 subjects were diagnosed with Alzheimer's disease within a year or two of testing. The other 20 remained symptom-free for several years, serving as a matched control group.

When the team compared the data from the cognitive performance tests, they noted more problems with cognitive skills of the subjects who went on to develop Alzheimer's than in the control group. The pre-Alzheimer's subjects had special problems with their ability to perform visual versus verbal tests. These changes occurred unevenly, affecting certain performance measures and not others, which indicated subtle patterns of deterioration in specific regions of the brain affected by Alzheimer's. Scientists noted a larger discrepancy between the results of the nonverbal spatial tests and the verbal tests in people who later were diagnosed with Alzheimer's. Since these changes are very slight, they are not noticeable if a clinician looks only in one area. This suggests that doctors should compare performance in different areas as they relate to one another if early changes in cognitive function are going to be detected.

For example, in the study subjects were asked to identify common items in a picture and reconstruct drawings of blocklike structures using actual building blocks. Those who would go on to develop Alzheimer's had a much larger discrepancy between their ability to name objects and their ability to reconstruct the block images. The control group was much more likely to perform both tasks equally well.

For this reason, scientists suspect that cognitive tests such as these might help detect early signs of Alzheimer's in people who have no symptoms, which would allow for early treatment at a time when drugs might really be able to slow the progression of the disease. This could be particularly helpful in those with a strong family history or who are considered at high risk for developing the disease.

See also ASSESSMENT TOOLS.

neuropsychologist A clinical psychologist with special training in neurology as well as intensive training in psychological assessment. The relationship of neuropsychology to other neurosciences is an evolving one, and may include not only diagnosing brain injuries and diseases such as Alzheimer's disease, but assessing treatment programs, patients' progress, and planning rehabilitation programs.

A clinical neuropsychologist may enter private practice and offer various forms of psychotherapy and cognitive rehabilitation to individuals, families, or groups, and can administer standardized psychological and neuropsychological tests and interpret and report on their results. Neuropsychologists may furnish legally recognized clinical and diagnostic opinions and conduct diagnostic interviews about the presence, scope, and treatment of cognitive/neuropsychological disorders, behavioral disorders, and mental illness.

A neuropsychologist and a neurologist differ in several ways. A neurologist is a physician (M.D.) who deals with the structural and physiological consequences of brain injury and organic brain disease, while the neuropsychologist (Ph.D.) investigates the cognitive and behavioral impact of these conditions. For example, for a person with Alzheimer's, the neuropsychologist might test the person's ability to think and reason clearly and check for memory loss or reading, learning, and comprehension problems.

neurotransmitter   A chemical released at the space between neurons (the synapse) that relays a signal from one nerve cell to another. When a neurotransmitter is released into the synapse, it moves across the space and attaches to a receptor in the membrane of a neighboring nerve cell.

Some neurotransmitters stimulate the release of neurotransmitters from other neurons, while others inhibit the release of neurotransmitters.

Neurotransmitters are made from the protein in food; this protein is first broken down in the stomach and intestines into smaller substances called amino acids. These amino acids enter the blood, where they are absorbed by the brain, which uses the amino acids to make neurotransmitters. It is the correct balance of neurotransmitters in the brain that is responsible for proper brain function. Any deficiencies in nutrients will upset the level of certain neurotransmitters, and interfere with the behaviors or actions for which they are responsible.

The most common neurotransmitters include ACETYLCHOLINE, norepinephrine, dopamine, GABA, and serotonin. Abnormal acetylcholine levels have been linked to the development of Alzheimer's disease; scientists have found that levels drop slightly in normal aging, but plummet by about 90 percent in people with Alzheimer's. Acetylcholine is a critical neurotransmitter in the process of forming memories, and it is the neurotransmitter commonly used by nerve cells in the HIPPOCAMPUS and CEREBRAL CORTEX—regions devastated by Alzheimer's disease.

In addition, serotonin, somatostatin, and noradrenaline levels are lower than normal in some Alzheimer's patients. Deficits in these substances may contribute to sensory disturbances, aggressive behavior, and nerve cell death. Most neurotransmitter research, however, continues to focus on acetylcholine because of its steep decline in Alzheimer's disease and its close ties to memory formation and reasoning.

neurotrophic factor   A protein, such as NERVE GROWTH FACTOR, that promotes nerve cell growth and survival. Growth factors elsewhere in the body support cell division. Although nerve cells cannot divide, they can regenerate after injury, and neurotrophic factors help in this regeneration. They also promote the growth of axons and dendrites, the neuron branches that form connections with other neurons.

Other neurotrophic factors that may be implicated in Alzheimer's include brain derived neurotrophic factor (BDNF) and neurotrophin-3. Studies have turned up a number of clues that link nerve growth factors specifically to the neurons that use ACETYLCHOLINE as a neurotransmitter.

nicotine   For years, researchers have been investigating a possible link between nicotine, smoking, and Alzheimer's disease. Some studies have found smoking increases the risk of Alzheimer's, while other studies have found the opposite.

A series of studies looked at the role of nicotine and nicotine-like substances on memory, learning, and response to stress. Researchers at Duke University found that a nicotine-like substance called AR-R 17779 improved memory and learning in rats. In July 1998, Netherlands researchers found that cigarette smokers are more than twice as likely to develop Alzheimer's disease as are nonsmokers; they also found that smokers also are more likely to develop vascular dementia, a common form of dementia caused by vascular disease and strokes. In the study, researchers followed 6,870 healthy men and women over age 55 for two years. During the study, 146 individuals developed dementia, of whom 105 were diagnosed as having Alzheimer's. Current smokers were more than twice as likely to develop dementia of any kind and Alzheimer's disease, and they also tended to develop dementia at a younger age. Former smokers had a slightly increased risk of developing Alzheimer's, when compared with people who had never smoked. In this study, the researchers observed that the type of apoE gene a person had modified the association between smoking and risk of dementia. In those without the APOE-4 version of the gene, smoking substantially increased the risk of dementia. However, there was no increased risk of dementia associated with smoking in those people who had the apoE-4 version.

In 1997 two contradictory studies about the impact of smoking and cognitive decline in healthy elderly were presented at the American Academy of Neurology meeting. One study, of 9,200 people over 65 in France, Denmark, the Netherlands, and England, found that current smokers had greater yearly cognitive decline compared to people who had never smoked and former smokers. But a second study, of 5,600 people over 65 in Italy, found that smoking had a protective effect against age-related cognitive decline.

While there is no evidence that nicotine will cure or prevent Alzheimer's disease, interest in using nicotine or nicotine-like substances was increased by reports from Dutch researchers in 1991 who found that smokers were less likely to develop Alzheimer's disease. Subsequent research in the United States found that smoking and Alzheimer's are not related, but that there may be genes that simultaneously decrease the predisposition to smoke and increase the risk of developing Alzheimer's.

In studies with laboratory animals, healthy volunteers, and patients with Alzheimer's disease, short-term administration of nicotine seems to improve memory or cognitive function. Theoretically, using nicotine to treat Alzheimer's disease has some scientific basis. Normally, acetylcholine serves as the chemical signal carrying messages between nerve cells in the brain. In Alzheimer's disease, this pathway is disrupted as brain cells die. The brain has two types of receptors for acetylcholine, one of which can be stimulated by nicotine. By stimulating these receptors, researchers hope to protect the brain cells by keeping them active and functioning and thereby slow the progression of the disease.

However, these studies are inconclusive and need to be confirmed. Furthermore, researchers have noticed that nicotine can adversely affect behavior. For instance, volunteers in one study tended to be awake at night more often, and some were more restless and agitated while in the study.

Because nicotine is an extremely toxic chemical, there may not be a safe dose for memory improvement. Experts warn that smoking or wearing a nicotine patch should not be considered as a way of treating or preventing Alzheimer's disease.

nimodipine (Nimotop)   A possible memory drug that has been used successfully to treat stroke patients and is being studied as a possible treatment for patients with Alzheimer's disease.

The drug is a CALCIUM CHANNEL BLOCKER, which means that it alters the flow of calcium ions through cell membranes, increasing brain blood flow and blocking excess calcium in the part of the brain associated with learning and memory. Nimodipine also seems to increase ACETYLCHOLINE levels, which are severely depleted in patients with Alzheimer's.

Nimodipine was approved by the U.S. Food and Drug Administration (FDA) in 1989 to treat hemorrhagic stroke, since it improves blood flow in the brain and lessens oxygen deprivation.

In recent studies, Italian researchers noted a 69.5 percent increase in mental performance among 40 patients aged 65 to 80 who were suffering from minor to medium signs of mental aging. Twenty percent showed no change, and 9.5 percent worsened. Vanderbilt University researchers found that nimodipine was effective in improving memory, depression, and general state of mind in 178 elderly patients they tested for cognitive decline.

Nimotop   See NIMODIPINE.

nitric oxide   A chemical that the body produces naturally to protect the heart, stimulate the brain, and kill bacteria, which—in high levels—may be linked with the onset of Alzheimer's disease. Nitric oxide causes blood vessels to dilate, and blood vessel inflammation has long been associated with Alzheimer's.

nomination   Naming objects. Poor nomination is the first symptom of Alzheimer's.

nonsteroidal anti-inflammatory drugs (NSAIDS)
A nonprescription pain reliever that reduces inflammation and may help protect against the onset of Alzheimer's disease. There is some limited evidence that people who regularly take NSAIDs for a long time, such as arthritis patients, also seem to have a lower incidence of Alzheimer's. If they do eventually develop Alzheimer's, patients who have taken NSAIDs seem to experience a slower rate of mental decline.

Since 1997, scientists have noted that some people who regularly take large amounts of ibuprofen and other NSAIDs run a lower risk of developing Alzheimer's. Initially, experts believed that anti-inflammatory drugs might lower the risk for Alzheimer's disease by decreasing brain inflammation commonly seen in the condition. However, new research suggests that ibuprofen (Advil and Motrin) appears to protect against Alzheimer's by interfering with the production of beta amyloid 42, a key protein found in the disease's brain-clogging deposits. The lowered protein level was found both in the test tube and in the brains of mice, but researchers did not report whether the mice showed fewer actual brain plaques.

Researchers who treated mice with ibuprofen and two other NSAIDs discovered the animals had as much as 80 percent less BETA AMYLOID protein. Several other pain relievers, including aspirin, had no such effect. However, NSAIDs have potentially serious effects on the kidneys and stomach; some 100,000 Americans are hospitalized each year for NSAID-induced ulcers, and more than 16,000 of them die. The doses used in the experiments were equal to more than 16 Advils a day—far more than what is typically recommended for pain. In addition, the potential Alzheimer's benefits of these drugs are not well understood, and are used only in cell cultures and lab animal experiments. This is why doctors don't prescribe NSAIDs for protection against Alzheimer's disease.

Researchers are working to develop a new kind of NSAID which protects the brain without causing such severe side effects. Research also suggests that anti-inflammatory drugs may only serve to prevent, not treat, the effects of Alzheimer's disease.

Scientists first noticed in the mid-1990s that regular use of these drugs for aches and pains may protect against Alzheimer's. More recently, a large Dutch study of people 55 or older concluded that those who took certain NSAIDs every day for at least two years were 80 percent less likely to develop Alzheimer's. The Dutch study drew information on the patients' drug use from a national database in Holland.

The U.S. NATIONAL INSTITUTE ON AGING is enrolling 2,500 patients in a new study comparing the potential protective effects of two widely used drugs—naproxen (Aleve) and Celebrex—with dummy pills; results are expected around 2008.

nonverbal memory   Memory for figures, spatial relationships, and so on. Nonverbal memory is assumed to be based in the deep structures of the right temporal lobe.

nootropics   A class of drugs designed to improve learning and memory without other central nervous system effects. The name *nootropics* was taken from the Greek *noos* (mind) and *tropein* (toward).

There is some disagreement about which drugs are considered nootropics, but experts usually agree that they include the pyrrolidone derivatives (piracetam and oxiracetam, pramiracetam, and aniracetam).

The mechanism by which these drugs seem to work is not known, although some studies suggest they affect the part of the nervous system that uses ACETYLCHOLINE as a NEUROTRANSMITTER. Acetylcholine levels are severely depleted in patients with Alzheimer's disease.

No nootropic drug has been approved by the U.S. Food and Drug Administration (FDA). They are only available to people outside of the United States.

normal pressure hydrocephalus   A type of hydrocephalus that usually occurs in older adults characterized by a buildup of fluid that causes the cavities of the brain to enlarge. As many as 250,000 Americans with some of the same symptoms as Alzheimer's disease, dementia, or Parkinson's disease, may actually have normal pressure hydrocephalus (NPH).

NPH normally occurs in adults over age 60, and in as many as 10 percent of all patients with symptoms of dementia. The disease causes a buildup of cerebrospinal fluid, which normally cushions the delicate brain and spinal cord tissue from injuries. Normally, the bloodstream absorbs most of this fluid that is produced each day. When an imbalance occurs, fluid builds up in a process known as hydrocephalus. Left untreated, hydrocephalus will create increased pressure in the head and may cause symptoms or brain damage.

Symptoms

The abnormal accumulation of fluid stretches the nerve tissue of the brain, causing three main symptoms: walking problems, dementia, and urinary incontinence.

Gait disturbances range from a mild imbalance to the inability to stand or walk at all. Many patients notice a wide-based, short, slow and shuffling gait. People may have trouble picking up their feet and often fall. Gait disturbance is often the most pronounced symptom and the first to become apparent.

NPH patients with mild dementia may experience a loss of interest in daily activities, FORGETFULNESS, problems with routine tasks, and short-term memory loss. Patients may deny that there are any problems, and not all NPH patients will have an obvious mental impairment.

Problems with bladder control are usually characterized by urinary frequency (sometimes as often as every one or two hours) and urgency in mild cases, whereas a complete loss of bladder control can occur in more severe cases. In very rare cases, fecal incontinence may occur. However, some patients never display signs of bladder problems.

Because these three symptoms are often associated with the aging process, people often assume that they must live with the problems or adapt to the changes occurring within their bodies.

Patients may struggle with symptoms for years before seeking treatment, usually because of a critical loss of function or disability. Unfortunately, the longer the symptoms have been apparent, the less likely that treatment will be successful.

Diagnosis

Unfortunately, NPH can be difficult to diagnose because it is so similar to the symptoms of other disorders, such as Alzheimer's or mild dementia. Many cases go completely unrecognized and are never treated. As a general rule, the earlier the diagnosis, the better the chance for successful treatment, but some people experiencing symptoms for years can improve with treatment.

Once symptoms of gait disturbance, mild dementia, or bladder control have been identified, a physician who suspects normal pressure hydrocephalus may recommend one or more additional tests that should include a neurologist and a neurosurgeon.

Diagnostic procedures for normal pressure hydrocephalus may include one or more of these tests: ultrasound, computerized tomography (CT), magnetic resonance imaging (MRI), lumbar puncture or tap, continuous lumbar CSF drainage, intracranial pressure (ICP) monitoring, measurement of cerebrospinal fluid outflow resistance or isotopic cisternography, and neuropsychological testing.

An ultrasound test uses sound to outline the structures within the skull. A CT scan creates a picture of the brain with X rays and a special scanner to show if the ventricles are enlarged or if there is obvious blockage. An MRI scan is safe and painless, and uses radio signals and a very powerful magnet to create a picture of the brain. This scan also will be able to detect if ventricles are enlarged as well as evaluate the CSF flow and provide information about the surrounding brain tissues. An MRI scan provides more information than a CT, and is therefore the test of choice in most cases.

However, patients with pacemakers or certain other metallic implants cannot have MRI scans because of potential interference.

A lumbar puncture (spinal tap) helps a doctor estimate CSF pressure and analyze the fluid. If the removal of some fluid dramatically improves symptoms, even temporarily, then surgical treatment may be successful. However, not all doctors advocate using a spinal tap as a screening test for NPH since many people who experience little or no improvement after the test may still improve with a shunt.

A lumbar catheter insertion is a variation of the lumbar puncture, which allows for continuous and more accurate recording of spinal fluid pressure, or for more continuous removal of spinal fluid over several days to imitate the effect that a shunt would have. Patients who respond dramatically to such spinal fluid drainage are likely to respond to shunt surgery.

Intracranial pressure monitoring requires admission to the hospital so that a small pressure monitor can be inserted through the skull into the brain or ventricles to measure the intracranial pressure.

Measuring CSF outflow resistance is a more involved test that requires a specialized hospital setting to assess the degree of blockage to CSF absorption back into the bloodstream. It requires the simultaneous infusion of artificial spinal fluid and measurement of CSF pressure. If the calculated resistance value is abnormally high, then there is a very good chance that the patient will improve with shunt surgery.

Isotopic cisternography involves injecting a radioactive isotope into the lower back through a spinal tap to allow the absorption of fluid to be evaluated over a period of time by periodic scanning. This will determine whether the isotope is being absorbed over the surface of the brain or remains trapped inside the ventricles. Isotopic cisternography involves a spinal puncture and is considerably more involved than either the CT or MRI.

Neuropsychological tests involve asking a series of questions used to determine if there is a loss of brain function due to hydrocephalus.

Cause

For most patients the cause of NPH cannot be determined, but in a few cases there is a history of previous brain injury or infection. In other cases, an imbalance in the production or absorption of CSF causes the hydrocephalus.

Treatment

One controversial treatment for patients who show a positive response to diagnostic testing is the placement of a CSF shunt, which is a device designed to drain fluid away from the brain. This allows the enlarged ventricles to return to normal.

As CSF fluid builds and the pressure in the ventricle increases, a one-way valve in the shunt opens, and the excess CSF fluid drains into the abdomen, where it is easily absorbed. This technique is very effective in improving the troubling symptoms of NPH.

If the cause of NPH is known, success rates can be as high as 80 percent; if the cause is not known, the success rate varies from 25 to 74 percent. Higher success rates have been reported from medical centers using the more demanding diagnostic tests such as lumbar catheters or the measurement of CSF outflow resistance.

The symptoms of gait disturbance, mild dementia, and bladder control problems may improve within days of shunt surgery, or they may take weeks to months to fade. However, there is no way to predict success. For patients who do improve, changes are seen in the first week in most cases. It is also not possible to make general predictions of how long the improvement will last, as the course of clinical improvement varies for each patient. Some patients seem to reach a plateau, while others improve for months but then seem to decline again.

However, because some patients do worse after having a shunt, many neurologists are reluctant to place them.

nucleus basalis of Meynert   An area near where the optic nerves cross that enters into the cerebral cortex. When this area is destroyed, it causes a drop in ACETYLCHOLINE activity similar to Alzheimer's disease. Scientists suspect that the beginning of Alzheimer's may be related to a slow death of cells in the nucleus basalis, which may lead to the formation of the plaques seen in the disease.

Nun Study   A longitudinal study of aging and Alzheimer's disease funded by the NATIONAL INSTITUTE ON AGING. In the 1980s, Kentucky researchers began to study 678 School Sisters of Notre Dame, aged 75 to 102 years, who had agreed to frequent physical and psychological tests and to have their brains studied after death. A number of important insights into Alzheimer's disease have already been gleaned from this ongoing project. In particular, scientists have found that traits in early, mid, and late life have strong relationships with the risk of

Alzheimer's disease, as well as the mental and cognitive disabilities of old age.

The Nun Study is directed by David Snowdon, Ph.D., neurology professor at the University of Kentucky's College of Medicine. The study began in 1986 as a pilot study on aging and disability using data collected from the older School Sisters of Notre Dame living in Mankato, Minnesota. In 1990, the Nun Study was expanded to include older Notre Dames living in the midwestern, eastern, and southern regions of the United States. The goal of the Nun Study is to determine the causes and prevention of Alzheimer's disease, other brain diseases, and the mental and physical disability associated with old age.

Participants are American Roman Catholic sisters who belong to the School Sisters of Notre Dame, an international religious congregation that began more than 150 years ago in Bavaria, Germany. The nuns range from sisters in their 90s who are highly functional with full-time jobs to sisters in their 70s who are severely disabled, unable to communicate, and bedridden. Each of the 678 participants in the Nun Study agreed to participate in annual assessments of their cognitive and physical function, medical exams, blood tests, and brain donation at death. The Nun Study represents the largest brain donor population in the world. In addition, the sisters have given investigators full access to their convent archives, including baptismal records, birth certificates, socioeconomic characteristics of each family, education documentation, autobiographies written in early, mid, and late life, as well as residential, social, and occupational data describing the nuns' mid and late lives. These archives are particularly useful in the study of Alzheimer's because they contain accurate risk factor data spanning the entire lifespan of the participants. Accurate information on early and midlife risk factors is difficult or impossible to obtain in most other studies on Alzheimer's, because these individuals cannot accurately recall their history.

Most sisters enrolled in the Nun Study because they believed their participation would help other women throughout the world. Many felt that they could continue teaching and helping others in their old age, and even after their death, by participating in this study.

The Nun Study is a collaborative effort between the University of Kentucky and the School Sisters of Notre Dame congregation. Scientists from other universities also are actively collaborating with this study, including the University of South Florida, University of Kansas, Medical College of Wisconsin, Duke University, Emory University, and Louisiana State University.

Several important findings have already been released as part of the ongoing study. Researchers have found that sisters with more NEUROFIBRILLARY TANGLES had more cognitive and memory problems. From the nuns with the least amounts of tangles to those in the latest stages of Alzheimer's, characterized by heavy and widespread tangles, the degree of neurofibrillary tangles was matched by increasingly poor performance on cognitive tests. The data also indicate that subjects with memory impairments in addition to other cognitive deficits had more of the tangles than subjects with non-memory cognitive deficits alone, and were more likely to be diagnosed with Alzheimer's disease over a four-year period.

Researchers also discovered that the better the nuns' linguistic ability—tested many years before their deaths—the less likely they were to develop Alzheimer's. For the study of linguistic ability, researchers concentrated on those nuns who joined the Milwaukee convent from 1931 through 1939 and who had written autobiographies at an average age of 22. The autobiographies were examined for linguistic ability as a test of cognitive function in early life. One component of linguistic ability, idea density, defined as the average number of ideas for each 10 written words, is associated with educational level, vocabulary, and general knowledge; while a second measure (grammatical complexity) is linked with working memory, performance on timed tests, and writing skills. About 58 years after they had written their autobiographies, the women took part in tests of cognitive abilities. For the 25 nuns who died, brain tissue was examined at autopsy.

The study found that low idea density shown in the writings of the young women was strongly linked with low cognitive test scores and the presence of Alzheimer's disease in late life. For example, the nuns with low idea density scores were 30 times more likely to do poorly on a standard measure of cognitive function, the MINI-MENTAL STATUS EXAM, than those with more complex writings. An even more dramatic difference was observed when cognitive ability and characteristics of brain tissue were compared in the nuns who died. Neurofibrillary tangles of Alzheimer's disease appeared in about 90 percent of those nuns who had low linguistic ability in early life.

The findings show that written linguistic performance—the study's measure of cognitive ability in early life—is a potent marker for cognitive problems, Alzheimer's disease, and brain lesions in late life.

Why there should be a relationship between the two is not clear. Snowdon and his colleagues have suspected that developing the brain and thinking abilities early in life might offer some type of reserve that protects people from Alzheimer's disease and cognitive problems later on.

Educational differences, however, did not explain the relationship between low linguistic ability in early life and poor cognitive function later on. Combining that with the study's findings on the nature of lesions in the brain, the scientists concluded that poor linguistic ability in early life could actually already be a subtle symptom of very early changes in the brain that ultimately lead to Alzheimer's disease.

Scientists note that the nun study is one of the first long-term studies in a well-controlled population to suggest that the process of Alzheimer's disease may begin earlier in life than previously thought. But linguistic ability in early life, while possibly a marker for Alzheimer's disease, needs to be examined further.

Researchers note that other factors could explain the link between early cognitive differences and disease in old age. The link might be related to inherited differences in cognitive ability, so that those with stronger linguistic ability early in life may be more resistant to later influences which lead to the disease, while those with poorer ability as young adults may be more at risk.

nursing homes Specialized facilities (also called skilled nursing facilities) designed for seniors who need 24-hour nursing care. Nursing facilities provide many of the same residential components of other senior care options including room and board, personal care, protection, and supervision. Some may offer other types of therapy, but it is their on-site medical staff that sets them apart from other types of senior housing. Around-the-clock nursing care is provided by registered nurses, licensed practical nurses, and nurses' aides. Nearly one out of every two women and one of four men over age 65 will enter a nursing facility some time in their lives; 25 percent of all nursing facility stays last more than a year and many last three years or more.

Standard services include a clean, furnished room, housekeeping and linen service, medically planned meals and snacks, trained medical staff, and professional service staff, such as an activity director, social worker, and so on.

Nursing homes usually charge extra for on-call physician and physician services; physical, respiratory, and speech therapists; medications; personal care items, and laundry service.

Basic Care

These services are required to maintain a resident's ACTIVITIES OF DAILY LIVING, and includes personal care, supervision, and safety. A nurse's aide, practical nurse, or a family member can provide this care.

Skilled Care

At this level of care, the regular services of a registered nurse are required for treatments and procedures. Skilled care also includes services provided by specially trained professionals, such as physical and respiratory therapists.

Subacute Care

This refers to comprehensive inpatient care designed for someone who has had an illness or injury. Subacute care is generally more intensive than traditional nursing facility care, but less than acute care. It requires frequent (daily to weekly) recurrent patient assessment and review.

Regulation

Nursing homes are licensed and regulated by the state public health department and the federal government, and are individually certified by the state for Medicare and Medicaid. Licensing standards in the state require that nursing homes maintain a staff of licensed and/or registered nurses, nursing aides, and administrators. The health care is supervised and authorized by a physician.

Payment Options

Nursing homes charge a basic daily or monthly fee. Families may buy long-term care insurance ahead of time, but others must depend on other forms of financing. Nursing home facilities accept a variety of MEDICARE, MEDICAID, and private insurance carriers.

In the meantime, a new six-state pilot project involving nursing homes serving Medicare and Medicaid beneficiaries released new information giving seniors and their families comparative information about local nursing homes' quality of care. The project involves nursing homes in Colorado, Florida, Maryland, Ohio, Rhode Island, and Washington as part of the federal government's Nursing Home Quality Initiative to improve the care received by the 2.9 million Americans who live in nursing homes. The complete quality data, along with other information about individual nursing homes, are available at Medicare's consumer website at http://www.medicare.gov, and through Medicare's help line at (800) 633-4227.

nutrition Eating nuts, leafy green vegetables, and other foods rich in antioxidants (such as vitamins E and C) may reduce the risk of Alzheimer's disease, according to two recent studies. The findings build on growing research into the effects of antioxidants on dementia.

Antioxidant vitamins have been shown to block the effects of harmful oxygen molecules called FREE RADICALS, which can damage cells and which have been linked to lesions in the brains of Alzheimer's patients.

One of the studies found strong effects from vitamins E and C. In the other, results from vitamin E foods were more conclusive, but researchers said there was a suggestion vitamin C also provided benefits. Previous research suggested that vitamin E pills could slow disease progression in people already diagnosed with Alzheimer's. The new studies examined people who had not developed the condition at the start of the study.

One study funded by the NATIONAL INSTITUTE ON AGING involved 815 Chicago residents over age 65 who had no initial symptoms of mental decline. Participants answered questions about their eating habits and were studied for about four years. Alzheimer's disease eventually was diagnosed in 131 participants. In particular, it was diagnosed in 14.3 percent of those with the lowest intake of vitamin E foods, compared with 5.9 percent of those with the highest intake. When factors such as age and education were taken into account, the group with the highest intake of vitamin E foods had a 70 percent lower risk of developing Alzheimer's. Participants with the highest vitamin E intake ate amounts that could be obtained from a diet including whole-grain cereal for breakfast, a sandwich with whole-grain bread for lunch, and a dinner including a green leafy salad sprinkled with nuts.

Intake of vitamin C (in foods such as citrus fruits) also appeared to offer some protection, but those results were not statistically significant.

Vitamin E did not protect participants who carry a gene variation called APOLIPOPROTEIN E-4 (apoE-4), which has been linked to the development of Alzheimer's.

The second study involved 5,395 people in the Netherlands over age 55 who were followed for an average of about six years. Alzheimer's developed in 146 of these participants. Those with high intakes of vitamins E and C were less likely to become afflicted, regardless of whether they had the gene variation.

On the other hand, eating a high-fat diet during early and mid-adulthood may be associated with an increased risk of developing Alzheimer's, especially in people with a marker called the apoE-4 version of the apoE gene. In one recent study, researchers found that people with the apoE-4 version who also ate the highest fat diets had a sevenfold higher risk of developing Alzheimer's than people with the marker who ate less fat.

Proper nutrition and a healthy diet are essential for maintaining overall good health and can be beneficial to people with Alzheimer's.

occipital lobe   One of four major pairs of lobes of the CEREBRAL CORTEX that include the center of the visual perception system. Although protected from injury because of its location at the back of the brain, any significant trauma can produce subtle changes to the visual-perceptual system, such as visual field defects.

The occipital lobe is involved in visuospatial processing, discrimination of movement, and color discrimination. Light reaches the sight centers in the occipital lobe through a complex pathway. After light hits the retina, the information is transmitted to the lateral geniculate nucleus in the thalamus. At this stage the brain interprets the light that the eye receives. From there, the axons then show the image in the visual association cortex that identifies what the eyes are seeing.

When the occipital lobe is damaged, it may lead to changes in sight and perception. When one side of the occipital lobe is damaged, sight is lost in half the visual field in both eyes. Lesions in the occipital lobe can cause unusual side effects, such as blindsight. A person with blindsight claims to have no vision at all, but when asked, the person can point to or identify objects at a distance unconsciously. Other lesions in the occipital lobe have been known to cause an inability to identify faces known as prospagnosia. Lesions can also cause writing impairments (agraphia) and an inability to recognize words (alexia). Disorders of the occipital lobe may cause illusions and visual hallucinations that can cause objects to appear larger or smaller than they really are, or make an object appear to be a different color. Lesions in the parietal-temporal-occipital association area can cause word blindness and alexia and agraphia.

occupational therapy   Skilled treatment that helps patients achieve independence in all facets of their lives. It can be effective in treating Alzheimer's disease. Services typically include customized treatment programs aimed at improving abilities to carry out the activities of daily living, comprehensive evaluation of home and job environments, and guidance for caregivers in safe and effective methods of caring for individuals.

Occupational therapy practitioners have studied human growth and development with specific emphasis on the social, emotional, and physiological effects of illness and injury. The occupational therapist enters the field with a bachelor's, master's, or doctoral degree; the occupational therapy assistant generally earns an associate's degree. Practitioners must complete supervised clinical internships in a variety of health care settings, and pass a national examination. Most states also regulate occupational therapy practice.

organic brain syndrome   A collection of symptoms involving disturbance of consciousness, intellect, or mental function that is of physical (organic) rather than psychiatric origin, but without a known physical cause. OBS is not a separate disease, but a general term used to categorize physical conditions that can cause mental changes.

However, with the growing recognition of the organic bases of many psychiatric disorders, the distinction between "organic" and "functional" has become blurred. As a result, the *Diagnostic and Statistical Manual of Mental Disorders, Fourth Edition* (DSM-IV), no longer recognizes OBS as a diagnostic entity.

OBS can be divided into two major subgroups: acute (DELIRIUM or acute confusional states) and chronic (DEMENTIA). A third group—encephalopathy (subacute OBS)—describes a gray zone between delirium and dementia; its early course may fluctuate, but it is often persistent and progressive.

The basic characteristic of all forms of OBS is a change in brain function caused either from an outside insult or an intrinsic process affecting the function of brain chemicals, or physical or structural damage to the cortex. Possible causes of OBS include degenerative diseases such as Alzheimer's disease, metabolic imbalances, hydrocephalus, infections, drugs, toxins, vitamin deficiencies, the effects of brain trauma, atrophy, STROKE (such as MULTI-INFARCT DEMENTIA), or tumor. The end result of these disruptions of function or structure is impairment of thinking that affects alertness, orientation, emotion, behavior, memory, perception, language, problem solving, or judgment. Knowledge of which areas are affected or spared guides both the workup and the diagnosis.

Delirium accounts for between 10 percent and 15 percent of admissions to hospitals (but usually is not the primary diagnosis). The incidence of dementia increases with age, from about 2 percent to 10 percent at age 65 to between 20 percent and 50 percent of those older than 85. About 60 percent of nursing home beds are occupied by a patient with dementia; Alzheimer's accounts for the majority of patients with dementia who are older than 55 (between 50 percent and 90 percent). Alzheimer's is less common and occurs at an older age in Japan, China, and parts of Scandinavia. In these countries, vascular causes of dementia may outnumber Alzheimer's.

Symptoms

In the acute phase of the condition, symptoms can range from a slight confusion to stupor or coma, and may include disorientation, memory impairment, hallucinations, and delusions. The chronic form of the syndrome causes a progressive decline in intellect, memory, and behavior.

Delirium begins with a sudden onset of impaired awareness, easy distraction, confusion, and perception disturbances, such as visual hallucinations. Recent memory is usually disrupted, and patients often are not sure where they are or what day it is. Patients may be agitated and the level of awareness may fluctuate over brief periods of time. They may be incoherent or repetitive.

Dementia, on the other hand, is characterized by a history of chronic, steady decline in short- and long-term memory and is associated with problems in social relationships, work, and ACTIVITIES OF DAILY LIFE. However, it is possible to be both delirious and demented. Earlier stages of dementia may be subtle, and patients may try to hide their impairments. Patients at this stage often have an associated depression.

Treatment

Treatment is more likely to be successful with the acute form of organic brain syndrome if the underlying cause can be identified; in chronic cases, irreversible brain damage may already have occurred.

Delirium is fully reversible in most cases if it is recognized and treated properly. Dementia is usually insidious and progressive, although between 20 percent and 30 percent of cases are due to reversible causes. On average, patients with Alzheimer's die within eight years of onset of symptoms, with a range of between two and 15 years. Subacute OBS (encephalopathy) may be reversible, persistent, or progressive.

organic mental syndrome Psychological or behavioral symptoms with unknown cause that are linked to brain dysfunction. A person would be diagnosed with an organic mental syndrome, for example, if he or she is delirious or demented from an unknown cause. Symptoms could be due to a wide variety of problems, such as a STROKE, substance abuse, poisoning, brain tumor, or neurological disease such as Alzheimer's disease. Once the source of brain dysfunction is discovered, the person's mental problems are rediagnosed.

pacing A behavior typical of patients with Alzheimer's disease, who may spend hours pacing up and down a room. Patients may pace because they are hungry, thirsty, constipated, in pain, or many simply want to use the toilet and are unable to express their wishes. Patients may feel sick or may be suffering the side effects of certain medicines. They may pace because they are bored or restless. They may be upset by noisy or busy surroundings, or they may be angry, distressed, or anxious. In some cases, pacing may be due to changes that have taken place in the brain.

If pacing cannot be prevented, the patient should be allowed to walk in a safe area without disturbing anyone else. Patients should wear comfortable clothes and supportive shoes, and feet should be checked regularly for any redness, swellings, or blisters.

paranoia Suspicion of others that is not based on fact. This is a common behavioral symptom of Alzheimer's disease, in which a patient may have unrealistic, blaming beliefs or become easily jealous and suspicious. For example, a person with Alzheimer's may misinterpret an unfamiliar face as a robber.

Paranoia is caused by damage to the part of the brain that makes judgments and separates truth from fiction. A person with Alzheimer's who becomes paranoid will not connect the unrealistic belief to reality, no matter how many explanations are provided. Caregivers should not argue with an Alzheimer's patient who makes accusations or becomes extremely suspicious, but should try distracting the person.

parietal lobes One of four major pairs of lobes of the cerebral cortex located at the upper middle part of the head above the temporal lobes. It includes the sensory cortex and the association areas involved in processing information about body sensation, touch, and spatial organization. The association areas in the parietal lobes are also involved in secondary language and visual processing.

Lesions in association areas in the parietal lobes can cause difficulties in learning tasks that require an understanding of spatial perception and the body's position in space.

parkinsonism Any condition that causes any combination of the types of movement abnormalities seen in Parkinson's disease, such as a masklike face, rigidity, and slowed movements. It causes a lack of muscle control because nerve cells can't transmit messages to the muscles. In addition to the loss of muscle control, some people with parkinsonism often become severely depressed. Scientists estimate that about 13.7 percent of patients with parkinsonism experience dementia.

Parkinson's disease is the most common cause of parkinsonism. In every age group, men are twice as likely to develop parkinsonism as women. Parkinsonism may be caused by disorders such as a STROKE, or by brain infections such as encephalitis, or meningitis. The influenza epidemic during the early part of the 20th century caused a number of cases of encephalitis and resulting parkinsonism. Other diseases of the brain that combine parkinsonism with additional nerve disorders include Wilson's disease, Huntington's disease, Shy–Drager Syndrome, corticalbasal ganglionic degeneration, PROGRESSIVE SUPRANUCLEAR PALSY, LEWY BODY DEMENTIA, CREUTZFELDT-JAKOB DISEASE, and even Alzheimer's disease. Alzheimer's patients can have movement problems just as Parkinson's patients can have dementia. It's a case of which is first and which is worse.

A few drugs used to treat blood pressure, vomiting, mental disorders, and seizures can cause or worsen parkinsonism. Other drugs causing parkinsonism include tranquilizers (such as HALOPERIDOL), metoclopramide, and phenothiazine medications, narcotics, or general anesthesia.

Poisons that can cause parkinsonism include manganese, carbon monoxide, carbon disulfide, the cycad nut, and the illicit drug MPTP (methylphenyl tetrahydropyridine).

Parkinsonism caused by medications is usually reversible. However, symptoms caused by toxins, infections, or disorders may or may not be reversible. When there is no underlying triggering cause, the condition is called Parkinson's disease, and is characterized by the depletion of chemicals that facilitate electrical transmission between nerve cells.

Symptoms

Initial symptoms may be mild and nonspecific, such as a mild tremor, or the feeling that one leg or foot is stiff or dragging. Other symptoms include muscle rigidity, stiffness, difficulty bending arms or legs, posture problems, movement difficulties, loss of balance, shuffling, slow movements, difficulty initiating any voluntary movement, freezing of movement when the movement is stopped, muscle aches and pains, shaking, tremors, finger-thumb rubbing, reduced ability to show facial expressions, masklike appearance, staring, inability to close mouth, slow speech, low-pitched voice, monotone, difficulty chewing or swallowing, loss of fine motor skills, difficulty writing, difficulty eating, frequent falls, mild decline in intellectual function, depression, confusion, or dementia.

Diagnosis

Examination may show increased muscle tone, tremors of the Parkinson's type, and difficulty initiating or completing voluntary movements. Reflexes are usually normal. Tests are not usually specific for parkinsonism but may be used to confirm or rule out other disorders that may cause similar symptoms.

Treatment

The treatment is aimed at control of symptoms. If the symptoms are mild, no treatment may be required. If the condition is caused by a medication, the benefits of the medication may be weighed against the severity of symptoms. If appropriate, medications may be stopped or changed. Treatment of underlying conditions may reduce symptoms.

When drugs such as levodopa (L-dopa) are taken orally, many of the worst symptoms are lessened. New drugs such as pramipexole (Mirapex) and ropinirole (Requip) can delay the need for levodopa. Future approaches to treatment include a focus on early detection and slowing progression of the disease. Encouraging results have been reported from certain experimental surgical treatments, such as transplantation of fetal dopamine-producing cells, and insertion of a pacemaker-like device deep in the brain to suppress uncontrolled movements. Traditional surgery can alleviate some tremors, and physical therapy may help mobility.

Good general nutrition and health are important. Exercise should continue. Regular rest periods and lack of stress are recommended, because tiredness or stress can make the symptoms worse. Physical therapy, speech therapy, and occupational therapy may help promote function and independence, and may help maintain skills and positive attitude, and minimize depression.

Parkinson's disease v. Alzheimer's While many people may not realize it, up to 70 percent of patients with Parkinson's disease will go on to develop dementia as the disease progresses. Parkinson's is caused by nerve cell death in a specific part of the brain, leading to muscle tremors, stiffness, and weakness—and memory and thinking problems. Scientists have found that Parkinson's patients with memory problems also have a smaller HIPPOCAMPUS, which may be the cause of verbal and visual memory problems.

More than half of people with Parkinson's disease have mild intellectual changes, and up to 20 percent have more serious cognitive problems.

Typically, however, the memory problems with these patients are not as severe as among those people with Alzheimer's disease. Instead, patients may have trouble concentrating, learning new information and recalling names. Although there is no specific test for Parkinson's, there are several ways to diagnose the condition.

Most doctors rely on a neurological exam. Brain scans may rule out other diseases whose symptoms mimic Parkinson's. There is no cure for Parkinson's disease, although medication and surgery may help in some cases. The most common drug (L-dopa) works well in treating the movement problems, but is not as effective in easing thinking and memory difficulties. A range of other drugs are often used to control symptoms, but these medications can cause side effects including confusion and even hallucinations.

perception   The process through which sensory information (hearing, sight, touch, movement, taste, smell) is recognized and interpreted. Perception involves both the intake of information through the senses, and the processing and making sense of information within cognition. While sensory experience itself is largely automatic for humans, perception also involves learned behavior and intellectual capacity.

perseveration   Persistent repetition of an activity, word, phrase, or movement, such as tapping, wiping, and picking that is quite typical of patients with Alzheimer's disease. Patients who are perseverating may use the same word over and over again, or take one piece of clothing out of a drawer and then unpack all the other clothes without a specific purpose. Damage to the outer surfaces of the frontal lobe can cause perseveration.

According to at least one British psychiatrist, the problem of perseveration may have begun to haunt French composer Maurice Ravel as he wrote his famous *Bolero*. The famous melody repeats 18 times without change during the course of the music, which suggests to some that the composer might have been experiencing symptoms of Alzheimer's disease, which began to trouble the composer at the age of 52. Some experts believe

that the repetitive nature of the score's principal theme is symptomatic of the degenerative condition. Others argue that it was not Alzheimer's disease but a growing tumor that later killed Ravel during brain surgery in 1937.

See also REPETITIVE BEHAVIORS.

personal care   See ACTIVITIES OF DAILY LIVING.

personal care homes   See BOARD AND CARE HOMES.

personality   An enduring tendency to act and feel in particular ways. Changes in personality are one of the most troubling aspects of Alzheimer's disease, which in later stages of the disease alters forever the very essence of a person's being. The concept of personality is complex and takes into account a whole range of a person's traits and behaviors, but most are irrevocably changed by the disease process.

There is evidence that part of the cerebral cortex known as the prefrontal cortex in the frontal lobe plays a role in personality traits, including planning and organizational ability, ethical and moral sense, and overall emotional control.

Alcohol appears to mimic this loss of prefrontal control over behavior, because intoxication can lead to similar personality changes as in Alzheimer's, including aggression, loss of sexual restraint, planning and organizational ability, and higher thinking.

pet therapy   The use of pets to calm a patient or reach an unresponsive individual, often used with patients with Alzheimer's disease. When introducing a pet to a person with Alzheimer's, caregivers should remember that not everyone will react positively to animals; those who owned pets previously tend to be more responsive.

phenserine   An experimental drug in the third generation of a class of drugs already used in the treatment of Alzheimer's disease called anti-cholinesterase (AchE) medications. Acetylcholinesterase breaks down ACETYLCHOLINE, a chemical responsible for learning and memory but which is deficient in the brains of people with Alzheimer's.

Therefore, a drug that interferes with acetylcholinesterase would boost acetylcholine levels. Phenserine has been shown to improve mental abilities in rats, and is currently in human trials.

In addition to blocking acetylcholinesterase, phenserine has also shown the ability to lower the formation of BETA AMYLOID, the toxic protein found in the brains of patients with Alzheimer's disease and thought to be associated with nerve cell death. Phenserine blocks the formation of beta amyloid by blocking its precursor, AMYLOID PRECURSOR PROTEIN (APP). This dual mechanism of action suggests that it not only has the potential to improve memory and cognition, but also to slow the progression of the disease. Uncovering this mechanism will now allow researchers to use phenserine as a building block in creating drugs that fight beta amyloid even more effectively.

The accumulation of so-called plaques and tangles in the brain is considered the hallmark of Alzheimer's disease. Beta amyloid is the principal component of brain plaques, and many researchers believe that if beta amyloid production can be slowed down in the early stages of Alzheimer's, this would also slow the progression of the disease. Much of the drug research in the Alzheimer's field is aimed at fighting beta amyloid.

Because phenserine rapidly disappears from the blood, researchers believe it would cause fewer side effects than drugs which remain longer in the body.

phosphatidylserine (PS)   A type of fat-soluble substance that is an essential component of cell membranes, found in highest concentrations in brain cells. Some experts believe it may help preserve (or even improve) some aspects of mental functioning in the elderly. Nerve cells depend on cell membranes to carry out their specialized functions. PS helps activate and regulate many of the proteins which play key roles in these membrane processes. Cell membrane support from PS supports the nerve cell as a whole, generating nerve impulses; accumulating, storing, and releasing nerve transmitters; and improving nerve transmitter action.

Some studies have shown mild benefits for patients with Alzheimer's disease and some haven't. Therefore, treatment with phosphatidylserine is still controversial.

However, this is certainly no cure; while it may reduce symptoms in the short term, at best it probably slows the rate of deterioration rather than stops the progression of the disease altogether. For example, in one six-month study, benefits began to disappear after the fourth month of treatment. PS also affects the levels of neurotransmitters in the brain related to mood; in one study, elderly depressed women who were given 300 mg of PS per day for a month experienced an average 70 percent reduction in the severity of their depression.

PS is found in only trace amounts in a typical diet; very small amounts are present in lecithin. Since the body makes all the phosphatidylserine it needs, the only way to get a therapeutic dosage is to take a supplement.

Phosphatidylserine was originally manufactured from the brains of cows, but it is no longer available due to current concerns about contaminated brain cells in animals (such as mad cow disease). Most phosphatidylserine today is made from soybeans. Many experts believe that soy-based phosphatidylserine is just as effective as products made from cows' brains. Phosphatidylserine also can be manufactured from cabbage, but in one study the results with this form of the supplement were not particularly effective.

Side Effects

Taken orally, PS is rapidly absorbed and readily crosses the blood-brain barrier to reach the brain. Doses of 100 mg to 300 mg per day are the usual recommended dose, preferably taken in three divided doses with meals. Phosphatidylserine is generally regarded as safe when used at recommended dosages. Side effects are rare, and when they do occur they usually consist of nothing much worse than mild stomach upset. No significant side effects associated with phosphatidylserine have been consistently reported.

There are no known drug interactions with phosphatidylserine, but the maximum safe dosage for young children, pregnant or nursing women, or those with severe liver or kidney disease have not been established.

Phosphatidylserine is sometimes taken with GINKGO BILOBA as a way of boosting memory, but because both products may thin the blood, some experts worry that combining the two might interfere with normal blood clotting. Some experts also believe that phosphatidylserine enhances the effect of prescription blood thinners such as heparin and coumadin (warfarin).

physostigmine A drug used as eyedrops in the treatment of glaucoma that also may produce mild memory improvement among patients with Alzheimer's disease. Physostigmine is believed to improve memory by inhibiting acetylcholinesterase, a substance that breaks down ACETYLCHOLINE, a neurotransmitter important in a range of memory processes. Low levels of acetylcholine have been linked with Alzheimer's disease.

In one study, scientists tested physostigmine with 20 Alzheimer's patients as they performed a range of cognitive tests. The chemical enhanced performance on recognition tests, but not on others. These findings are typical of studies that found only modest improvements in memory with physostigmine. Moreover, the action of physostigmine was of very short duration, so scientists began studying other longer-acting drugs for the treatment of Alzheimer's.

The drug improves efficiency and reduces the effort needed to perform working memory tasks while altering the activity of some of the brain regions activated by this memory task, according to a study by the NATIONAL INSTITUTE ON AGING. The drug may enhance efficiency during the processing of information by focusing attention on the task at hand or it could help minimize the effects of distracting stimuli. Either way, a more efficient working memory could be a great advantage for Alzheimer's disease patients and other memory-impaired people.

TACRINE, no longer used for treatment of Alzheimer's disease, acts on the acetylcholine system in a way similar to physostigmine. Some scientists believe that since physostigmine improves the brain's response to memory tasks, similar drugs that enhance the cholinergic system might help relieve symptoms in Alzheimer's disease patients.

Pick's disease Pick's disease is a form of DEMENTIA characterized by a slowly progressive deterioration of social skills and changes in personality leading to impairment of intellect, memory, and language. It may be difficult to distinguish from Alzheimer's disease except on autopsy, although it is much less common. Alzheimer's disease causes 50 percent to 60 percent of dementia cases, whereas Pick's disease accounts for about 5 percent of cognitive deterioration.

The disease is characterized by Pick's bodies in the brain cells—miscellaneous bits of parts of the normal cell. Although the parts are recognizable, their normal relationships have been disrupted. The cause is unknown.

Pick's disease was first identified in 1892 by Dr. Arnold Pick, who described the progressive mental deterioration in a 71-year-old man. On autopsy, the brain showed an unusually shrunken frontal cortex, the region involved in reasoning and other higher mental functions. This shrinkage is different from the brain changes associated with Alzheimer's disease.

Symptoms

The disorder, which begins in the frontal lobes, does not cause memory problems at first. Instead, like Alzheimer's, the patient begins to first experience changes in personality and social behavior. Memory problems later appear, until eventually patients become mute, incontinent, and immobile. The condition is more common in women than men; patients contract this disease at about 55 years of age, with death following in about seven years.

Diagnosis

Pick's disease is diagnosed in a process similar to Alzheimer's. Often a patient is diagnosed with probable Alzheimer's, and later the diagnosis is changed to Pick's.

Treatment

There is no cure or specific treatment for Pick's disease, and its progress cannot be slowed down. However, some of the symptoms of the disease may be treated effectively. The course of Pick's disease is an inevitable progressive deterioration that may take anywhere from less than two years to more than 10 years. Death is usually caused by infection.

pillaging Taking items that belong to someone else. Pillaging is a common behavioral symptom of patients with Alzheimer's disease. Patients with Alzheimer's may take an object, believing that it belongs to them.

piracetam A nootropic drug that may improve cognitive functions, although studies have failed to demonstrate a clear benefit for the treatment of Alzheimer's disease.

Piracetam was developed in the mid-1960s by a Belgian pharmaceutical company and originally used to treat motion sickness. Since then, piracetam has been used experimentally or clinically to treat a wide range of diseases and conditions, primarily in Europe. Between 1968 and 1972, however, there was an explosion of research into its possible ability to facilitate learning and prevent amnesia.

plaques See AMYLOID PLAQUES.

positron emission tomography (PET) A type of brain scan technique that allows scientists to visualize the activity and interactions of particular brain regions as they are used during cognitive operations such as memorizing, recalling, speaking, reading, learning, and other sorts of information processing.

This peek into the living brain can help scientists measure early changes in brain function or structure to identify those individuals who are at risk of Alzheimer's disease even before they develop the symptoms of the disease. These various imaging techniques are still used primarily as research tools. PET is not widely available outside large urban areas, and it is not routinely used because health insurers balk at reimbursement.

power of attorney The means by which one person gives another the power to handle his or her personal affairs. However, the power ends at death.

The powers granted to another individual can be quite specific or very broad, but they allow someone to step in and handle personal affairs in the event of incapacitation or incompetence. If no POA has been granted for someone with Alzheimer's disease, for example, the court must appoint a guardian, who might not be someone the patient would have chosen. Even two people who are married can't make certain decisions for the other without a POA.

In the case of a patient with Alzheimer's, it would be important to obtain a full POA while the patient is still competent; a more restricted POA, for example, might not include permission to make decisions about health care. Without a standard POA (or at least a medical POA), a patient who needs health care but does not want it cannot legally be forced to accept care unless it is an emergency. (In fact, forcing a patient to submit in such situations is probably illegal.) In some cases, it is definitely illegal.

A patient who is still legally competent should be encouraged to assign a durable power of attorney for health care to a trusted friend or family member. If the patient is not legally competent, the only option is to establish a conservatorship or guardianship. While this step is intimidating and has some associated expenses, it is absolutely necessary for a patient who is already incompetent.

A *personal power of attorney* gives a patient's appointed agent the right to make decisions about medical care, entering a nursing home, nonfinancial matters, and so on.

A *financial power of attorney* gives an agent the power to handle financial decisions. For example, if a patient with Alzheimer's became mentally incapacitated, his wife could not access his personal checking account to pay bills without a financial POA.

A *medical power of attorney* grants authority to someone the patient trusts to make decisions with a physician about medical care options.

A *standard power of attorney* gives a patient's agent the right to make decisions in all areas of the patient's life. Every spouse should have a standard POA for the other.

The power of all types of POA ends at the patient's death, however. At that point, the patient's assets become part of a probate estate, and an executor must receive authorization from the local courts to act in that capacity.

A *nondurable power of attorney* is only a temporary, specific POA used for a limited transaction, such as to settle a real estate sale if a person is out of town, or bill payment while a person is out of the country. A *durable power of attorney,* on the other hand, is permanent, and allows an appointed agent to take appropriate legal action if the authorizing person becomes incapacitated.

See Appendix V for a sample POA form.

prefrontal cortex   Brain structure important in judgment, planning, impulse control, and abstract thinking, that may be affected in Alzheimer's disease. The prefrontal cortex is also intimately connected with the limbic system, and receives input from other brain areas about the internal emotional and motivational states. These influences, together with other information synthesized by the prefrontal cortex from incoming sensory information, help to give meaning and significance to external events.

Researchers suspect that the prefrontal cortex plays a role in structuring behavior by helping prepare sensory and motor systems for action. Relatively more developed in humans than any other species, this area has an enormously complex interaction with other parts of the brain. When this area is damaged, doctors can't point to any one particular skill or function that is lost; rather, it appears as if an essential quality of being human is lost.

preimplantation genetic diagnosis (PGD)   A technique in which a woman's eggs are screened and selected in the lab to avoid a particular genetic disease. For the first time, in 2000 a woman with a gene that is all but certain to cause Alzheimer's disease in midlife gave birth to a baby free of the defect after having her eggs screened and selected in the laboratory. The case appears to be the first time PGD has been used to eliminate the genetic chance of early onset Alzheimer's. There is no similar test for the more typical form of Alzheimer's, which strikes older people.

In the past, PGD, which can also involve the testing of early embryos, has been used to screen for other devastating diseases such as Tay-Sachs and sickle-cell anemia, which strike in early childhood. It is less commonly used to detect diseases that strike adults.

The patient, a married woman who was 30 when she had the procedure, desperately wanted children, even though Alzheimer's will probably steal her mind long before her daughter grows up. The patient, whose name was not released, has a brother and sister who developed Alzheimer's in their 30s. Tests showed that she has a mutation called V717L that has been found to lead to the formation of the brain-clogging protein deposits that are a hallmark of Alzheimer's. This flaw is probably present in only a dozen or so families worldwide; afflicted patients are virtually assured of developing early onset Alzheimer's.

The woman, who has a background in genetics and was well-informed of the ramifications, underwent in-vitro fertilization, in which eggs are fertilized in the lab and implanted in the womb. But in this case, before the eggs were fertilized, they were examined to find those that were free of the mutant gene. She had to undergo two rounds of tests because eggs tested the first time had the V717L flaw.

Her doctor, geneticist Yury Verlinsky, a PGD pioneer at Chicago's Reproductive Genetics Institute, says that using PGD for early onset Alzheimer's is the only relief for at-risk couples. However, he notes that he will not screen for gender or other cosmetic factors, but otherwise does not pass judgment on which patients he will test. Verlinsky's clinic has done about 2,000 PGD procedures, resulting in more than 200 babies, in the past 10 years. The procedure is not widely available, in part because the defects it tests for are generally rare. It is also difficult to perform.

The procedure costs about $2,500 at Verlinsky's clinic. The cost does not include the clinic's $7,500 fee for in-vitro fertilization.

Some experts warn that such procedures are certain to prove highly controversial, especially since in this case it involves testing for diseases that are not going to appear until 30 or 40 years later.

However, testing for early onset Alzheimer's falls within guidelines from the American Society of Reproductive Medicine, which sets standards for fertility clinics. The group supports PGD when used for medical reasons, although clinics can decide for themselves which conditions to test for.

presenilins Proteins that may be linked to EARLY ONSET ALZHEIMER'S DISEASE. Genes that code for presenilin 1 and presenilin 2 have been found on chromosomes 14 and 1, respectively, and are linked to early onset familial Alzheimer's disease. Scientific interest in the presenilin proteins heightened dramatically when scientists discovered that mutations in the genes that code for presenilin 1 and presenilin 2 account for approximately 40 percent of cases of inherited Alzheimer's disease. Presenilin 1 on CHROMOSOME 14 is more common, with an age at onset ranging from 28 to 50. More recently, scientists have linked presenilin 1 to the more common, noninherited forms of Alzheimer's as well. Presenilin 2 on CHROMOSOME 1 accounts for fewer cases, whose onset begins in a person's 40s to 50s.

Both of these genes are dominant (a child who received just one gene from either parent would inevitably get the disease). Experts believe that anyone with a defect in either gene will probably develop the illness before age 65.

Since the genes were first discovered in 1995, scientists have discovered that the mutated forms of the genes may cause Alzheimer's by boosting production of BETA AMYLOID, a protein that causes the plaques typically found in the brains of Alzheimer's patients. Scientists believe that a buildup of beta amyloid damages cells, and that the presenilins also participate in cellular suicide, sending precise chemical messages to cells urging them to die. This mechanism of cell death begins in healthy people at around age 45. People with the mutated form of the presenilin gene are far more sensitive to these enzymes.

Scientists recently discovered that presenilin 1 may be one of the enzymes that clip a larger protein into beta amyloid. In addition, presenilins have a number of other possible functions besides clipping the larger AMYLOID-PRECURSOR PROTEIN. Understanding more about the functions of the prese-

nilins will shed further light on the nature and development of Alzheimer's, possibly leading to new targets for prevention or treatment strategies.

Scientists believe that presenilins may be involved in cellular death. Studies conducted by a number of researchers indicate that in mice, neurons expressing presenilin 1 mutations are more vulnerable to stress-related cell death. Neurons in these mice can be rescued by treating them with substances that interfere with programmed cell death (APOPTOSIS). Proper regulation of cellular CALCIUM levels is essential because abnormal increases in calcium can lead to cell death.

Presenilins also may be involved in cell-cell communication by maintaining healthy cellular connections. A study conducted by scientists at Mt. Sinai Medical Center in New York showed that presenilin 1 is located at the communication point of a cell (synapse) and that it may be necessary for proper connections between neurons. It could be that presenilin mutations linked to Alzheimer's affect presenilin function at the connection points between brain cells.

pressure sore A reddened painful spot on the skin caused by continuous pressure in bedridden or demented patients, also known as decubitus ulcers or bedsores. As people age, their skin becomes increasingly delicate, so that even quite mild friction on the skin can produce pressure sores, which may appear over any bony prominence (especially on the heels, base of the spine, and elbows). The continual pressure on the skin interferes with blood flow, and is further affected by a patient's age, nutritional level, and general physical shape.

Pressure sores tend to occur in patients with a significant degree of physical or mental impairment or both. A severely demented patient with Alzheimer's will not be able to complain if a particular area of the skin is uncomfortable.

People normally move around in bed, even during sleep. However, in the later stages of dementia, the person may not move for long periods. This may be because of the lack of motivation associated with dementia in the later stages or a physical disability, or a combination of the two. This lack of movement can lead to pressure sores.

Patients who lie on their backs may develop pressure sores on the heels and buttocks, or any area of the body which presses against the bed or chair for a prolonged period. Areas such as the shoulders, shoulder blades, hips, and ankles are especially at risk, because there is less protective tissue in these areas.

Likewise, most people move around naturally when they are sitting down. However, in the later stages of dementia, people may remain seated for long periods in one position because of the lack of motivation, physical disability, or both. As a result, pressure sores may occur. Caregivers should encourage patients to move from side to side in the chair from time to time, or to change position while they are sitting. They should stand up and walk around at least once every couple of hours.

Treatment

Any reddened area of the skin should receive special attention, because untreated sores can be dangerous. Any broken skin will need to be promptly dressed. Any reddened areas of skin should never be rubbed or massaged, because this could cause further damage.

Prevention

Skilled, vigilant nursing care can prevent most of these ulcers from forming. Bedridden patients should be turned every two hours to distribute their weight, and the skin should be kept clean and dry. Urine and feces should be promptly removed before they irritate the skin; dusting powder also may help. Other preventive aids may include sheepskins on the bed, air or water mattresses, and foam rings. Patients with Alzheimer's should be encouraged to get up from bed during the day and to move around as much as possible, either independently or with help.

Caregivers should make sure there are no rough seams in clothes, or any objects which could cause friction left in pockets. Bedding should be smooth; even wrinkles in the sheets can contribute to pressure sores, and a person in the later stages of dementia will not be able to alert caregivers if they can feel wrinkles.

Tight clothing or tight bedding should be avoided (especially over the feet). Because too much heat and moisture can also contribute to pressure sores, it's important to keep the patient from becoming hot and sweaty. The patient should be completely dry after washing, especially in the skin folds. The skin should be patted dry rather than rubbed.

Overall health is an important means to prevent bedsores. Good nutrition means that the skin will be healthier and more resistant to the development of sores, and regular exercise improves circulation and helps relieve any pressure on the skin.

prion diseases A family of diseases that causes a DEMENTIA that in some respects resembles Alzheimer's disease. They include CREUTZFELDT-JAKOB DISEASE, mad cow disease, and sheep scrapie and are all caused by an abnormal folding of a prion protein, which then can infect an animal with disease.

Although Alzheimer's disease is not infectious, there are similarities between prion diseases and Alzheimer's, including the fact that both prions and BETA AMYLOID form amyloid structures in the brain.

prions A shortened name for "proteinaceous infectious particle," this is a mutant form of a protein first identified by the brash and controversial California neurologist Stanley B. Prusiner. In 1982, Prusiner first identified the radical new infectious particle that was neither virus nor bacteria, but that somehow can pass on its mutated shape by nudging up against a healthy cell's normal prions to alter their shape.

Basically a protein, the prion is capable of causing a range of brain diseases, such as CREUTZFELDT-JAKOB DISEASE, that may be confused with Alzheimer's disease.

About 60 years ago scientists discovered that sheep were contracting a disease (scrapie) that transformed their brains into pitted sponges, but researchers could never identify the virus responsible. Then neurobiologists discovered a strange movement disorder among New Guinea tribesmen. Both, many scientists now believe, are caused by prions.

This protein arises from cells it may one day destroy. Normally, it can be found harmlessly sitting on the surfaces of nerve cells, until something induces it to infect a new cell and replicate by transforming the cell's normal prion protein molecule (PrP) into a mutant version. About 10 percent of prion diseases are hereditary; that is, the gene for PrP mutates, which leads to substitutions or alterations among the other amino acids that make up PrP. Somehow, these slight differences induce the protein to switch its shape. Different diseases will result depending on the makeup of the rest of the gene.

Some scientists think that accumulation of toxic forms of PrP cause cellular destruction, but others believe that imbalances in normal PrP concentrations can hurt cells. Others suspect that the loss of functional PrP can lead to the disintegration of the brain; they also believe that normal PrP helps produce synapses, without which nerve cells cannot communicate.

progressive supranuclear palsy (PSP) A rare brain disorder that causes serious and permanent problems with control of gait and balance. The most obvious sign of the disease is an inability to move the eyes properly, caused by lesions in the area of the brain that coordinates eye movements. PSP is often misdiagnosed because some of its symptoms are so much like those of Alzheimer's disease, Parkinson's disease, and more rare neurodegenerative disorders, such as CREUTZFELDT-JAKOB DISEASE.

Symptoms
In addition to the vision difficulties caused by problems in moving the eyes, PSP patients often exhibit changes in mood and behavior, including depression and apathy, in addition to mild DEMENTIA. However, the pattern of symptoms can vary considerably from one person to the next. Although PSP is a progressive disease, the disease isn't fatal in itself. PSP is a progressive disease but is not itself directly life-threatening. Patients do tend to have serious complications such as pneumonia as a result of swallowing problems. The most common complications are choking and pneumonia, head injury, and fractures from falls, and the most common cause of death is pneumonia. With good attention to medical and nutritional needs, however, some PSP patients live well into their 70s and beyond.

Cause
The symptoms of PSP are caused by a gradual deterioration of brain cells in a few tiny, important places in the brainstem.

Diagnosis
The key to establishing a diagnosis is to identify early gait instability and problems moving the eyes, as well as ruling out other similar disorders.

Treatment
There is currently no effective treatment, although scientists are searching for better ways to manage the disease. In some patients the slowness, stiffness, and balance problems may respond to antiparkinsonian drugs such as levodopa, or levodopa combined with anticholinergic agents, but the effect is usually temporary. The speech, vision, and swallowing difficulties usually don't respond to any drug treatment. Antidepressants such as Prozac, Elavil or Tofranil may be of some modest help. Nondrug treatment for PSP may include weighted walking aids to offset the tendency to fall backward, and bifocals or special prism glasses to ease the problem of looking down. Physical therapy has not been proven to help, but certain exercises can help keep the joints limber. A surgical procedure, a gastrostomy, may be necessary to improve swallowing problems. This surgery involves placing a tube through the skin of the abdomen into the intestine to avoid having to eat by mouth.

In the Future
Scientists are studying the use of FREE RADICAL scavengers (drugs that can get rid of potentially harmful free radicals). In addition, better understanding of the related diseases of Parkinson's and Alzheimer's diseases will help solve the problem of PSP.

ProMem See METRIFONATE.

pseudodementia A disorder that mimics DEMENTIA and Alzheimer's disease but that includes no evidence of brain dysfunction. Nearly one out of 10 patients thought to be suffering from true dementia in fact have a pseudodementia linked to depressive illness. Unlike dementia, depression is treatable; many people respond well to antidepressant drugs. Pseudodementia is found most often among elderly patients.

psychometric tests   See MENTAL STATUS TESTING.

psychotic symptoms   Between 40 percent and 60 percent of patients with Alzheimer's disease experience psychotic symptoms as their disease worsens, including PARANOIA, HALLUCINATIONS, misidentification, and DELUSIONS. The presence of psychotic symptoms in Alzheimer's patients is linked to more aggressive behavior, more rapid functional decline, and early institutionalization. About 30 percent of people with Alzheimer's exhibit some type of paranoia in the early stages of the disease; by the late stages, about half of all patients have at least some psychotic symptoms.

One recent study suggests that the development of psychotic symptoms may be determined in part by genetic factors, since there is a significant association between psychosis in family members and the occurrence of Alzheimer's plus psychosis of siblings. In the study, the odds of exhibiting psychosis were more than double among siblings of Alzheimer's patients who themselves exhibited psychosis. Scientists suspect that there may be a set of genes that each contribute a modest risk to psychosis. The researchers did not rule out the possibility that environmental factors in the patients' early lives might make the Alzheimer's patients more susceptible to psychosis.

The study included families with two or more members diagnosed with definite, probable, or possible Alzheimer's. The 371 family members diagnosed with Alzheimer's and psychotic behaviors had a total of 461 siblings, also diagnosed with Alzheimer's.

Sibling age and the age at which they developed Alzheimer's were ruled out as factors in the development of psychosis.

race and Alzheimer's disease   African Americans and Hispanic Americans appear to have a higher overall risk of Alzheimer's disease than do Caucasians. However, differences in socioeconomic status, health care, education, prenatal events, and life history all may influence a person's eventual risk of Alzheimer's. Even certain diagnostic tests that measure language, memory, and thought processes may cause some people to be diagnosed with Alzheimer's depending on their educational level or cultural background.

A five-year study of more than 2,100 people found the APOE-4 gene associated with an increased risk of Alzheimer's disease in African Americans, Hispanics and Caucasians, but among people with apoE-2 or apoE-3 genes instead of apoE-4, Hispanics were twice as likely and African Americans were four times as likely, to develop Alzheimer's disease by age 90 as were Caucasians of the same gender and education level. The reasons for these different rates of risk are still unclear.

REACH   The acronym for Resources for Enhancing Alzheimer's Caregiver Health, a major five-year initiative established in 1995 to carry out research in ways to help caregivers of patients with Alzheimer's disease and related disorders. REACH is cosponsored by the NATIONAL INSTITUTE ON AGING and the National Institute of Nursing Research (NINR).

REACH projects focus on characterizing and testing the most promising home- and community-based interventions for caregivers (particularly in minority families). The interventions include support groups, behavioral skills training programs, family-based interventions, environmental modifications, and computer-based information and communication services.

An important outcome of this initiative will be a shared database that will enable investigators to answer key questions about the best way to maintain and improve the health and quality of life of caregivers of dementia patients. Investigators are particularly interested in exploring issues related to depression among caregivers, but they are also assessing the effects of caregiving on health status, health practices, and use of health care services.

So far more than 1,000 families with diverse ethnic backgrounds have entered the study.

For more information about the project, see the REACH website (http://www.edc.gsph.pitt.edu/reach/).

reality orientation   A type of therapy for patients with Alzheimer's disease in which continual, repetitive reminders are given to keep the patient stimulated and oriented. In order for reality orientation to be effective, the techniques must be applied consistently by all of the people who come into contact with the patient. When applying reality orientation, caregivers should address the confused patient as though the person can understand everything.

The technique requires that caregivers mention names of familiar people and objects, as well as the current date, the week, and the time of day, in all conversations with the patient. Personal care efforts should be encouraged, because maintaining the basic ACTIVITIES OF DAILY LIVING helps keep a confused person in touch with reality.

In an environment focusing on reality orientation, a large clock and a calendar should be visible at all times. Earlier-stage Alzheimer's patients should be encouraged to use a watch that also includes dates. Stimulating materials such as magazines or newspapers should be available for the patient, and a schedule of daily activities should be posted that includes the time and the date.

Signs, directional arrows, night-lights, or color-coded doors may help keep patients from getting lost. Many nursing homes use a reality orientation board that includes information about today's date, year, weather, next meal, and next holiday. Other materials that can help patients remain oriented in place and time include a clock with moveable hands, photo albums, large print books, maps, and a world globe.

recall   A term used to denote the ability to retrieve information from long-term memory. Recall is involved in a broad range of tasks and specific tests, from remembering a phone number to calling up information for a school exam. While useful as a descriptive term, it does not refer to a specific area of cognitive function.

Difficulty recalling information may be caused by a number of different learning problems. This may include problems imprinting information during processing because of poor attention or short-term memory, as well as difficulty with rapid retrieval tasks that are typically found in expressive language disorders.

receptor   A specialized component of a cell that is embedded in the membrane of nerve cells, that can detect mechanical changes in the environment, triggering impulses in the sensory nervous system. Certain receptors bind neurotransmitters, which trigger electrochemical changes in nerve function. Receptors are found on the axon's dendrites and cell bodies of nerve cells.

Reminyl   See GALANTAMINE.

repetitive behaviors   Repeated questions, stories, and outbursts or specific activities done over and over again are typical of people with Alzheimer's disease. Some patients constantly repeat the same behavior, such as packing and unpacking a bag or rearranging the chairs in a room. This behavior may relate to a former activity or job, such as cleaning the house or organizing an office. The person may be bored and need more activities to stimulate them or more contact with other people.

Sometimes patients repeat the same phrase or movement many times (PERSEVERATION). This may happen if the person is too hot or too cold, hungry or thirsty. Otherwise, these patients may find their environment too noisy or stressful; they may be bored. Some patients find that stroking a pet, going for a walk, or listening to favorite music is a good way of soothing themselves.

Some patients may ask the same question over and over again, either because they do not remember asking or they have forgotten what the answer was due to short-term memory loss. Feelings of insecurity or anxiety about their ability to cope may also play a part in patients' repetitive questioning.

Caregivers should not get angry but should either try to get the patient to find the answer for themselves, or distract the person with an activity. People with dementia often become anxious about future events, which can lead to repetitive questioning. If this is the problem, the patient should not be told about an upcoming event until just before it happens.

residential care facilities   See BOARD AND CARE HOMES.

respite care   Services that provide people with temporary relief from tasks associated with taking care of a family member with Alzheimer's disease. Caring for a patient with Alzheimer's is a 24-hour-a-day job that can be physically and emotionally exhausting, triggering feelings of anger, frustration, loneliness, and depression. Without a break from the daily responsibility, a caregiver's health can deteriorate, reducing the quality of care the Alzheimer's patient receives. Family caregivers often develop stress-related illnesses such as heart disease, hypertension, or ulcers; an occasional break allows an exhausted caregiver to regroup.

Respite care services include in-home help, short nursing home stays, or ADULT DAY SERVICES to allow caregivers to go on vacations, business travel, or a weekend getaway.

In-home services offer a range of options, including companion services, personal care, household assistance, and skilled care services. Helpers can be hired privately, through an agency, or as part of a government program. The in-home respite care worker or volunteer comes into the home one or two times a week for four hours or less during each visit. These workers sit and visit with the patient so that the caregiver can leave the house without worrying about leaving the patient alone. In-home respite workers might play games, read, or walk around the house with the patient. These workers do not bathe the patient, clean the house, or cook a large meal, although some workers may prepare a simple lunch or do light housework.

Adult day services provide participants with opportunities to interact with others, usually in a community center or facility. Staff members at the service lead various activities such as music programs and support groups. Transportation and meals are often provided.

With financial assistance, many family caregivers who would not otherwise use this service will have the opportunity to obtain temporary relief. As a result, the individual with DEMENTIA may remain at home for much longer than would otherwise be possible.

restraints Devices used to ensure safety by restricting and controlling a person's movement. They are sometimes used to control patients with Alzheimer's disease who may wander or be aggressive.

However, because using restraints can interfere with a patient's dignity, many facilities are restraint-free or use alternative methods to help modify behavior. Indeed, studies have demonstrated that effective programming can eliminate the need for restraints, according to the Joint Commission on Accreditation of Health Care Organizations (JCAHO), an organization that accredits health care organizations.

Because physical restraints restrict a person's ability to move, they can lead to INCONTINENCE, loss of muscle tone, PRESSURE SORES, DEPRESSION, and appetite loss. Instead of physical or chemical restraints, experts recommend that patients be given a safe place to wander and distractions when they become agitated.

retirement communities See CONTINUING CARE RETIREMENT COMMUNITY.

retrieval The searching and finding process that leads to recognition and recall of information out of long-term memory.

risk factors Several risk factors have been identified with Alzheimer's disease: the most significant are age, family history, and genetics. The risk of getting Alzheimer's disease rises with age, doubling in each decade after age 65. Still, only one or two people in 100 have Alzheimer's at age 65, but that risk increases to about one in five by age 80, when the average patient is diagnosed. By age 90, half of all Americans have some symptoms. It's also true that people with relatives who develop Alzheimer's disease are more likely to develop the disease themselves.

Some studies have found that traumatic head injuries earlier in life seem to be linked to Alzheimer's. Statistics also indicate that the more years of formal education people have, the less likely they are to develop Alzheimer's later in life. Other studies have found that good linguistic ability is linked to a lower chance of developing Alzheimer's, as does a high level of FOLIC ACID (folate) and ACETYLCHOLINE in the blood.

rivastigmine (Exelon) Drug that was approved as a treatment for mild to moderate Alzheimer's disease in 2000. Rivastigmine works by blocking enzymes that break down ACETYLCHOLINE, a brain chemical that carries messages between brain cells. Patients with Alzheimer's appear to produce smaller amounts of acetylcholine in their brains. According to some studies, patients who took this drug showed greater improvement in thinking and remembering, in the ability to carry on ACTIVITIES OF DAILY LIVING, and in overall functioning.

Normally, the human brain produces acetylcholine, it carries messages, and then it is broken down by a special enzyme called acetylcholinesterase. Like other drugs designed to treat Alzheimer's, Exelon prevents the last part of the cycle so that acetylcholine is not broken down. As a result, there is more acetylcholine available to carry messages in the brain.

According to the manufacturer (Novartis), studies show that between 25 percent and 30 percent of people who take the medication score better on tests of memory, understanding, and activities of daily living after six months than they did before starting therapy. However, between 10 percent and 20 percent of patients taking the placebo also scored better on the same tests at the end of six months. Another 20 percent of patients who took the drug were more or less the same after six months on the drug as when they started, whereas about another 10 percent of those on the placebo were no worse. (Normally most people with Alzheimer's disease would decline noticeably over this period of time.) The drug had no clear effect on the remaining patients.

Rivastigmine has received approval for use against Alzheimer's in 60 countries around the world. It is normally taken twice a day with food, beginning with a low dose of 1.5 mg twice a day, building to a total of 6 to 12 mg a day.

Side Effects

The drug causes side effects including nausea, vomiting, loss of appetite, fatigue, and weight loss. In most cases, these side effects were temporary and declined with continuing treatment, but sometimes the nausea and vomiting are severe enough that patients lose weight. In clinical trials, 26 percent of women and 18 percent of men who took high-dose Exelon lost at least 7 percent of their initial body weight due to nausea and vomiting. Because of the nausea, the drug should be taken with meals.

Side effects are more common when treatment first starts or when the dose is increased, but often fade with time. It is not possible to tell who will have side effects and who will not.

Ronald and Nancy Reagan Research Institute

An expansion of the existing research program of the ALZHEIMER'S ASSOCIATION launched by the association and the Reagan family in 1995 to accelerate efforts to delay the onset of, and eventually to prevent, Alzheimer's disease.

Former president Ronald Reagan and First Lady Nancy Reagan announced the formation of the new institute on November 1, 1995, to unite the leading scientific minds from around the world with drug and biotechnical companies to boost the exchange of information and find treatments, preventions, and cures.

Nancy Reagan explained that the institute was established to serve as a symbol of hope to all those who share the Reagans' dream of finding a cure for Alzheimer's disease. President Reagan had announced in a letter to the American people on November 5, 1994, that he was suffering from the early stages of Alzheimer's disease.

While major strides have been made recently in Alzheimer's research, there still is no cure, prevention, or truly effective treatment. Potential cutbacks in federal funding threaten to slow continued progress. The Reagan Institute allows experts who now work separately to focus together on priorities, and help bring effective treatments to market more quickly. Alzheimer's expert Zaven Khachaturian serves as the primary consultant to the association for the Reagan Institute.

The primary focus of the Reagan Institute is to provide grants for innovative research, and to promote cooperative working relationships among the association, scientists, pharmaceutical and biotechnology companies, universities and medical centers, private foundations, and the federal government.

For contact information see Appendix I.

Safe Return See ALZHEIMER'S ASSOCIATION SAFE RETURN PROGRAM.

safety Because patients with Alzheimer's disease often feel confused and frightened, it is vital that caregivers create safe and comfortable surroundings to help patients feel more relaxed and less overwhelmed.

A person with Alzheimer's can't understand the meaning of many actions and behaviors. For example, patients might not remember why they must wear warm coats in cold weather or why eating spoiled food is unsafe. However, because of the cognitive limits of patients with Alzheimer's, it is often easier to prevent accidents rather than trying to teach someone safety skills.

For example, to protect patients from being burned, caregivers might remove knobs from the stove and keep matches and cigarettes locked away. Because many accidents happen when a patient is rushed, it is important to allow patients to travel at their own pace. Many accidents also occur during personal care activities such as bathing or eating. Accidents can be avoided if the patient is given a simple, step-by-step direction with enough time to complete each task.

It is especially important that caregivers monitor everything the patient may ingest, since many don't understand the danger in eating tainted food or foreign objects. Poisoning and choking, especially in the latter stages of Alzheimer's, is a real danger. Medication is also dangerous, since patients may not remember which medication was taken or which pill to take. A list of emergency numbers for police, fire, and poison control should be posted beside all phones.

Homes should be safety-proofed for patients with Alzheimer's in much the same way that a home would be made safe for toddlers. All cabinets that contain dangerous substances and toxic chemicals should be locked, if the substances can't be moved out of reach. Garages, basements, and workrooms where toxic chemicals are kept should be locked at all times.

Because patients can't differentiate between safe and tainted food, everything in the refrigerator should be fresh and clean. Because patients may eat small rocks, dirt, plants, flowers, or bulbs, toxic plants such as mistletoe or oleander should be removed.

Guns have no place in a home with an Alzheimer's patient, even someone who might have once been able to handle a gun. Patients should never be given unsupervised access to a gun.

Because alcohol can have a negative effects on a patient with Alzheimer's, drinking should be carefully monitored. Alcohol should not be mixed at all with certain medicines.

The kitchen can be a dangerous place with an Alzheimer's patient in the home, who may no longer remember how to safely operate appliances such as a toaster oven, stove, coffeemaker, or barbecue.

Because patients with Alzheimer's can't judge temperature, they may forget that stoves, curling irons, or space heaters can be hot and dangerous, and they may not feel heat until they have been scalded. To avoid accidents, caregivers should set the home water heater below 140 degrees Fahrenheit.

Bathrooms are also highly dangerous places for patients with Alzheimer's, who may be frightened by the shiny surfaces of glass and polished tile. To minimize the risk of electric shock, all electrical appliances should be removed from the bathroom.

To prevent falls, grab bars, bath seats, and commode chairs should be installed.

See also SAFETY ASSESSMENT SCALE FOR PEOPLE WITH DEMENTIA LIVING AT HOME.

Safety Assessment Scale for People with Dementia Living at Home (SAS)   A test that can help CAREGIVERS make a more objective assessment of the risk of domestic accidents that may result from the declining mental ability of a patient with Alzheimer's disease. The test was designed by a Canadian team of researchers who tested and validated the scale among 175 patients in English and French, in both urban and rural areas of the country.

The assessment scale is not a simple checklist. Whether answering the 32 questions of the scale's long version, or the 19 questions of the abridged version, health care workers answer questions such as "Is this person alone at home," by picking "Always," "Most of the time," "Occasionally," or "Never."

With the SAS, caregivers can determine precisely the level of care and services needed to make sure that the person with memory and cognitive deficits can safely stay at home for a longer period of time. Physicians, nurses, family helpers, social workers, and occupational therapists can evaluate in a few minutes the risks of accidents in any particular home. When comparing the results of the assessment, caregivers can intervene to diminish potential risks.

See also SAFETY.

SAM-e S-adenosylmethionine (SAM-e)   A naturally occurring compound that increases the body's levels of SEROTONIN, melatonin, and dopamine. SAM-e is produced naturally in the body from a substance called adenosine triphosphate and the amino acid methionine, which is found in protein-rich foods and is long thought to have properties that affect mood and mental functions. SAM-e's major role in the body is to release an essential substance that fuels dozens of biochemical reactions.

Discovered in 1952, SAM-e has been extensively studied, and few researchers dismiss its therapeutic potential. But doctors are wary of advising patients to try SAM-e because most studies are European, with few large, long-term, randomized clinical trials. Moreover, little is known about dosage, long-term effects, and comparisons with other medications.

Clinical studies suggest that people with Alzheimer's disease and depression have lower levels of SAM-e in their brain tissue. While it has been reported that some people with Alzheimer's who take SAM-e supplements have better cognitive function, further studies are needed to determine how safe and effective this supplement may be for individuals with the disease.

selective serotonin reuptake inhibitors   The newest and most successful class of antidepressants that prevent brain cells from reabsorbing SEROTONIN, effectively raising the level of this neurotransmitter and easing depression. SSRIs may be prescribed to ease the depression common among patients with Alzheimer's disease. SSRIs include Prozac (fluoxetine), Zoloft (sertraline), Paxil (paroxetine),+ and Celexa. Two other new antidepressants also affect serotonin—Serzone (nefazadone) and Luvox (fluvoxamine). A malfunctioning serotonin system has been implicated in the development of DEPRESSION.

These new drugs have moved to the forefront of modern psychiatric treatment because they work as well as any of the older antidepressants while causing far fewer serious side effects. The lack of side effects is primarily due to the fact that they are relatively selective, primarily affecting only one neurotransmitter system (serotonin) instead of others throughout the brain.

Although SSRIs lack many of the more serious side effects, they do cause some problems, such as nausea, dizziness, or dry mouth, in addition to a wide variety of sexual side effects such as decreased or increased sexual interest, ejaculation or orgasm problems, and impotence. Many doctors now estimate that as many as 70 percent of people who take SSRIs may experience some type of mild sexual problem.

The main difference among the SSRIs is the side effects they produce. Paxil seems to produce the most drowsiness, which means it can improve sleep among Alzheimer's patients with insomnia. Zoloft and Luvox seem to cause more stomach problems. Paxil, Prozac, and Zoloft seem to lessen appetite, whereas Luvox does not affect a person's interest in food. Paxil has been linked to more complaints of constipation and dry mouth, and seems to trigger more pronounced withdrawal symptoms when medication is stopped. All SSRIs seem to cause problems with sexual interest or performance.

Unlike older antidepressants, SSRIs are not very dangerous even in high doses, and most are available in single daily doses. And unlike many older antidepressants, the SSRIs don't seem to cause weight gain in many people, and may even trigger a mild weight loss.

If a patient decides to stop taking an SSRI, the dosage should be gradually diminished. Abruptly stopping the medication may lead to dizziness, dry mouth, insomnia, nausea, nervousness, and sweating.

All SSRIs work well for elderly patients, but research suggests that older patients taking Paxil or Luvox will have much higher blood levels of the medication than would a younger patient. For this reason, some doctors prescribe lower doses of these drugs for older people, or monitor their response more closely.

Some studies also suggest that SSRIs may be beneficial to cognitive performance in the elderly, although they have not been approved by the U.S. Food and Drug Administration for this use.

selegiline (Eldepryl) A medication that may slow certain symptoms of Alzheimer's disease for up to seven months, according to at least one study sponsored by the NATIONAL INSTITUTE ON AGING. Eldepryl, which was approved in 1989, is currently used to help treat Parkinson's disease.

In the study, scientists at 23 Alzheimer's Disease Cooperative Study (ADCS) sites in the United States assessed 341 patients with moderate Alzheimer's disease to determine if Eldepryl or alpha-tocopherol (vitamin E) slowed the progression of the condition. Patients were assessed throughout the study to determine the progression of the disease, as measured by loss of ability to perform basic daily activities, institutionalization, progression to severe dementia, or death. Both Eldepryl and vitamin E delayed the progression of the disease by about seven months, but Eldepryl had more side effects.

semantic memory Memory for facts, such as the information that would be contained in a dictionary or encyclopedia with no connection to time or place. People don't remember when or where they learn this type of information.

Semantic memory registers and stores knowledge about the world in the broadest sense; it allows people to represent and mentally operate on situations, objects, and relations in the world that aren't present to the senses. A person with an intact semantic memory system can think about things that are not here now.

Because semantic memory develops first in childhood—before episodic memory—children are able to learn facts before they can remember their own experiences.

The seat of semantic memory is believed to be located in the medial temporal lobe and diencephalic structures of the brain.

See also MEMORY.

senile dementia An older term for Alzheimer's disease. In the past, DEMENTIA was divided into two forms: presenile (affecting people under age 65) and senile (over age 65). Those designations are not used today.

Senile dementia (or senility) was a catchword that for many years had been used to label almost any eccentric behavior in older people. It was equated with such terms as chronic brain failure, chronic brain syndrome, organic brain syndrome, or Alzheimer's.

There are a number of reasons for confusion, forgetfulness, and disorientation besides Alzheimer's disease. Symptoms could be caused by overmedication or medication interaction, chemical imbalances such a lack of potassium, DEPRESSION, sudden illness, malnutrition and dehydration, or social isolation.

senile plaque See BETA AMYLOID PLAQUE.

senility A term that once referred to changes in mental ability caused by old age. However, the term "senile" simply means "old" and therefore, senility does not really describe a disease. It is considered by many people to be a derogatory or prejudicial term.

Most people over age 70 suffer from some amount of impaired memory and reduced ability to concentrate. As a person ages, the risk of DEMENTIA rises, affecting about one of every five people over age 80. Depressive illness and confusion due to physical disease are also common.

serotonin   A chemical found in many tissues of the body that, in the brain, helps transmit nerve signals between nerve cells. It is believed to be involved in mood (especially DEPRESSION) and influences the function of the heart, kidney, immune, and gastrointestinal systems. Any disruption in the synthesis, metabolism, or uptake of serotonin may be partly responsible for a range of mental health problems, including depression and, perhaps, Alzheimer's disease.

Serotonin originates in neurons deep in the brain stem and is found throughout the brain, where it affects a variety of brain functions such as the regulation of anxiety, mood, thought, aggression, appetite, sex drive, and the sleep/wake cycle.

Unfortunately, the serotonin system declines substantially as people get older. In fact, one study noted a 55-percent decline in serotonin receptors in several areas of the brain that persisted even after normal aging changes in the brain were taken into account.

sexual activity   The need for closeness, intimacy, and affection is a very important and natural part of life that involves caring touch, understanding, comfort, and a feeling of safety in relationships. Sexuality is also a natural expression of human need, but for many people sexuality means more than sex—it also involves a broader expression of intimacy.

People with Alzheimer's disease continue to need caring, safe relationships, but they will vary in the ways they can give and receive affection, and the way their dementia affects that ability. Some patients may become demanding and insensitive to the needs of others, and less able to provide caring support. They may also experience changes in their expression of sexuality. While some continue to want sexual contact, others may lose interest; still others may engage in inappropriate sexual behaviors.

Many caregivers may have complicated feelings about continuing a sexual relationship with a partner who has Alzheimer's, ranging from distaste to rejection to guilt.

A patient with Alzheimer's may no longer know how to handle sexual desire, or what is socially acceptable sexual behavior. Some partners find that a patient's desire for sex increases as a result of Alzheimer's, resulting in unreasonable demands at odd times or inappropriate places. Occasionally, a patient may become aggressive if sexual needs are not met. Some caregivers complain they feel like a sexual object because their partner no longer relates to them in an intimate, caring way. Once people with Alzheimer's have had sex, they may immediately forget what has occurred.

On the other hand, many patients lose interest in a physical relationship and may become very withdrawn, refusing to express affection. This can be hurtful to the healthy partner.

Still other patients may lose their inhibitions, make sexual advances to others, or undress or fondle themselves in public. Sometimes patients make a sexual advance because they mistake a stranger for their partner. Sometimes, an action that seems sexual—such as a woman who suddenly lifts her skirt—may simply mean she has to go to the bathroom.

Treatment

Inappropriate behavior should be gently discouraged; distracting the patient or redirecting them to another activity can help. It can be helpful for caregivers to find ways to include different types of touching in everyday life so that the patient gets some physical contact. Massage, holding hands, and embracing are ways caregivers and family members can continue to provide loving touch.

Brain damage can increase a person's desire for sexual activity and decrease inhibitions. The loss of intimacy that occurs as the disease gradually erodes the patient's personality may make it hard for the caregiver to sustain a sexual relationship.

The patient may continue to be sexually satisfied while the partner is no longer emotionally satisfied. Despite these problems, sexual relations can continue to be important. Caregivers can rely on touching, being caressed, and other physical contact as a substitute for the sex act.

shadowing A behavioral problem typical of patients with Alzheimer's disease characterized by following or mimicking the caregiver, or talking, interrupting, and asking questions repeatedly. At times, the patient may become upset if the caregiver wants to be alone. Clinging behavior is especially common in an overwhelming environment.

Treatment

To avoid shadowing, it is important to keep the patient calm, since agitation may trigger episodes of shadowing. Simple, repetitive activities such as folding wash or stuffing envelopes can keep a patient occupied and calm. Headphones for listening to calming music—especially music from the patient's past—are a good idea.

Allowing a patient to snack on low-sugar cereal or sugarless gum may cut down on the endless talking and questions, provided the patient is not prone to choking. A substitute—such as a pet— may provide a friendly distraction and be a source and an object of affection. Support groups can be a good source of innovative ways to handle shadowing and SUNDOWNING.

Short Portable Mental Status Questionnaire (SPMSQ) A series of 10 questions aimed at probing memory, computational ability, and present orientation. It is sometimes used to help diagnose Alzheimer's disease. Questions include such basics as the patient's phone number, name of the current president, and the patient's mother's maiden name.

shouting and screaming It is not unusual for patients with Alzheimer's disease to constantly call for someone or shout the same word over and over again. Patients who constantly scream may feel sick, lonely, or depressed, or they may be experiencing hallucinations.

Patients who shout at night may be reassured if the caregiver installs a night-light in the bedroom. If the patient is anxious about a failing memory, reassuring or distracting may help. Patients who call out for someone from their past may be reassured if the caregiver talks to them about the past. Boredom may trigger some shouting episodes; listening to music may help. If the patient is shouting because there is too much noise in the environment, a quieter room may help.

single photon emission computed tomography (SPECT) A type of brain scan that tracks blood flow and measures brain activity. Less expensive than POSITRON EMISSION TOMOGRAPHY (PET) scans, SPECTs can increase the likelihood of an accurate diagnosis of Alzheimer's disease.

SPECT is a type of radionuclide scanning, a diagnostic technique based on the detection of radiation emitted by radioactive substances introduced into the body. Different radioactive substances (radionuclides) are taken up in greater concentrations by different types of tissues. This gives a clearer picture of organ function than do other scanners.

A classic finding of Alzheimer's via a SPECT study often shows a marked suppression of activity across the entire brain, but especially in the frontal lobes, the parietal lobes, and temporal lobes.

The radioactive substance is swallowed or injected into the bloodstream, where it accumulates in the brain. Gamma radiation (similar to, but shorter than, X rays) is emitted from the brain, detected by a gamma camera, which emits light, and used to produce an image on a screen. Using a principle similar to CT scanning, cross-sectional images can be constructed by a computer from radiation detected by a gamma camera rotating around the patient.

It is also possible to create moving images by using a computer to record a series of images right after the administration of the radionuclide.

This is a safe procedure, requiring only tiny doses of radiation. Because the radioactive substance is ingested or injected, it avoids the risks of some X-ray procedures in which a radiopaque dye is inserted through a catheter into the organ, and unlike radiopaque dyes, radionuclides carry almost no risk of allergy or toxicity.

Using SPECT to increase the chance of a correct diagnosis of Alzheimer's may be essential because some potential treatment options such as drugs or neural transplants might be associated with high risks.

skilled nursing care   A level of care that must be given or supervised by licensed nurses under the general direction of a doctor. Skilled nursing care might include intravenous injections, tube feeding, or changing dressings.

Any service that could be safely performed by the average nonmedical person without the direct supervision of a licensed nurse would not be considered skilled nursing care.

sleep apnea   Episodes of failure to breathe during sleep that may last for 10 seconds or longer, and may be caused either by a failure of the brain's regulation of breathing during sleep, or by excessive muscular relaxation. It is common among patients with Alzheimer's disease.

In central sleep apnea, the patient's airway stays open, but the diaphragm and chest muscles don't work because of a disturbance in the brain's regulation of breathing during sleep.

Obstructive sleep apnea, on the other hand, is more common, and is caused by excessive relaxation during sleep of the muscles of the soft palate at the base of the throat and the uvula. These muscles block the airway, making breathing labored and causing loud snoring. A complete blockage will halt breathing, making the sleeper stop snoring. The pressure to breathe makes muscles of the diaphragm and chest work harder, the blockage is opened, and the patient gasps and briefly wakes. This type of sleep apnea may also be caused by enlarged tonsils and adenoids, a large tongue, or a small airway.

Often, patients experience a combination of central and obstructive sleep apnea, which is characterized by a brief period of central apnea followed by a longer period of obstructive apnea. Snoring is common in this condition.

The periods of arousal during the night are brief and aren't usually remembered; people who experience them will often complain of being sleepy during the day.

Because most people with severe sleep apnea are overweight, the condition is eased with weight loss. In addition, people subject to sleep apnea should not drink alcohol within two hours of going to sleep, and should not take sleeping pills. Both substances slow down the breathing muscle activity, and may worsen the condition.

Patients can find relief by using a continuous positive airway pressure mask worn over the nose and mouth during sleep, which forces oxygen into both nasal passages and the airway to keep them open.

See also SLEEP PROBLEMS.

sleeping pills   Although sleep disturbances can be a frustrating problem for the family of patients with Alzheimer's disease, in general sleeping pills or tranquilizers should be kept to a minimum because they can cause increased confusion in patients.

Barbiturates (such as Seconal or Nembutal) were formerly the preferred sleeping pill, but they can depress breathing and heart function, and lethal overdose is fairly frequent. Combination with alcohol is particularly hazardous.

The drugs used to induce drowsiness (hypnotics and sedatives) are often the same as those used to relieve anxiety (anxiolytics). Although hypnotic medications may worsen the situation by increasing daytime confusion and causing dependence, brief use of short-acting hypnotics may help some patients, as part of a program including keeping the patient awake during the daytime, and late afternoon or early evening walks.

Today, the most popular anxiety relievers and sleep inducers are the benzodiazepines, which enhance the effect of the inhibitory neurotransmitter gamma-aminobutyric acid (GABA). In prescription form, benzodiazepines are relatives of diazepam (Valium) and are marketed as sleeping aids. The three most common are Dalmane, Halcion, and Restoril, which have little effect on breathing or on heart function. The side effects of using this drug include poor coordination, reduced reaction time, and impaired memory. These "hangover" effects occur when the blood level is at its peak and will vary depending on how long the drug remains in the body. They may become ineffective within a few weeks because of tolerance.

Zolpidem (Ambien) is a short-acting drug that is not a benzodiazepine but has a similar mechanism of action.

Preparations containing antihistamines are sold over the counter under such names as Nytol and Sominex. They are fairly safe and may be useful, but tolerance may develop quickly.

For depression associated with disturbed sleep, sedative antidepressant drugs such as amitripty-line (Elavil) and trazodone (Desyrel), are often prescribed.

Antipsychotic drugs (neuroleptics) may provoke sleep in anxious, hallucinating manic, or schizo-phrenic patients.

Many practitioners prescribe diphenhydramine because its side effects are relatively mild, although even this medication can contribute to confusion and may have other undesirable side effects.

sleep problems People with Alzheimer's disease tend to have a variety of sleep problems that may be so severe they lead to placement in a nursing home. Patients with early Alzheimer's often awaken at night and may be extremely confused, wanting to wander outside or act on some delusion.

Sundowning
The most common sleep problem is SUNDOWNING, characterized by pacing, AGITATION, WANDERING, and confusion at night. No one knows what causes sundowning, but some experts suspect it may be related to the lack of sensory input due to darkness or quiet, or changes in biological rhythms.

Indeed, control of the sleep-wake cycle occurs in a small area of the brain called the suprachias-matic nucleus, which tends to deteriorate with age—especially in patients with Alzheimer's. As control of the sleep-wake cycle fades, the patient begins to have problems with sleep patterns. Most doctors prescribe strong sedatives such as thorazine or Mellaril, but these drugs are not consistently effective and can have serious side effects.

Since the biological sleep center becomes defective in Alzheimer's, boosting the response from the sleep center can be useful. The best way to do this is with bright light—especially sunlight. Providing sunlight to the patient in the morning hours can help establish a more normal sleep time around 10 P.M. or 11 P.M. Using this technique while avoiding daytime naps can help normalize the sleep center.

Depression
Depression is also very common in patients with Alzheimer's, which can lead to a major cause of insomnia, trouble staying asleep, and early morning awakening. Treating depression with the appropriate medication is highly effective in helping sleep, and can also help behavior.

Sleep Apnea
Sleep apnea is also more common among Alzheimer's patients. This condition is caused by the obstruction of the air passage into the lungs during sleep. The problem may occur anywhere from 30 to 300 times a night. Snoring and daytime sleepiness are the chief symptoms. Left untreated, the disorder lowers oxygen levels throughout the night that can lead to high blood pressure, heart disease, and strokes. It can also cause fragmented sleep, leading to deteriorating memory problems, depression, and fatigue. The condition can be diagnosed at a sleep center, and treatment is aimed at keeping the airway open by wearing a mask that supplies pressure to the airway, minor surgical operations that open the airway, and dental devices that pull the jaw and tongue forward to open the airway.

Restless Legs
Other sleep disorders that are more common in patients include restless legs syndrome and leg movements during sleep. The movements often interrupt sleep enough to cause daytime sleepiness. Restless legs syndrome, on the other hand, produces uncomfortable sensations in the legs when at rest. The problem occurs mainly in the evening, and relief is obtained by moving the legs. It has a tendency to be more problematic at night, and since walking around or moving or massaging the legs helps, the person often has a difficult time getting to sleep.

Treatments

There are a number of ways to help ease a patient's sleeplessness. First of all, a regular sleeping schedule with no daytime naps and a lot of stimulating activities just before bedtime can improve the problem. Substances such as caffeine, nicotine, and alcohol should be avoided, especially right before going to bed.

Exercise is important, but patients should exercise during the day, not in late evening, because exercise can actually be stimulating. A cup of warm milk right before bed can help soothe patients and induce sleep, especially if background noise is masked in the bedroom throughout the night. A sleep mask and earplugs also may help. Any medications that might be stimulating should be taken long before bedtime.

Some behavioral techniques also can help with sleep problems among patients. Relaxation therapy, sleep restriction, reconditioning, and bright-light therapy are all good methods that can improve sleep problems.

Relaxation therapy tries to help patients ease anxiety and body tension. Sleep restriction is a technique that begins by allowing a person to sleep only for a few hours a night; over time, the hours of sleep are increased until a more normal night's sleep is achieved. Another treatment that may help some patients is to recondition them to associate their bed with sleep. This means a patient may not use a bed for any activity other than sleep and sex.

Bright-light therapy can help patients whose internal clocks have gone awry. In the wintertime, commercial lights provide necessary light exposure to readjust the internal circadian rhythm. People who wake too early may benefit from bright-light therapy in the evening, avoiding sunlight in the morning. Because experts must synchronize the time of light exposure to the patient's body temperature, medical supervision is required.

Sleep problems in patients with Alzheimer's can be a problem as well to the caregiver, who loses sleep by staying up making sure the patient doesn't leave the house. In these cases, inexpensive alarms can be set around the house so that if the patient walks outside a designated area, alarms ring. Simple alarms activated by stepping on a pad or breaking a light beam are available in electronics supply stores. More elaborate sensors are available that can connect with household burglar alarm systems.

small head size The risk of developing Alzheimer's disease is higher for people with small head sizes who also carry an Alzheimer's-related gene, according to a recent study. People with a small head and the gene variant APOLIPOPROTEIN E-4 (apoE-4) are 14 times more likely to develop Alzheimer's than are people without that combination. Having a small head size without the gene did not significantly increase the risk of developing Alzheimer's.

Scientists suggest that this could mean that having a large brain reserve protects against Alzheimer's. Head circumference is one way to measure brain reserve. In this theory, symptoms appear when the loss of brain cells falls below a critical threshold of brain reserve. People with apoE-4 are likely to have more rapid brain cell damage, but people with large brain reserves may have the same changes in their brains, but won't experience symptoms until much later.

The study of head size involved 1,869 healthy Japanese Americans over age 65 in King County, Washington. The study participants were followed for an average of 3.8 years. During that time, 59 people developed Alzheimer's disease. The people who developed Alzheimer's were also older, less educated, shorter, lighter, and had lower estimated verbal IQ scores than those who did not develop Alzheimer's during the study period.

Some scientists wonder if it might be possible to prevent the onset of disease by boosting brain reserves throughout life. In the study, 18 percent of the risk of Alzheimer's was attributable solely to small head size. Therefore, researchers suggest if it were possible to increase brain reserve by preventing brain damage over a lifetime, nearly 20 percent of the disease might be preventable.

Study participants were divided into three groups, based on head circumference. Only the group with the smallest head circumference (less than 21.4 inches) who also had the gene version apoE-4, had a significantly greater risk of Alzheimer's.

smell, sense of Many patients with Alzheimer's disease have problems with their sense of smell, which can affect their appetite and lead to WEIGHT LOSS.

A person is able to smell because odors travel up the nasal cavity to the olfactory nerves, which send electrical signals to the brain where the interpretation of smell occurs. Any glitch along this path will interfere with a person's ability to detect or identify odors.

The sense of smell is made possible because of the presence of smell receptors (specialized nerve cell endings) in a small area of mucous membrane lining the roof of the nose. These receptor cells have cilia that reach down to the surface of the mucous membrane, and are stimulated by odor molecules. When the molecule "keys" fit into the receptor "locks," the process triggers nerve impulses in the olfactory nerve that are transmitted to the brain, where they are translated in parts of the limbic system and frontal lobes.

Because the senses of smell and taste are so intricately intertwined, problems in smell usually affect the ability to taste as well. This is why Alzheimer's patients complain that food has lost its taste.

social withdrawal A behavioral symptom typical of patients with Alzheimer's disease in which they become less interested in interacting socially with those around them.

Society for Neuroscience A nonprofit professional organization of basic scientists and physicians who study the brain and nervous system, including Alzheimer's disease. Founded in 1970, the society has grown from 500 members to more than 29,000 and is the world's largest organization of scientists devoted to the study of the brain.

The society's primary goal is to promote the exchange of information among researchers. For this purpose, the society publishes *The Journal of Neuroscience* and holds an annual meeting each fall. The society is also devoted to education about the latest advances in brain research and the need to make neuroscience research a funding priority.

For contact information, see Appendix I.

special care unit Specialized facilities or areas within an existing nursing home or hospital that offer residential care for patients with Alzheimer's disease and other patients with DEMENTIA. Some BOARD AND CARE HOMES and ASSISTED LIVING FACILITIES also cater to individuals with dementia. Special care units provide an environment, activities, and trained staff designed to address the special needs of people with memory loss and related behavioral problems.

First appearing in the 1980s, special care units have spread quickly over the past 10 years. As of 1996, nearly one in four nursing homes had at least one organized dementia care unit, wing, or program. Dementia-oriented programs include small group activities, short programs, and activities arranged by functional or cognitive ability levels. Dementia-oriented design features include secured exits, small dining rooms, single-occupancy rooms, and special indoor or outdoor areas for wandering.

The most important part of a special care unit is the security, so that residents cannot wander away from the premises. Special care units should have alarms at all exits, and locks on windows. The unit should be uncluttered and well lit, with particularly easy access to toilets (including the use of color coding or pictures on doors), good acoustics to lessen noise, and short distances between bedrooms and activity rooms to minimize confusion.

All staff on the unit should be trained in how to relate to a person with dementia. There should be a minimum ratio of six residents to one staff person. In addition, a special care unit should have staff available who can help residents with cueing during mealtimes, so as to lessen the chance of choking.

Different levels of activities should be available, since higher functioning individuals may resent some activities as childish. Music, exercise, and art projects are good choices for all levels. PET THERAPY and tactile activities are generally designed for later-stage dementia residents.

Staff must be trained in basic safety measures for confused residents to ensure that dangerous substances such as cleaning products, medication, and other products are kept safe. A special care unit should have a process for family input and suggestions, as well as grievances and dispute resolution.

Yet these special units vary widely in quality. Some offer only one special feature, such as a sheltered area for pacing, or specialized staff training. Most have several special features, such as family counseling, support groups, and therapeutic activities for patients. However, the ALZHEIMER'S ASSOCI-ATION cautions that the trend to special care units in nursing homes specifically for people with Alzheimer's may too often be a marketing tool that segregates memory-impaired patients but fails to provide for their special needs.

Because special care units are unregulated in most states, the Alzheimer's Association conducted its own investigation of the quality of care in these units. The association surveyed 112 state ombudspersons, 61 directors of state nursing home licensing agencies, and 453 family members on their experiences with special care units. According to their results, family members are generally satisfied with the special care units. However, more than 20 percent of families report that no efforts were made to adapt the environment to the special needs of patients, or advise the family about alternatives to nursing home placement. In addition, advocates who were surveyed report there is little difference between the care provided in most special care units and that in traditional nursing homes in several important areas.

While there isn't much information about the comparative cost of special care units and more traditional nursing homes, one-third of the families surveyed say they paid more for a special care unit than a conventional nursing home would cost.

There are no definitive studies that prove that either way of providing care to residents with dementia is superior.

Although there are no other regulatory policies covering SCUs, concerns about quality led the Joint Commission on Accreditation of Healthcare Organizations to develop and implement a set of standards for these special units. The Joint Commission is a private, nonprofit organization dedicated to improving quality of care in a variety of healthcare settings. Since 1994, nursing homes have been able to voluntarily submit to a survey process for SCUs using specific standards in hopes of getting accredited by the Joint Commission. A small percentage of nursing homes have thus far sought accreditation.

speech The ability to speak is gradually lost among patients with Alzheimer's disease. In severe Alzheimer's, the ability to speak ends, and communication may drop to about six or seven intelligible words. By late dementia, all verbal abilities are lost.

spongiform encephalopathies A group of rare diseases (including CREUTZFELDT-JAKOB DISEASE) characterized by the spongy appearance of the cortex, diffuse degeneration of neurons in the cerebrum, basal ganglion, and spinal cord, and the proliferation of glial cells in the brain. The diseases cause a rapid, progressive DEMENTIA similar to Alzheimer's disease, but also accompanied by striking rigidity, weakness, and muscle spasms. In addition, there is usually a characteristic brain wave pattern.

There is no specific treatment; the muscle spasms may respond to benzodiazepines such as clonazepam or diazepam.

See also PRION DISEASES.

stages of Alzheimer's disease Most experts divide Alzheimer's disease into three stages: early, middle, and late. Each stage is referenced by degrees of memory loss, activity, sleep disturbance, and other characteristics. While the condition is marked by a slow and gradual decline, not all patients experience the same symptoms and level of function. This variability is one reason why diagnosis can be so challenging in this disease.

For example, experts have found that while AGI-TATION occurs more often in the late stage, 35 percent of the time it also occurs in the first stages of the disease. Therefore, describing agitation as a characteristic of late-stage Alzheimer's could be misleading. WANDERING also occurs across the stages, most often in late disease, but appears in 12 percent of people in the early stages.

While it is fairly certain that in the late stage of disease patients will not be able to take care of themselves, almost any individual characteristic of the condition can occur at any stage.

Early Stage

In the beginning period of the disease, patients typically begin to experience purposeless activity and awaken at night. There may be mild cognitive decline with problems in finding the right word or name. The patient may get lost when traveling to an unfamiliar location, and coworkers become aware of the patient's problems on the job. The patient may read a passage of a book and retain relatively little material, or may lose or misplace valuable objects.

Clinical tests may reveal a problem in concentration, but objective evidence of a memory problem can be discovered only with an intensive interview.

At this point, patients will often deny their illness and experience mild to moderate anxiety. As cognitive abilities continue to decline as this first stage progresses, the person remembers less and less about current and recent events and may show some memory loss for personal history. The person will have more problems in traveling, handling a checkbook, and so on.

Usually patients in this stage know where they are and what day it is, and can recognize familiar persons and faces.

Middle Stage

In the middle stage of Alzheimer's, patients tend to begin forgetting people's names, develop PACING and restless activity, and are often awake half the night. By this stage, patients can no longer survive without some help. Many patients become unable to remember major aspects of their lives, such as their address or telephone number, the names of close family members, or where they went to college.

There is often some confusion as to the date, day of week, and season. In this stage, even an educated person may have trouble counting backward from 40 by fours or from 20 by twos.

People at this stage still remember many major facts about themselves and others, usually knowing their own names and generally remembering the names of their spouse and children. They require no assistance with toileting and eating, but may have some trouble choosing the proper clothing to wear.

As the stage continues, cognitive decline worsens and patients may occasionally forget the name of their spouse. The patient begins to lose the ability to remember recent events and life experiences.

As the stage continues, patients may retain some sketchy knowledge of their past lives, and by now are usually unaware of their surroundings, the year, the season, and so on. They may have trouble counting from 10, both backward and sometimes forward, and they will need some help with ACTIVITIES OF DAILY LIVING. They may become incontinent and need help traveling, although they may still be able to find their way in familiar locations.

Still, patients almost always recall their own names, and they can usually tell the difference between familiar and unfamiliar persons, although most names may elude them in the middle stage.

They may experience significant personality and emotional changes, such as delusional behavior, such as thinking their spouse is an impostor, or talking to imaginary figures in the environment. They may become obsessive and anxious. Some patients may become violent, even if they were never violent before in their life.

Late Stage

By the late stage, patients may forget how to perform basic activities of daily living, even as basic as how to eat. They may mutilate themselves. Sleep patterns are often reversed, so that they sleep during the day and remain awake all night.

In this stage there is very severe cognitive decline, and all verbal abilities will eventually be lost, so that there is no speech at all—only grunting.

Patients are incontinent and require help in eating and toileting. Basic motor skills of walking, sitting, and head control, are lost. The brain appears to no longer be able to tell the body what to do.

statins   See CHOLESTEROL-LOWERING DRUGS.

statistics   About 4 million Americans have Alzheimer's disease, and that number is expected to triple by the middle of this century unless a cure or prevention is found. The likelihood of Alzheimer's increases with age; one in 10 people over 65 and nearly half of those over 85 have the condition. A small percentage of people as young as their 30s and 40s get the disease.

A person with Alzheimer's disease will live an average of eight years, up to as many as 20 years or more from the onset of symptoms.

It is an expensive condition: The disease costs the United States at least $100 billion a year, and neither Medicare nor most private health insurance covers the long-term care most patients need. Yet more than seven of 10 people with Alzheimer's disease live at home, and almost 75 percent of home care is provided by family and friends. The remainder is paid care that costs an average of $12,500 per year. Families pay almost all of that themselves.

Eventually, the burden of caring for a patient with Alzheimer's becomes too great, and many patients must be institutionalized. Half of all nursing home residents suffer from Alzheimer's disease or a related disorder. The average cost for nursing home care is $42,000 per year, but this can quickly exceed $70,000 a year in some areas of the country.

Hoping to find a cure or prevention, the federal government estimates it spent about $466 million for Alzheimer's disease research in 2000. Among that research were at least 17 medicines under development to treat or prevent Alzheimer's disease.

stroke   An interruption of blood to the brain that can damage an area of the brain tissue. A stroke occurs when a blood clot blocks a blood vessel or artery, or when a blood vessel breaks, interrupting blood flow to an area of the brain. When this happens, brain cells die in the immediate area, usually within a few minutes to a few hours after the stroke starts. Doctors call this area of dead cells an infarct.

In the United States, stroke will occur in about 200 out of every 10,000 people each year; incidence rises quickly with age, and is higher in men than in women.

When brain cells die, they release chemicals that set off a chain reaction, endangering brain cells in the surrounding area for which the blood supply is not completely cut off. Without prompt medical treatment, this larger area of brain cells also will die.

When brain cells die, abilities controlled by that area of the brain are lost. Someone who has a small stroke may experience only minor effects, such as weakness of an arm or leg, but a larger stroke may cause partial paralysis or loss of the ability to speak. Some people recover completely from less serious strokes, while others die after very severe strokes.

The brain damage caused by strokes may play a role in determining the onset and severity of Alzheimer's disease symptoms, according to research.

In one study of 102 college-educated nuns over age 67, 61 of the women on autopsy were found to have brain lesions characteristic of Alzheimer's disease. Nearly half of those with Alzheimer's also had one or more areas of brain damage caused by strokes. Those who had this damage plus Alzheimer's lesions had been more demented and had performed significantly worse on tests of mental functioning than those nuns who did not have stroke damage.

Researchers suggest that having these areas of stroke damage in certain key areas of the brain may produce dementia symptoms in those people made susceptible by the brain cell damage caused by their Alzheimer's disease.

Previous research had suggested a relationship between the brain's blood supply and DEMENTIA. More research is needed to clarify the relationship between problems with the blood vessels in the brain and Alzheimer's disease.

About 30 percent of stroke survivors experience dementia, destroying memory and other intellectual abilities. Stroke dementia is common and is found more often among older individuals, smokers, and those with lower levels of education. Stroke survivors who have trouble understanding speech or speaking, who have had a major disability, or who have had other strokes, are most likely to have memory problems as well. Memory loss after a stroke is also linked to people who have had a stroke on the left side of the brain, or whose stroke affects their ability to walk or maintain urinary continence.

Stroke survivors may have dramatically shortened attention spans or they may experience deficits in short-term memory. Survivors also may lose their ability to make plans, understand meaning, learn new tasks, or engage in other complex mental activities. Stroke survivors who develop apraxia lose their ability to plan the steps involved in a complex task and to carry out the steps in the proper sequence. Stroke survivors with apraxia may also have problems following a set of instructions. Apraxia appears to be caused by a disruption of the subtle connections that exist between thought and action.

Cause

A stroke may be caused by any of three mechanisms: cerebral thrombosis, a cerebral embolism, or hemorrhage. Cerebral thrombosis is a blockage by a clot that has built up on the wall of a brain artery, depriving the brain of blood; it is responsible for almost half of all strokes.

Cerebral embolism is a blockage by material that is swept into an artery in the brain from somewhere else in the body, depriving the brain of oxygen. It accounts for up to 30 to 35 percent of strokes.

Less common is a cerebral hemorrhage, the most serious type of stroke. It is caused by the rupture of a blood vessel and bleeding within or over the surface of the brain. Hemorrhages account for about a quarter of all strokes. The hemorrhage is usually from a vessel at the base of the brain, where blood leaks into the brain substance itself, often resulting in coma and paralysis. Death is almost inevitable if the hemorrhage is large.

Symptoms

A stroke that affects the dominant of the two cerebral hemispheres in the brain (usually the left) may cause disturbance of language and speech. Symptoms that last for less than 24 hours followed by a full recovery are known as transient ischemic attacks; such an attack is a warning that a sufficient supply of blood is not reaching part of the brain. If circulation through smaller vessels is not enough, brain tissue may die.

Blockage of the anterior cerebral artery on one side of the brain usually causes paralysis and sensory loss in the limb on the opposite side. If the artery of the dominant hemisphere is affected, mental confusion and speech impairment also may occur.

A blockage of the main branch of the middle cerebral artery on one side produces paralysis and sensory loss on the opposite side, mainly affecting the face and arm. Speech impairment also can occur when the area is in the dominant hemisphere. Blockage of smaller vessels of the middle cerebral artery produces one-sided blindness, inability to read, or to recognize sensory stimuli, or to perform skilled movements in combination or as isolated symptoms.

Blockage in the main part of the posterior cerebral artery on one side causes damage to the thalamus and the visual cortex, with muscular weakness and sensory loss accompanied by burning pain.

Blocking the basilar artery on the underside of the brain is serious, often causing paralysis and sensory loss in all extremities and in the muscles supplied by the brain stem. Blockage of the vertebral artery that runs toward the spinal cord is not usually fatal, although symptoms can be disabling.

A brain hemorrhage of any size is likely to be fatal, whereas the majority of patients with a clot are likely to recover from the initial damage. A number of patients do die in the first weeks after a stroke as a result of complications, such as pneumonia.

Treatment

While there are no proven treatments to reverse memory loss related to stroke, some personality or psychological problems associated with stroke dementia—such as DEPRESSION—may be treated or improved through counseling and social support. Additional progression of the dementia may be halted by preventing a second stroke.

Risk Factors

Certain things can increase the risk of stroke: high blood pressure that weakens the walls of arteries or atherosclerosis (thickening of the lining of arterial walls). Stroke can also be caused by conditions that cause blood clots in the heart that may migrate to the brain: irregular heartbeat, damaged heart valves, or heart attack. Conditions that increase the risk of high blood pressure or atherosclerosis can also cause stroke, such as fatty substances in the blood, high level of red blood cells in the blood. Diabetes mellitus is a risk factor; people with diabetes are five times as likely to have a stroke as nondiabetics. Smokers also have higher risk; those who smoke more than 25 cigarettes a day have three times higher risk of stroke from a clot, and 10 times higher risk of stroke from a burst blood vessel. Those who quit smoking, however, can cut the risk to that of a nonsmoker in just two years.

Oral contraceptives also increase the risk of stroke in women under age 50, but the older high-dose pills were far more dangerous than today's low-dose versions. Women who smoke, use birth control pills, and have migraines appear to have an even greater chance of having a stroke.

African Americans and Hispanics are also at higher risk of stroke, as are pregnant women; stroke is 13 times more common during pregnancy because of changes in blood consistency.

substance P   A small peptide found in high concentrations in areas of the brain that regulate emotional behavior and the biochemical response to stress and that is depleted in patients with Alzheimer's disease. Levels of substance P also rise in the brain and spinal cord in response to pain.

Scientists believe that in the brain, substance P may act on the AMYGDALA, (a pivotal neural area that triggers fear and fear-related memories) and the hypothalamus, important in the stress response.

sundowning   A term used to describe the delirium or worsening of delirium in the late afternoon, often seen in patients with Alzheimer's disease. Patients may become more animated, more confused, more agitated, or hallucinate more aggressively. Often, this behavior continues through the evening and fades away later at night, only to return the next day at about the same time.

While frequently observed, the syndrome is not well researched. The best explanation is that by late in the afternoon fatigue or the accumulated stresses of the day are setting in for patients and they are less able to control their symptoms. Hormonal levels, which rise and fall during the day, don't seem to be related. Nor does the loss of light or change in lighting seem to be a factor.

The problem can be managed with increased support from staff, activities to keep patients involved, and appropriate use of neuroleptic or benzodiazepine medications begun an hour before the uncomfortable behavior is expected to occur.

support groups   Groups aimed at caregivers of patients with Alzheimer's disease can offer valuable support to family members engaged in the stressful responsibility of patient care. Typically, Alzheimer's support groups consist of caregivers and a trained staffer who monitors the group.

To find support groups, caregivers can begin by contacting elder agencies or searching the Internet for Alzheimer's disease news groups, message boards, and online support groups.

suspiciousness   A behavioral trait common among patients in the latter stages of Alzheimer's disease in which they may worry that other people are taking advantage of them or want to hurt them in some way.

For example, when patients with Alzheimer's lose something, they may accuse someone else of stealing from them, or they may imagine that a friend is out to destroy them. Such paranoid ideas may be related in part to a faltering memory or an inability to recognize friends.

When faced with these types of suspicions, caregivers and friends should try to avoid arguing with the patient, but simply state the facts and then reassure or distract the person.

symptoms   While the primary symptom of Alzheimer's disease is memory loss, there are a variety of other signs that most patients exhibit; however, not all patients will experience all symptoms.

In addition to memory loss, about 70 percent of patients experience AGITATION, 60 percent to 70 percent become apathetic, 40 percent to 50 percent develop delusional disorders and psychosis, half are depressed, anxious, or irritable, 30 percent become disinhibited, and 10 percent have HALLUCINATIONS.

At first, Alzheimer's disease destroys brain cells in parts of the brain that control memory, including the HIPPOCAMPUS (a structure deep in the brain that helps to encode short-term memories). As nerve cells in the hippocampus stop working properly, short-term memory fails, and the person's ability to complete familiar tasks begins to decline.

There are a range of simple signs of impending Alzheimer's disease that doctors can identify during the earliest beginning stage of the condition. Repeating stories, forgetting relatives' names and having trouble balancing a checkbook are all early signals of Alzheimer's that doctors should be looking for.

Next, the disease attacks the areas responsible for language and reasoning in the CEREBRAL CORTEX, interfering with language skills, judgment, and personality. Emotional outbursts and behavior such as WANDERING and agitation become more frequent as the disease continues. Eventually, many other areas of the brain shrink and die, and the patient becomes bedridden, incontinent, totally helpless, and unresponsive to the outside world.

Memory Loss

One of the problems with the symptoms of memory loss is that many of them are quite normal, and yet many mimic the early symptoms of Alzheimer's. Of course, not all memory complaints in later life signal Alzheimer's disease or even a mental disorder. Many memory changes are only temporary, such as those that occur during any stressful situation that makes it hard to concentrate. There are major differences between normal behavior and Alzheimer's symptoms:

- *Memory loss:* the memory loss of Alzheimer's often affects daily life and job skills. It's normal to occasionally forget a task or a person's name, but frequent forgetfulness or unexplainable confusion at home or in the workplace may signal something's wrong. It's normal for people to forget where they placed their glasses, but not that they wear glasses.
- *Problems with familiar tasks:* It's normal to forget a pan on the stove, but patients with Alzheimer's might forget to serve an entire meal or even that they made it.
- *Language problems:* It's normal to forget a word sometimes, but a person with Alzheimer's disease forgets many words and also substitutes inappropriate words so that sentences become hard to understand.
- *Disorientation:* It's normal to momentarily forget what day of the week it is, but people with Alzheimer's disease not only forget the day, they get lost on their own street.
- *Poor judgment:* A person with Alzheimer's often exhibits bad judgment; for example, dressing inappropriately or making poor financial decisions.
- *Abstract thinking problems:* Most everyone occasionally forgets a multiplication fact now and then, but people with Alzheimer's forget how to recognize numbers, and can no longer add or subtract.
- *Misplacing things:* It's normal for people to forget their keys, but to forget they have a car is more likely to be indicative of Alzheimer's.
- *Personality changes:* Occasional bad moods are normal, but the personality of a person with Alzheimer's can change dramatically and become suspicious or fearful.

Alzheimer's disease begins slowly with mild forgetfulness that leads to problems finding the right word. Ever so gradually, it progresses to an inability to recognize objects, and ultimately, to an inability to use even the simplest of things, such as a hairbrush. This gradual degeneration often lasts more than 10 years.

People with mild dementia can usually live independently with only minor problems in work or social activities. As the dementia continues, patients may seem capable, but independent living becomes increasingly dangerous. They may begin to dress carelessly and neglect work and family responsibilities, leave the stove or iron turned on, or become lost while away from home. As short-term memory falters, Alzheimer's patients can no longer perform everyday tasks such as zipping a zipper. Behavioral symptoms are also quite common, since the damage to the brain can cause a person to act in different or unpredictable ways. Some people become anxious or aggressive, while others engage in repetitive behavior. Other behavioral symptoms may include AGITATION, COMBATIVENESS,

DELUSIONS, DEPRESSION, HALLUCINATIONS, INSOMNIA, and WANDERING.

As the dementia becomes severe, patients must be constantly supervised. Their language ability disintegrates, and they may string together unrelated words into meaningless sentences. Eventually the failing nervous system affects the entire body and they become completely incapacitated—even unable to eat. Death usually follows as the result of pneumonia or an infection.

Early Identification of Symptoms

When Ohio researchers at the University of Cincinnati Medical Center looked at the records of 50 patients with memory loss or personality changes, scientists found that patients had demonstrated a pattern of symptoms that may be common signs of early Alzheimer's. In fact, 60 percent of the patients had had problems managing their finances or balancing their checkbooks, and a fifth of the family members were concerned by the patient's poor judgment, such as wearing dirty clothes or poor personal cleanliness. Up to 16 percent of family members reported that patients could not perform tasks such as cooking or grocery shopping without some help. Many families also complained that the patients often repeated stories or statements, got lost while driving in familiar areas, and forgot the names of relatives or neighbors.

Although some of the patients had been referred to the center by their doctors, there was no evidence that their doctors had questioned them or their families about any of these symptoms. Patients tend to try to hide these symptoms from their doctors.

Therefore, it may be important for family members to watch for early warning signs such as forgetting names and birthdays, missing appointments, and mismanaging personal finances, since normal memory loss in the elderly should not interfere with a person's ability to carry out these activities.

Although there is no cure for Alzheimer's disease, diagnosing it early may spare patients some of the medical complications, accidents, and financial problems that unrecognized Alzheimer's can bring.

synapse   The point at which a nerve impulse passes from the axon of one nerve cell to a dendrite of another. To send a message, one nerve cell transmits an electrical signal to another by firing across the synapse gap between nerve cells. This triggers the release of neurotransmitters that diffuse across the space between cells, attaching themselves to receptors on the neighboring nerve cell. The receiving cell has receptors that recognize the chemical transmitter and speeds the signal through the nerve cell. The human brain contains about 10 billion nerve cells joined by about 60 trillion synapses.

synuclein   A protein (full name: alpha-synuclein) known to accumulate abnormally in the plaques found in patients with Alzheimer's disease, LEWY BODY DEMENTIA, Parkinson's disease, and in a number of other diseases that are collectively called synucleinopathies.

A rare form of inherited Parkinson's is caused by a mutation in the gene that directs the production of synuclein, triggering the mutated synuclein to clump together. This finding strengthens the idea that abnormal protein deposits are one common thread that links dementing diseases. When abnormal proteins such as synuclein build up on synapses, the chemical information between cells might not be transmitted properly and the circuit might be interrupted.

tacrine (Cognex) The first drug approved by the U.S. Food and Drug Administration (FDA) to treat some of the symptoms of mild to moderate Alzheimer's disease. However, it is now rarely used in the United States and has been replaced by safer drugs.

It works by preventing the breakdown of ACETYLCHOLINE, a brain chemical important to memory. Acetylcholine deficiency is thought to result in memory loss associated with Alzheimer's disease. The drug has been shown to increase cognition in about a third of patients with mild to moderately demented Alzheimer's disease; unfortunately, the drug does not stop the degeneration of brain tissue, and so it cannot cure the disease.

The FDA approved tacrine largely because a 30-week study showed that high doses improve cognition in people with mild to moderate Alzheimer's. Since its approval, clinical experience has been disappointing. Depending on the study, tacrine helps only 20 percent to 40 percent of those who take it. Doctors can't predict who will respond to tacrine, to what extent, and for how long. Tacrine may help somewhat, but only for a minority of people with Alzheimer's.

Side Effects

Side effects are related to the fact that tacrine boosts an enzyme that can lead to liver damage; the long-term effects of this rise remain unclear. About half of patients give up on the drug because of the side effects. Of those who continue, less than half of patients with mild to moderate stages of the disease notice a slight improvement. Patients taking very high dosages of the drug (more than 160 mg per day) show the most improvement, but they also have the high-

est risk for liver damage; discontinuing the drug reverses any liver problems. Other frequent side effects include nausea, vomiting, diarrhea, abdominal pain, indigestion, and skin rash.

Although tacrine can harm liver function during treatment, the risk of permanent damage from long-term treatment is not known. Patients should have their blood tested every other week for at least 16 weeks when first taking tacrine to make sure it's not affecting the liver. If any abnormality in liver function occurs, doctors must adjust the dosage accordingly or discontinue administration of this drug.

tardive dyskinesia A type of movement disorder that occurs in more than 20 percent of patients after continuous medication with neuroleptic drugs, which are sometimes used to treat behavioral symptoms of Alzheimer's disease.

Scientists believe that the disorder appears more often in those who have had acute reactions to neuroleptic drugs. The dyskinesias include facial and limb movements, writing or involuntary movements, and dystonia (posture disorder with spasm in the muscles of the shoulder, neck, and trunk). The involuntary movements are often restricted to the head and neck, such as chewing or tongue-thrusting. Symptoms may fluctuate, taking months or years to disappear after drug withdrawal. About half of the cases are reversible within five years, but some people may never improve. The movements do not typically worsen once a plateau has been reached.

Stopping and starting neuroleptic drugs is not effective, and may even be associated with increased risk of developing tardive dyskinesia.

Treatment is difficult, and many medicines have been suggested, including tetrabenazine and reserpine. Other drugs that have been tried with varying success including baclofen, valproic acid, diazepam, alpha antagonists, amantadine, clonidine, and carbidopa-L-dopa.

tau protein   A kind of protein that plays a critical role in the brain. In healthy nerve cells, the internal support structure (called microtubules) is shaped like two train rails, whose parallel tracks are joined together by crosspieces made of tau protein. These crosspieces function like rungs of a ladder to hold the microtubule "train tracks" apart. Microtubules are essential to healthy cells, since they carry nutrients from the body of the cells down to the ends of axons.

In cells affected by Alzheimer's disease, the tau protein that normally forms the crosspieces between the microtubules begins to twist, like two threads wound around each other, until the entire microtubule collapses and becomes hopelessly entangled. Eventually, the entangled axons shrivel and die.

When scientists look at the brain of a person who has died from Alzheimer's disease, neurofibrillary tangles typically appear throughout the brain. Researchers from the University of Kentucky's Sanders-Brown Center on Aging in Lexington, Kentucky, found a close correlation between the degree of memory problems and the levels of these neurofibrillary tangles.

Together, tau and the protein BETA AMYLOID form the tangles and plaques that have been the hallmarks of the disease since it was first described in 1907 by Alois Alzheimer. Scientists disagree about whether it's the sticky plaques of beta amyloid in the brain or the tangles of tau protein inside brain nerve fibers that play a more central role in the destruction of brain cells. While tangles of tau have been found in the brain of people with Alzheimer's, many scientists believed that tangles were probably a secondary part of the disease. Most Alzheimer's researchers have focused attention on beta amyloid as the substance that kills brain cells.

Others think the mutant protein plaques and tangles are really a marker left by nerve cells killed by some other cause. The key question scientists need to resolve is the relationship between beta amyloid and tau. It's also important to discover if these substances are the triggers of the disease, or merely the by-product of some neurological process gone terribly awry.

television   Although exercising the brain can help prevent Alzheimer's disease, TV watching is not the kind of protective behavior that exercises the brain; in fact, some researchers believe it may even be a risk factor for Alzheimer's. Other research has shown that the onset of Alzheimer's is delayed by education and by intellectually demanding professions.

temporal lobe   The part of the brain that forms much of the lower side of each half of the main mass of the brain (cerebrum). The temporal lobes are concerned with the smell, taste, hearing, visual associations, some aspects of memory, and a person's sense of self. Any interference in the normal function of the temporal lobes may cause peculiarities in any of these functions.

testosterone   A male hormone associated with masculine behavior, aggression, and increased sex drive that also may play a role in fighting Alzheimer's disease. In a recent study conducted with female rats at the University of Texas Medical School at Houston, testosterone injections prevented a key biochemical abnormality occurring in the disease. Alzheimer's occurs in one of 10 people over age 65, nearly half of those over age 85, and about twice as many women as men. The fact that women live longer only partly explains why this occurs.

Animal studies hint that ESTROGEN plays many roles in brain tissue, including the modulation of chemicals involved in relaying messages between nerve cells. Because researchers believe the sudden drop in estrogen in postmenopausal women may trigger Alzheimer's, Estrogen Replacement Therapy has been examined as a potential treatment. However, estrogen's effects on Alzheimer's remain controversial. Some women seem to benefit from ERT, but in one study reported in 2000, patients with mild to moderate Alzheimer's who took estrogen for four months did no better than those taking placebo.

As men get older, they experience only a gradual decline in levels of testosterone, which may be converted to estrogen in certain areas of the brain. Until recently, no one had looked at what testosterone might do for the Alzheimer's brain, because there are a number of problems linked to prescribing testosterone. Testosterone supplements are often abused by body builders, and doctors are less comfortable prescribing testosterone because it is a drug of abuse and extensive safety data are lacking. In addition, testosterone has been studied as a possible cause for aggression in Alzheimer's patients, especially men. As a treatment, experts fear it could have undesirable side effects in people.

Yet other evidence suggests that stress plays a role in the development of Alzheimer's, and hormones such as testosterone have been shown to regulate the brain's stress response. Studies have found that stress leads to a biochemical change in a brain protein that is a primary culprit in Alzheimer's disease.

In one study, rats were stressed and then given daily injections of estrogen or testosterone. The rats who got testosterone showed no sign of the brain changes linked to Alzheimer's in humans. Scientists believe the findings suggest that giving testosterone to aging men or to postmenopausal women may help to delay, prevent, and possibly treat Alzheimer's disease. However, Alzheimer's experts caution that the experiments using rats are a long way from research that can be applied to humans.

Other research suggests that when doctors suppress testosterone levels in men with prostate cancer, they may inadvertently be increasing the level of a substance implicated in Alzheimer's disease. A separate study indicates that when testosterone levels drop, there is a dramatic increase in levels of amyloid protein, the prime suspect in the death of nerve cells in Alzheimer's disease. Some scientists believe that this phenomenon may explain why Alzheimer's disease occurs in late life. People with a genetic predisposition to Alzheimer's may have borderline high amyloid levels until menopause (or the male equivalent, andropause) reduces hormone secretion. Brain amyloid levels may then rise enough to cause amyloid accumulation to begin.

A number of studies have found that hormone replacement therapy in postmenopausal women cuts the risk for Alzheimer's disease in half, leading scientists to speculate that hormones such as estrogen and testosterone might help to break down amyloid.

tetrahydroaminoacridine (THA) Another name for the drug TACRINE (Cognex), which interferes with cholinesterase, an enzyme that breaks down ACETYLCHOLINE, a chemical important in learning and memory that is deficient in the brains of patients with Alzheimer's disease. While THA has helped some patients, its impact on the disease in general has proved disappointing. Three other cholinesterase inhibitors have been approved by the U.S. Food and Drug Administration and work about as well as tacrine.

THA See TETRAHYDROAMINOACRIDINE.

thalamus A crucial brain structure that first receives messages from the body about heat and cold, pain and pressure, smell and taste, and which is active in memory. The thalamus is involved in many cases of memory disorders; tumors in this area can lead to DEMENTIA. The thalamus also seems to regulate cycles of sleep and wakefulness, which is often disordered among patients with Alzheimer's disease.

Named for the Greek word for "chamber" or "inner room," the thalamus is important in the factual memory circuit and serves as the entrance chamber to the perceptual cortex. All sensations except for smell enter the cortex via the thalamus.

thioridazine (Mellaril) One of a major group of antipsychotic drugs, formerly known as major tranquilizers, that are sometimes given to a patient with Alzheimer's disease. It belongs to a group of drugs called phenothiazines that are effective for treating psychoses (such as schizophrenia) but that should not be used to treat anxiety, the loss of mental abilities in nonpsychotic people, to sedate, or to control restless behavior or other problems in nonpsychotic people.

Side Effects
These antipsychotics can cause serious adverse effects, including tardive dyskinesia, drug-induced

parkinsonism, weakness, and muscle fatigue. All antipsychotic drugs tend to exhibit more side effects than antianxiety drugs and are reserved for more severe situations.

toileting problems Eventually, many patients with Alzheimer's disease experience loss of bladder or bowel control due to drugs, stress, environment, or clothing. When incontinence first appears, a doctor should be consulted to rule out a urinary tract infection, weak pelvic muscles, or medications.

If the problem continues, there are a number of things caregivers can do to address the issue. Visual clues such as signs, colorful rugs, or bright lid covers can help a patient find the bathroom. Nearby items that can be mistaken for a toilet, such as a trash can, should be avoided. Caregivers should identify when accidents occur and plan for them. For example, if a patient has an accident after each meal, the caregiver should promptly get the person to the bathroom after eating. Incontinence at night can be avoided by limiting liquids (especially caffeine) after dinner. Clothing should be easy for the individual to remove; Velcro instead of buttons or zippers may help.

Because a person with Alzheimer's may forget to use the bathroom, caregivers should remind the patient from time to time, in addition to noticing cues such as restlessness or facial expressions that may indicate the person needs to use the bathroom.

Touch-Tone telephones Automated touch-tone phone answering systems may one day help screen older callers for early signs of DEMENTIA and Alzheimer's disease. In a study of 155 patients, a Touch-Tone system identified warning signs in 80 percent of patients who had been diagnosed with mental impairments by their doctors. It also gave passing grades to 80 percent of patients diagnosed as normal.

Participants were given recorded instructions such as: "Spell 'fun' on the Touch-Tone pad," and "Press '1' if the following sentence makes sense . . ."

The program is designed as a toll-free telephone triage center for people who may wonder if their forgetfulness is a sign of something more serious.

The research was funded by the NATIONAL INSTITUTE ON AGING.

Many experts suspect there are significant numbers of people with early symptoms of Alzheimer's who could be getting help, and an automated system might be a good, low-cost way to track them down. The system is similar to one used a few years ago on National Depression Screening Day to encourage depressed people to seek treatment.

Experts believe that automated Touch-Tone systems have advantages for people who think they might be losing their mental abilities, because consumers might prefer to take a test themselves before consulting a doctor.

toxins A number of toxins have come under suspicion as a possible cause of Alzheimer's disease or DEMENTIA.

Two amino acids found in seeds of certain legumes in Africa, India, and Guam are known to cause neurological damage. Both enhance the action of the neurotransmitter GLUTAMATE, which is also linked to Alzheimer's disease. In Canada, an outbreak of a brain disorder much like Alzheimer's occurred among people who had eaten mussels contaminated with DEMOIC ACID. This chemical, like the legume amino acids, also stimulates glutamate. While these toxins may not be a common cause of dementia, they could eventually shed some light on the mechanisms that lead to neuron degeneration.

trailing Behavior exhibited by patients in the beginning stages of Alzheimer's disease who may feel extremely insecure and anxious, and who constantly follow a caregiver or family member. Memory loss and confusion about time means that a few moments may seem like hours to a person with dementia; they may feel safe only if a caregiver is nearby.

No matter how frustrating, caregivers should try not to speak sharply to the patient, which will only increase the person's anxiety. Instead, distracting the person with a pet or a familiar toy may be reassuring.

tranquilizers A class of medications only rarely used to treat behavior problems caused by

Alzheimer's disease. These drugs should be used only after other nondrug approaches have failed to improve a person's symptoms. Medication may be needed when patients are in danger of harming themselves or if the caregiver is unable to deal with the situation. Tranquilizers sometimes are divided into major or minor tranquilizers, depending on what they do and how strong they are.

Major Tranquilizers

Also called antipsychotic drugs, these may help relieve more severe AGITATION or psychosis. Low doses of these medications may make the person more comfortable by reducing certain symptoms, such as delusions, suspicion of others (PARANOIA), HALLUCINATIONS, hostility, or AGITATION. These medications also may improve sleep.

However, the side effects of these medications may worsen some symptoms of Alzheimer's disease, such as apathy, withdrawal from family and friends, and the ability to think clearly.

Examples of major tranquilizers sometimes used to treat hallucinations, paranoia, and severe agitation in people with Alzheimer's disease include HALOPERIDOL (Haldol), risperidone (Risperdal), quetiapine (Seroquel), and olanzapine (Zyprexa). Risperidone and olanzapine have fewer side effects than haloperidol.

Men are more likely to receive more potent tranquilizers than women in nursing homes, in part because they experience more behavior problems such as WANDERING, abusiveness, and social impropriety.

Minor Tranquilizers

Minor tranquilizers (antianxiety drugs) relieve anxiety and mild agitation and may help calm the person. However, they can cause drowsiness if the dose is too high. When minor tranquilizers are needed, short-term or occasional use often is better than continuous use. These medications may increase confusion and upset the person's balance, increasing the risk of falls.

In addition, patients may become dependent on these medications over time, worsening symptoms when patients suddenly stop taking them. To avoid this problem, these medications usually are stopped gradually.

Part of a class of drugs called BENZODIAZEPINES, alprazolam (Xanax), and lorazepam (Ativan) are two minor tranquilizers sometimes used in Alzheimer's disease. Another antianxiety medication called buspirone (BuSpar) also can be tried.

treatment There have been four drugs approved for the treatment of Alzheimer's disease. Patients also can be treated by ANTIOXIDANTS and psychotropic drugs to slow the progression of the disease, improve cognition, and reduce behavioral disturbances.

A growing consensus indicates that Alzheimer's is caused by an increase in the production or accumulation of BETA AMYLOID protein that eventually kills brain cells either by oxidative damage or inflammation. Loss of neurons in strategic areas leads to low levels of neurotransmitters, including ACETYLCHOLINE, norepinephrine, and SEROTONIN. The death of brain cells in the HIPPOCAMPUS, temporal, and posterior parietal cortex produces the memory loss, aphasia, and hallucinations. A low level of acetylcholine-producing cells in the basal forebrain contributes to the cognitive and behavioral problems; low levels of serotonin and norepinephrine may play a role in the behavioral problems.

Drug treatment in Alzheimer's has focused on three types of agents: ANTIOXIDANTS such as vitamin E and selegiline; approved Alzheimer's drugs called CHOLINESTERASE INHIBITORS that compensate for transmitter deficits, and psychotropic drugs that ease behavioral symptoms. Various other drugs have been used to treat Alzheimer's, including GINKGO BILOBA and NONSTEROIDAL ANTI-INFLAMMATORY DRUGS, but research has not yet proven these effective.

Managing patients with antioxidants, Alzheimer's drugs, and psychotropic drugs can slow the progression of the disease, improve cognition, and reduce behavioral disturbances, which may enhance patient and caregiver quality of life and put off institutionalization.

Cholinesterase Inhibitors

There are four drugs that have been approved by the U.S. Food and Drug Administration (FDA) for the treatment of Alzheimer's; all other drugs used in this condition are prescribed on an off-label basis. That means it is legal for doctors to prescribe them, but the use has not been officially approved by the FDA for Alzheimer's.

The four drugs that have been approved include TACRINE, DONEPEZIL, RIVASTIGMINE, and GALANTAMINE. These drugs work to offset the drop in acetylcholine that occurs after the death of brain cells that produce it (choline acetyltransferase). These four drugs block the enzyme responsible for the elimination of acetylcholine in the synapse; this boosts the level of available acetylcholine, which improves cell-to-cell communication in the brain.

Unfortunately, these four drugs are only modestly effective in mild to moderate Alzheimer's, and no studies have compared these four drugs among themselves to find out which one works best. Available data do not suggest major differences among them.

The primary differences among them are related to their side effects, half-life and related dosing regimens, and how they are metabolized.

Principal side effects are gastrointestinal and include nausea, vomiting, cramping, and diarrhea. Tacrine is the only drug associated with liver toxicity, which is why this drug requires careful monitoring of liver function tests.

Rivastigmine has been associated with WEIGHT LOSS, so patients must be carefully weighed when on this drug. The appearance of side effects is related to the rate of dose increase.

These drugs should be started at low doses and gradually increased; if side effects appear, the interval between dose increases may be extended or the dose reduced. With this approach to dose, between 75 percent and 90 percent of patients should be able to tolerate the medications.

Evidence suggests that the earlier drug treatment is begun, the better the response. Although the disease will progress and cognitive decline continue after treatment has begun, the level of function remains better than it would have been if untreated. Research suggests that patients should be treated for three to five years until the condition significantly worsens.

Because studies show that nursing home patients with moderately severe dementia continue to respond to the drugs, institutionalization or moderately severe dementia do not mean drugs

must be stopped. When the doctor suggests stopping the drug, it should be withdrawn slowly; if there is clear deterioration in thinking, function, or behavior, the doses should be increased again.

Experts do not recommend combining these drugs, which could be toxic. However, anecdotal evidence suggests that patients who don't respond to one drug may respond to another of the four.

Studies suggest about half of treated patients are restored to the functional level of the previous six months, and about another quarter improve to levels of a year before. Some patients show no benefit at all, while others exhibit marked benefits.

In addition, these drugs improve ACTIVITIES OF DAILY LIVING and behavior, including apathy, visual hallucinations, depression, anxiety, disinhibition, wandering, pacing, rummaging, and delusions.

Antioxidants

Brain cells are injured in part by FREE RADICALS, and scientists suspect that antioxidants may therefore help prevent some of this damage. Two antioxidants—SELEGILINE and vitamin E—have both been shown to slow down the progression of Alzheimer's in patients with mild to moderate dementia.

The principal side effects of high-dose vitamin E are stomach upset and prolonged clotting time with easy bruising or bleeding. Patients who experience these symptoms should reduce their vitamin E dosage. Selegiline may cause anxiety or insomnia, and in rare cases may trigger psychosis.

Alternative Therapy

The efficacy of GINKGO BILOBA and other alternative drugs used to treat Alzheimer's has not been established. ESTROGEN Replacement Therapy in postmenopausal women has been associated with a lessened chance of developing Alzheimer's, which suggests that estrogens might be beneficial in the treatment of women with established Alzheimer's. Recent clinical trials of ERT, however, found no cognitive or behavioral benefits in women with symptoms of Alzheimer's.

Studies also suggest that anti-inflammatory agents lessen the chance of developing Alzheimer's, but it is not clear if nonsteroidal anti-inflammatory drugs (such as ibuprofen) improve thinking clarity in Alzheimer's. Giving the anti-inflammatory steroid prednisone to patients with Alzheimer's produced no cognitive improvement and worsened behavioral disturbances compared with placebo.

Psychotropic Drugs

Psychotropic drugs are used to treat behavioral disturbances in Alzheimer's, such as AGITATION, psychosis, DEPRESSION, ANXIETY, and INSOMNIA. Major TRANQUILIZERS including risperidone (Risperdal), olanzapine (Zyprexa), quetiapine (Seroquel), and haloperidol (Haldol), all significantly reduce behavioral problems.

Agitation occurs in up to 70 percent of patients and is more likely as the disease advances, triggered by pain, environmental disturbances, delusions, or depression. Because agitation may lead to aggression, it often requires drug treatment. Classes of drugs used to treat agitation include antipsychotics, mood-stabilizing anticonvulsants, the antidepressant trazodone (Desyrel), anti-anxiety medications, and beta blockers. Evidence suggests that the best choices for easing agitation are neuroleptics, trazodone, or anticonvulsants. Side effects (such as tardive dyskinesia and parkinsonism) are more common with haloperidol than with antipsychotics or trazodone, and neuroleptics may worsen cognitive problems. Carbamazepine and valproic acid also have been shown to reduce agitation in patients with Alzheimer's.

About half of all patients become psychotic, experiencing delusions of theft and infidelity, and by misidentification. Hallucinations are relatively rare, occurring in only about 10 percent of patients. Atypical antipsychotics are the treatment of choice for patients with psychotic symptoms, including risperidone, olanzapine, quetiapine, and ziprasidone. Clozapine requires weekly monitoring of white blood cell counts and is not normally used to treat Alzheimer's patients. Although neuroleptics such as haloperidol also reduce psychotic symptoms, they carry a greater risk of side effects.

Up to half of all patients also become depressed, but major depression is more unusual, occurring in just 6 percent to 10 percent of patients. Depression in Alzheimer's disease is usually treated with the newer antidepressant class—selective serotonin reuptake inhibitors (SSRIs such as sertraline, citalopram, or fluoxetine). Alternatively, antidepressants such as nortriptyline or venlafaxine have been used. However, there have been few studies that have established the usefulness of antidepressants in the treatment of mood symptoms among patients with Alzheimer's.

Up to half of all patients also experience anxiety at some point in the course of the illness, but most patients do not need drug treatment for this. For those who do, benzodiazepines are not a good choice because of their negative effects on thinking and memory. Anti-anxiety drugs such as buspirone (BuSpar) are preferred.

Insomnia occurs at some point in the course of the illness in many patients with Alzheimer's, and many patients totally reverse their day and nighttime hours. This may disturb the sleep of caregivers, thus increasing the family stress. Drugs such as temazepam, zolpidem, or zaleplon, or sedating antidepressants such as trazodone, may help manage insomnia. It may also be helpful to limit daytime naps and morning exposure to sunlight, manage pain, and restrict fluids at night.

tube feeding   Patients with advanced DEMENTIA (including Alzheimer's disease) often develop eating problems and lose weight. Feeding tubes are often used in this situation, even though the benefits and risk of this therapy are not clear.

Families face enormous pressure to use all available medical technology to keep their relatives alive, often leading them to make decisions that may not be in the best interests of the patient. Many people with dementia may express wishes ahead of time not to be kept alive artificially.

Researchers at Johns Hopkins Geriatrics Center in Baltimore found that tube feeding does not prevent aspiration pneumonia, prolong survival, reduce the risk of sores or infections, improve function, or keep the patient comfortable. Instead, researchers discovered there are substantial risks with tube feeding.

Instead, researchers say a comprehensive, conscientious program of hand feeding is the best treatment for severely demented patients with eating problems.

The official position of the ALZHEIMER'S ASSOCIATION is that when a severely demented patient has previously made his or her wishes known and when there is coexisting illness, it is ethically permissible for the physician to withhold treatment that would serve mainly to prolong the dying process. When there is no prior expression or a living will, responsible family members or the patient's guardian should indicate their wishes about treatment.

The association further believes that severely and irreversibly demented patients need only care given to make them comfortable, and if such a patient rejects food and water by mouth, it is ethically permissible to withhold nutrition and hydration artificially administered by vein or gastric tube.

tyrosine An amino acid that is associated with alertness. Scientists have found that tyrosine supplements may improve alertness and boost cognitive performance. However, some scientists caution that taking large doses of any amino acid may eventually disrupt the body's metabolic system.

vacations Vacations are a good way to relax and escape some of the stress of caregiving. But before taking a patient with Alzheimer's disease on a trip, it's important for family members to consider the person's level of impairment, and what adaptations might need to be made so that a vacation can be relaxing and enjoyable for everyone.

First, family members should think carefully about what the patient can handle. The responsibilities of caring for a patient with Alzheimer's won't disappear on vacation, so there may be a limit to how restful and relaxing the getaway would be. Some families decide instead to arrange respite care at home for the patient with Alzheimer's. Although some family members might feel guilty, in fact it may well be that the patient would be more comfortable at home in a secure environment.

If the patient is going along on vacation, it's a good idea to take the sort of trip the patient is used to taking. If the patient has never flown on an airplane, it's probably not a good idea to start now. It's also a good idea to vacation somewhere fairly close to home so the patient won't have to be traveling for long periods of time.

Quiet, calm destinations are usually a better choice than a busy, noisy, overstimulating location such as a large city, that may cause a patient to feel anxious. Even large amusement parks or visiting a large, noisy family can trigger anxious moments for a patient with Alzheimer's.

Caregivers traveling with a patient for the first time may want to consider a short trip to see how the person reacts to traveling. If it works out well, then a longer trip can be planned later. Likewise, it's a good idea to plan a vacation with a safety net, in case it doesn't work out. Vacation packages should allow you to leave early without financial penalty if the person becomes ill or wants to return home. Alternatively, trip insurance is another good way to protect your investment.

Caregivers should advise airlines, hotels, and tour operators of the patient's condition. Identification tags are a must for a traveling patient, with the names of the caregiver and patient. The caregiver should handle all credit cards, travelers' checks, and passports.

A patient should never be left alone or with a stranger. Even if the stranger seems well intentioned, a person who is not familiar with the disease may not understand how to react in a difficult situation.

When to tell the patient of the upcoming trip depends on the person's condition. Some patients can be told in advance so as to feel a part of the preparations. Others can simply be told shortly before leaving with a simple explanation. Still others may deal with the trip best by being told on the day of the trip itself.

When traveling, caregivers should plan plenty of breaks for snacks, and anticipate delays. It's a good idea to call ahead to see if there will be any delays in departure, and to avoid having to drive or handle luggage if possible. Items such as magazines or tapes may help keep the patient relaxed during travel.

Restroom use can be a problem if the patient and caregiver are of the opposite sex. If possible, the patient should always be accompanied into the bathroom with someone, either a friend or staff member.

While traveling it's a good idea to maintain a typical routine as much as possible, keeping eating and sleeping patterns the same as at home. Quiet, calm restaurants and hotels are helpful. Search for the same types of food the patient is used to at home. If the patient showers each night, the same pattern should be maintained while traveling.

vaccine Studies of a vaccine treatment for Alzheimer's disease were stopped in 2002 when 12 Alzheimer's patients injected with the experimental vaccine began to suffer with serious brain inflammation. Elan Corp., Ireland's largest pharmaceutical company which manufactures the vaccine, halted the experiment when it discovered that the first four patients (all from France) suffered an encephalitis-like reaction. Since then, doctors have discovered eight more people with the apparent side effect, which can be hard to distinguish from worsening Alzheimer's. All 12 were stable or improving after the vaccine was stopped.

The negative reactions raised serious questions about the future of Elan's highly touted vaccine, which had excited researchers in 2000 when it was discovered that in mice, the compound could ward off and even reduce the brain-clogging plaques that are a hallmark of Alzheimer's.

Initial safety tests in British patients showed no signs of serious side effects, but because the vaccine works by inducing the immune system to attack the BETA AMYLOID protein making up those plaques, some scientists warned that inflammation was a potentially serious side effect. It was a serious enough concern that participants in the latest 360-patient study were warned about the potential risk.

The study might be able to continue if there were some way to identify who is at highest risk of the reaction, but Elan's oversight panel and government regulators would have to agree.

In 1999, researchers at Elan Corporation of south San Francisco reported that they had used a fragment of beta amyloid protein to vaccinate mice genetically engineered to develop plaques. Experts theorized that the vaccine would stimulate a person's immune system to recognize and attack the harmful beta amyloid protein. A year after the vaccination, seven out of nine mice remained plaque free. Then scientists vaccinated year-old mice whose brains were already riddled with plaques and discovered that the plaques started to melt away!

A recent study by NIA-funded researchers at Harvard Medical School provided a second approach to using the immune response to remove amyloid plaques. These researchers used the same amyloid as that used in the vaccine but administered it nasally rather than through injections. They found that the nasal administration induced an immune response in the mice; when young mice were given the human beta amyloid by this route, they had a much lower amyloid burden at middle age than did animals that did not receive the vaccine. Although the nasal administration was not as effective as the original vaccination method, these results open the door to an alternative approach that may be better tolerated long-term than the injected amyloid vaccine.

vagus nerve stimulation (VNS) A type of treatment that early research suggests may help treat mild to moderate Alzheimer's disease.

The vagus nerve is also known as the 10th cranial nerve, which is responsible for breathing, swallowing, taste, circulation, and digestion. It is a primary component of the parasympathetic nervous system, and affects other organs by releasing ACETYLCHOLINE, which is deficient in patients with Alzheimer's. Some experts think that stimulating this nerve might boost levels of acetylcholine, easing Alzheimer's symptoms.

In one study, after three months of VNS treatment, eight of the 10 patients with Alzheimer's either improved, or had no worsening of symptoms. Of the eight responders, six had improved symptoms and two had no worsening. After six months of VNS, seven of the eight initial responders continued to maintain improvements in symptoms compared to their baseline assessments. Normally, Alzheimer's patients would worsen each year.

VNS has been used for years to treat epilepsy, in which side effects are mild and well-tolerated.

Alzheimer's is considered a "forgetful dementia" because its most common first symptom is the rapid forgetting of recently learned material. Scientists wondered if VNS might be effective because of treatment-related improvements in memory reported both in animal research and in patients with epilepsy.

Animal studies in 1998 showed that stimulating the vagus nerve enhanced memory storage; 1999 studies found that VNS enhanced recognition memory or verbal learning by 35 percent. Many epilepsy patients and their physicians have also reported an improvement in memory following VNS.

As of September 30, 2001, the VNS Patient Outcome Registry had data on 3,351 epilepsy patients treated with VNS for three months and 1,721 patients treated with VNS for one year; 26 percent of those patients treated for three months and 33 percent of those treated for a year reported that their memory was better or much better. Alertness was better or much better in 56 percent of patients after three months of VNS and 61 percent of patients after one year of VNS.

vasopressin Another name for ADH (antidiuretic hormone), this chemical functions as a neurotransmitter in the brain that some consider to be the ink with which memories are written.

Vasopressin is released from the pituitary gland and acts on the kidneys to increase their reabsorption of water into the blood. External vasopressin is approved for treatment of diabetes as a way to prevent the frequent urination common in the disease. It is given via the nose or by injection, and has also been studied as a possible treatment for Alzheimer's disease.

Research has shown that when subjects are given vasopressin, they remember long lists of words better and seem to encode better.

Vasopressin is available by prescription in the United States, and is available in a nasal spray bottle. However, it can produce a range of side effects from congestion to headache, and increased bowel movements, abdominal cramps, nausea, drowsiness, and confusion. Because it temporarily constricts blood vessels, it should not be used by anyone with high blood pressure, angina, or atherosclerosis, and should be used cautiously by patients with epilepsy.

verbal memory Memory for verbal information. Verbal memory is assumed to reflect functioning of the deep structures of the left temporal lobe.

vinpocetine A compound derived from vincamine, a chemical found in the leaves of periwinkle as well as the seeds of various African plants, that may enhance memory. Developed in Hungary more than 20 years ago, vinpocetine is sold in Europe as a drug under the name Cavinton. In the United States, vinpocetine is available as a dietary supplement.

Vinpocetine doesn't exist to any significant extent in nature, and producing it requires significant chemical work. A significant volume of evidence supports the idea that vinpocetine can enhance memory and mental function, especially in those with Alzheimer's disease and related conditions. It might help those with ordinary age-related memory loss as well, although this has not been proven.

Vinpocetine is available in 10 mg capsules, usually taken three times a day, and is absorbed best when taken with meals. It should not be combined with blood-thinning drugs such as Coumadin (warfarin), heparin, aspirin, or Trental (pentoxifylline), except on the advice of a doctor. Vinpocetine might also interact with natural substances that thin the blood as well, including ginkgo, phosphatidylserine (PS), garlic, and high-dose vitamin E. Safety in pregnant women or people with severe liver or kidney disease has not been established.

viruses and Alzheimer's disease Various researchers have suggested that suspicious brain tissue changes in Alzheimer's disease may be caused by a virus, because a slow-acting viruslike particle has been identified as a cause of some brain disorders that closely resemble Alzheimer's disease (such as CREUTZFELDT-JAKOB DISEASE). However, no virus has ever been isolated from the brains of those with Alzheimer's disease, and no immune reaction has been found in the brains of Alzheimer's patients like that found in patients with other viral dementias.

Still, the theory persists that a slow virus, which lurks in the body for decades before being stimulated into action, may be linked to the development of Alzheimer's. Some scientists think that people with a genetic susceptibility to Alzheimer's may be vulnerable to certain viruses, particularly under circumstances when the immune system is weakened.

In one study, researchers discovered that the risk for Alzheimer's was very high in people with both the APOE-4 gene (a gene version linked to Alzheimer's) and evidence of herpes virus (HSV) 1, a form of herpes that causes cold sores. Furthermore, research is finding that parts of the HSV-1 protein strongly resemble BETA AMYLOID, a protein found throughout the brain plaques so common in the disease. Most Americans are infected during childhood with HSV-1, and while most people who are exposed to HSV-1 do not develop Alzheimer's, it appears that those genetically disposed to Alzheimer's are more likely to develop the disease if they are exposed to herpes.

visiting   Maintaining social contacts can be beneficial for patients with Alzheimer's disease, but arranging social visits takes extra planning and effort.

Many times, friends, acquaintances, and even family members may hesitate to spend time with a patient because they worry about not knowing what to do or say. Others may not understand the behavior changes that are caused by the disease, and feel uncomfortable about visiting.

By addressing each of these concerns, caregivers can maintain important social interactions for patients with Alzheimer's.

Caregivers should be the first to invite visitors to the home, because friends and family may be reluctant to take the first step. Caregivers should explain why social visits are important and suggest a specific date that would be convenient.

To make the most of social occasions, caregivers should discuss the patient's condition with visitors beforehand, warning that the person might look or act differently than before the diagnosis. Visitors should be warned about specific behavior changes, such as fidgeting or WANDERING. Caregivers should also suggest ways to communicate more easily with the patient. Visitors should understand that one-on-one visits are better than large crowds, and that the patient may repeat things or ask repetitive questions. Knowing what to expect beforehand can ease a visitor's nervousness.

Visitors should understand that the visit is to provide a social interaction for the patient, not because the caregiver wants some time off. Rather than simply sitting around the living room, many caregivers find that specific activities such as going

to lunch, taking a walk, or looking through photos enrich the social interaction and help ease discomfort for visitors. Reading from a book or singing a song that is special to the patient may be other helpful activities.

If the patient is invited to someone else's home, the visit should be kept relatively short. It may be a good idea to bring along a favorite photo album, book, or music tape to help occupy the patient during the visit.

Visits at the Nursing Home

Putting a family member in a nursing home because of Alzheimer's is a stressful situation, but frequent visits from friends and family members are still appreciated by the patient. Family members should get to know the staff and ask questions about special problems. Visitors should be apprised of the patient's condition, and told how long a visit is possible. Simple activities such as giving the person a small gift, reading a poem, or singing a story can be enjoyable.

Visitors should leave a card or note when they have visited, or sign a guest book in the person's room.

visual memory   The ability to take in, store, and retrieve information presented visually. Short-term visual memory is the ability to hold visual information in short-term memory in order to process it, either moving it into long-term memory or shifting focus.

Visual working memory (or nonverbal working memory) involves the ability to hold visual information in mind while considering it, reflecting on it, or in some other fashion processing it.

Long-term memory also involves visual forms, in which images are stored on a long-term basis and available for recall.

vitamins   All communication in the brain depends on the function of NEUROTRANSMITTERS— chemicals that relay signals throughout the brain. To manufacture these important neurotransmitters, the brain needs supplies of at least three B vitamins: FOLIC ACID, B_6, and B_{12}.

While the link between vitamins and cognition and memory has been controversial, some studies have shown that better nutrition can lead to improved learning and IQ. Several other studies suggest that getting too little of these vitamins (especially folic acid and B_{12}) may interfere with mental well-being.

Nutritionists have known for some time that severe deficiencies of the B vitamins can lead to memory problems. While many cases of poor memory are not eased by popping extra vitamins, it is true that nutrition can influence the health of the brain. In particular, if the body's level of B vitamins drops, memory performance can falter.

About 5 percent of dementia cases are caused by poor nutrition, especially of the B vitamins: thiamin (B_1), niacin (B_3), folate (folic acid), and vitamin B_{12}. Of these, folate and B_{12} deficiencies are most common. For this reason, blood tests to assess B vitamin levels are a standard part of the clinical assessment for Alzheimer's disease. The best sources of B vitamins are kidney beans, chickpeas, lentils, green leafy vegetables, grains, and orange juice. B_6 is found in beef, poultry, and seafood.

Though it was previously thought that age-related cognitive decline was inevitable, research now suggests that deficiencies of folate or vitamin B_{12} and high levels of HOMOCYSTEINE are associated with cognitive impairment and DEMENTIA. One study found significant negative effects on cognition in the elderly subjects who had deficiencies of folic acid or vitamin B_{12} and high levels of homocysteine.

Niacin (B_3)

Niacin (B_3) may be a memory enhancer, according to some research; in one study subjects improved their memory between 10 percent and 40 percent simply by taking 140 mg of niacin a day.

B_12

B_{12} is important to memory, but it can't be absorbed by up to 20 percent of people over age 60 and up to 40 percent of those over age 80. For this reason, older people should eat cereals fortified with B_{12}, or take a multivitamin supplement—this way, the vitamin is more easily absorbed by the body. Vitamin B_{12} problems also appear in those vegetarians who don't eat eggs, fish, or dairy products, and therefore don't get vitamin B_{12}.

Choline

Scientists at the University of North Carolina discovered that rat mothers who don't get enough of the B vitamin choline may permanently affect the development of learning and memory centers in the brains of their developing infants. Whether this is true in pregnant humans is not known.

Folic Acid

Folic acid has been closely linked to dementia in the elderly; among healthy people, low levels of folic acid have been linked to lower scores on memory tests. This vitamin is contained in a wide variety of foods, especially liver and raw vegetables, legumes, nuts, avocados, cereals, and spinach and other leafy greens. Normally, a well-balanced diet provides enough folic acid, but low-dose supplements (200–500 micrograms) seem safe. However, taking high doses of folic acid requires medical supervision.

Antioxidant Vitamins

Taking vitamin C and E supplements may help protect memory with age by absorbing harmful FREE RADICALS—highly reactive compounds that are released during normal chemical reactions in the body, attacking other cell substances and damaging the cell wall, metabolic machinery, and genetic material. Cells have natural defenses against this damage, which include the antioxidants vitamins C and E, but with age some of these protective mechanisms decline.

Research clearly shows that free radicals damage the brain during normal aging, and also in Alzheimer's disease. Therefore, antioxidants—which can neutralize cell-damaging free radicals—could theoretically help improve memory. In fact, vitamin E has been tested primarily in Alzheimer's disease patients and has been shown to slow the progression of the disease by about seven months.

In one study, vitamins C and E were more effective as a preventive to memory loss, helping men perform better on tests of memory, creativity, and mental sharpness. The vitamins did seem to help prevent men from developing two types of dementia, but not the dementia related to Alzheimer's disease. In addition, studies have found that men who took vitamins for many years showed a much better improvement, which suggests that long-term use of vitamins is needed to boost memory later in life. Vitamin E acts as a blood thinner, and should not be combined with blood-thinning medications or substances such as ginkgo biloba. Patients should consult a doctor before taking vitamin E, especially if they are at risk for bleeding problems.

Columbia University researchers found that patients in the early stages of Alzheimer's who took vitamin E for two years were able to fight off more advanced stages of the disease for a longer period than those who took a placebo. Participants who took vitamin E took significantly longer to reach one of these points than the placebo group, although they didn't demonstrate an improvement in symptoms.

In one Columbia University study, moderate-stage Alzheimer patients who for two years ingested either vitamin E or SELEGILINE, a drug normally prescribed for Parkinson's disease, took a significantly longer time to reach more advanced stages of the disease than those who took a placebo. The research was funded by the NATIONAL INSTITUTE ON AGING and is reported in the April 24, 1997, issue of the *New England Journal of Medicine*.

Although the research is encouraging, experts say it is premature to actually recommend vitamin E or selegiline as a specific treatment for Alzheimer's disease without additional confirming research. However, since previous research has demonstrated that vitamin E has other health benefits, there seems to be no reason not to take vitamin E in moderation.

The Recommended Dietary Allowance for vitamin E is 30 International Units (I.U.) a day. Previous research has shown that vitamin E can help prevent cardiovascular disease, increase immune response capability and possibly help protect against some cancers, though some studies did not show these positive effects. Natural sources of vitamin E include green, leafy vegetables, vegetable oils, nuts, seeds, seed oils, whole grains, wheat germ, rice, sweet potatoes, and avocados.

In the Alzheimer's disease study, participants received significantly larger amounts of vitamin E than are available with normal dietary intake. Vitamin E is available in vitamin supplements, but

little is known about the effects of high doses or possible interactions with other drugs. Vitamin E may be associated with increased bleeding and may cause muscle weakness, headaches, nausea, and vomiting.

In the study, 341 moderate stage Alzheimer patients received selegiline (10 mg per day), vitamin E (2,000 IU per day), both, or a placebo for two years, and were followed to see when they either died, were institutionalized, became unable to do certain basic ACTIVITIES OF DAILY LIVING, or developed severe dementia. Those who took vitamin E or selegiline took significantly longer to reach one of these outcomes. There was no evidence of added benefit with combined treatment using both drugs.

According to the researchers, it is not clear yet if the drugs were having an effect specifically on the disease process or on the overall health of the participants. While the study was not designed to measure whether the people in the trial got better, it did show that it took them longer to get worse.

Vitamin E costs less and worked at least as well as selegiline on Alzheimer's progression, with fewer side effects. For these reasons it is preferred over selegiline in Alzheimer's disease treatment. Vitamin E is considered to be a harmless medication that most people can take without side effects.

People taking blood thinners such as warfarin (Coumadin) or ticlopidine (Ticlid) may not be able to take vitamin E.

Doctors aren't sure what the best dose of vitamin E may be, but the doses of vitamin E in the study were 1,200 IU twice daily. Many doctors recommend 400 IU twice daily because they believe this dosage to be safe for most individuals and it should have the antioxidant effect desired in the brain.

Supplements

Although patients who have thinking problems may not eat well and could therefore have a vitamin deficiency as a result of their dementia, several studies have shown that people with both dementia and B_{12} deficiencies recover when given the vitamin by injection. Other studies have shown that when people with folate and niacin deficiencies have experienced mental improvement when they received supplemental vitamins. Unfortunately, only about 25 percent of those with dementia due to thiamine deficiency recover completely when given supplements; another 50 percent show partial recovery. Thiamine deficiency is usually seen in alcoholic patients, but it also can be found among depressed people and pregnant women suffering from chronic vomiting.

wandering   One of the hallmarks of Alzheimer's disease in which the patient paces around a room, follows a caregiver from room to room, or wanders away from home. Up to 60 percent of patients with Alzheimer's disease will wander and become lost at least once during the course of the disease, and up to 46 percent of those wanderers may die if they are not found within the first 24 hours.

For this reason, patients should wear Medic-Alert bracelets with their address in case they do get lost. The outlook for patients who do wander away from home is not good. Less than 4 percent of memory-impaired adults who wander away from home are able to return unassisted, according to a University of Florida study.

Wandering happens even in the best caregiving situations, especially if the patient becomes angry or agitated. In fact, from 675 missing and discovery incidents reported nationwide to ALZHEIMER'S ASSOCIATION SAFE RETURN over a 13-month period, nearly 20 percent of the memory-impaired adults found wandering in communities left from nursing homes. Too often, caregivers are embarrassed to call for help, but it is critical that a missing-person report be filed as soon as the patient has been discovered as missing.

Law enforcement searches should begin immediately and be concentrated within a five-mile radius of the person's home. It is also crucial to continue searching throughout the night because these adults often will not stop to sleep, but will continue to wander. Wandering into the community without supervision is a major problem among people who are memory impaired, and can cause injury or death.

In a recent Florida study, about 82 percent of memory-impaired wanderers were found within the first 12 hours after they were last seen, with 43 percent found between noon and 6 P.M. Although afternoon was the most likely time for these wanderers to be discovered, 19.6 percent were located between 6 and 9 P.M. and 17.8 percent between 9 P.M. and 7 A.M. Nearly half (46.1 percent) were found in under five hours, with only 9.2 percent missing more than 24 hours. One person was missing four days. Almost one-fourth of these individuals left during evening and nighttime hours. Nearly half (49 percent) were found between one and five miles away from where they were last seen, while 37 percent were found less than one mile from home. The remaining 14 percent were found more than five miles away.

Places where the memory-impaired wanderers have been found highlight their unpredictable behavior. More than a fourth were found in residential yards, and 22 percent were found standing in the middle of streets. In addition, 11.8 percent were found in businesses, 9.2 percent at health-care facilities, 5.8 percent at public access areas, 3.9 percent in shopping centers, 3.7 percent standing on sidewalks, 3.4 percent along highways, 3.1 percent at convenience stores and 3.1 percent in restaurants. Only 1.8 percent were found in remote natural areas, 1.6 percent in parking lots, 1.6 percent in food stores, 1 percent in banks, 0.8 percent along railroad tracks and 0.8 percent in senior care centers. Of those found in remote areas, all were found dead.

Most wanderers (84 percent) in the study walked away from their caregivers, with only 5.6 percent driving away. The remainder used public transportation. All those who drove a car were found within 24 hours. All those missing for more than 24 hours were on foot with the exception of one who had taken a train. In this study, only four wanderers were found dead.

Wanderers were most likely to be found by Good Samaritans or law enforcement officials, despite the lack of missing-person reports in most cases. However, when a report was filed, the wanderer was much more likely to be found by police.

To prevent a patient from leaving the house at night, deadbolt locks should be installed on the main doors. Wandering that occurs at a certain time of the day may be reduced by involving the patient in strenuous activity right before that time. Discouraging naps during the day and evening intake of liquids can help reduce wandering. Encouraging movement and exercise can help reduce wandering. Wandering that occurs at night may be avoided by having the patient get more exercise during the day. The patient should be allowed to walk around in a secured environment such as a fenced yard as a part of the daily routine.

Safety gates should be installed across doors and on openings at the top and bottom of stairs to help keep patients in a limited area where they can wander safely. It is also a good idea to set up a place in the home where the patient can wander safely.

See also ALZHEIMER'S ASSOCIATION SAFE RETURN.

weight loss   Some amount of weight loss is typical in patients with Alzheimer's disease as the condition progresses. The weight loss occurs for a number of reasons; first, calories can be burned due to the constant restless activity typical of the condition. Most patients also don't smell as well as they did before, so food is less appealing. Patients in the early stages of disease who may be suffering with DEPRESSION may lose their appetite. Eventually, patients in more advanced stages of Alzheimer's may forget how to eat and have a decreased response to hunger.

While weight loss is a typical part of the disease process, the sight of the patient gradually losing weight can trigger guilt among caregivers and family members. Family members who aren't around the patient on a daily basis may interpret weight loss as the result of poor care.

Patients who are losing weight should be evaluated to make sure there is no other medical cause of the problem; if there is none, then the loss is considered to be part of the disease process. Nutritional supplements can be given to reverse a weight loss trend.

Patients with significant weight loss to the point where they are malnourished should not continue to follow a low cholesterol, low salt, or any other restrictive diet, unless absolutely necessary. Even "junk food" is acceptable if it can stimulate a patient's appetite.

Wernicke's area   A part of the brain located in the TEMPORAL LOBE near the primary auditory cortex that is critical to language comprehension, especially at the level of the meaning of individual words (rather than syntax, which is regulated by Broca's area.) Damage to this part of the brain results in Wernicke's aphasia, which makes individuals unable to understand words while listening, and unable to produce meaningful sentences.

wine   There is a possible relationship between moderate consumption of wine and a reduced risk of Alzheimer's disease, according to a 1997 French study of more than 3,600 people over age 65 that compared the amount of wine they drank with testing for Alzheimer's disease. (Wine represents 97 percent of alcohol consumption in Bordeaux, France, where the study was done.)

The researchers found that those people who drank moderate amounts of wine were less likely to have Alzheimer's disease than were people who drank only a little, or who drank a lot. For this study's purpose, moderate consumption was defined as three to four glasses per day.

However, just because those who drank moderate amounts of wine had less chance of having Alzheimer's does not mean there is a direct, cause-and-effect relationship. More research is needed to investigate and explain the results.

The ALZHEIMER'S ASSOCIATION does not support the consumption of alcoholic beverages to fight Alzheimer's disease. Although moderate alcohol consumption has been recognized as protection against cardiovascular disorders, it is also well known that alcohol is toxic to the brain when used in excess.

zinc A toxic chemical that some experts suspect might be related to Alzheimer's disease since recent studies found that zinc triggered clumping of the BETA AMYLOID protein. Beta amyloid is found in the plaques typical of Alzheimer's disease.

APPENDIXES

APPENDIX I
ALZHEIMER'S DISEASE RESOURCES

ADVANCE DIRECTIVES

American Association for Retired Persons
AARP Foundation
Room B4-240
Washington, DC 20049

Offers a state-specific advance directive guide, "Planning for Incapacity: A Self-Help Guide," by mail order; enclose a $5 check payable to AARP Foundation. Information on obtaining and completing advance directives is also available at the AARP website address below.
http://www.aarp.org/endoflife

American Medical Association
Booklet on advance directives
http://www.ama-assn.org/public/booklets/livgwill.htm

Legal Services for the Elderly
17th Floor
130 West 42nd Street
New York, NY 10036
(212) 391-0120

Partnership for Caring
Free, state-specific living wills
(800) 989-9455 (toll-free)
http://www.partnershipforcaring.org.

U.S. Department of Health and Human Services
Guidelines on advance directives
http://www.hcfa.gov/pubforms/advdir.htm

AGING

American Association of Retired Persons (AARP)
601 East Street, NW
Washington, DC 20049
(202) 434-AARP

American Society on Aging
833 Market Street
Suite 511
San Francisco, CA 94103-1824
(415) 974-9600
http://www.asaging.org

Asociacion Nacional pro Personas Mayores (National Association for Hispanic Elderly)
234 E. Colorado Boulevard, #300
Pasadena, CA 91104
(800) 953-8553 (toll-free in-state only)
or (213) 487-1922
http://www.health.gov/nhic/NHICScripts/
Entry.cfm?HRCode=HR0853

National Alliance of Senior Citizens
1700 18th Street, NW
Suite 401
Washington, DC 20009
(202) 986-0117

National Association of Area Agencies on Aging
927 15th Street, NW
Sixth floor
Washington, DC 20005
(202) 296-8130
http://www.n4a.org

National Council on the Aging, Inc.
409 Third Street, SW
Suite 200
Washington, DC 20024
(202) 479-1200

National Council of Senior Citizens
1331 F Street, NW
Washington, DC 20004
(202) 347-8800

National Indian Council on Aging
10501 Montgomery Boulevard, NE
Suite 210
Albuquerque, NM 87111
(505) 292-2001
http://www.nicoa.org

United Seniors Health Cooperative
1331 H Street, NW, #500
Washington, DC 20005
(202) 393-6222

ALZHEIMER'S DISEASE

Alzheimer's Association
919 N. Michigan Avenue
Suite 1000
Chicago, IL 60611-1676
(800) 272-3900 (toll-free)
http://www.alz.org

This nonprofit group supports families and caregivers of Alzheimer's patients. Chapters nationwide provide referrals to local resources and services, and sponsor support groups and educational programs.

Alzheimer's Disease Education and Referral Center
P.O. Box 8250
Silver Spring, MD 20907-8250
(800) 438-4380 (toll-free)
adear@alzheimers.org
http://www.alzheimers.org/adear

ADEAR responds to requests from health professionals and the public. The center collects and disseminates information about Alzheimer's disease and related disorders and about recent research into the causes of and potential treatments for the disorder.

The Alzheimer's Foundation
8177 South Harvard
M/C-114
Tulsa, OK 74137
(918) 481-6031

Alzheimer's Foundation of the South
3401 Medical Park Drive
Building One, Suite 101
P.O. Box 9693
Mobile, AL 36691
(334) 438-9590
http://www.alzfoundation.com

John Douglas French Alzheimer's Foundation
11620 Wilshire Boulevard
Suite 270
Los Angeles, CA 90025
http://www.jdfaf.org

APHASIA

National Aphasia Association
156 Fifth Avenue
Suite 707
New York, NY 10010
http://www.aphasia.org/
(800) 922-4622 (toll-free)

Education, research, rehabilitation, and support services to assist people with aphasia and their families.

ASSISTED LIVING

See NURSING HOMES

CAREGIVERS

See also FAMILY SUPPORT

National Association of Professional Geriatric Care Managers
1604 N. Country Club Road
Tucson, AZ 85716-3102
(520) 881-8008
http://www.caremanager.org

Professional Geriatric Care Managers: Mid-Atlantic Chapter
Delaware, Maryland, Virginia, District of Columbia, West Virginia
http://www.gcmonline.org

Professional Geriatric Care Managers: New England Chapter
Connecticut, Maine, Massachusetts, New Hampshire, Rhode Island, Vermont
http://www.lexingtonweb.com/gcm-ne/

Professional Geriatric Care Managers: Western Region
Alaska, Arizona, California, Colorado, Hawaii, Idaho, Montana, Nevada, New Mexico, Oregon, Utah, Washington, Wyoming
http://www.gcmwest.com

CLINICAL TRIALS

CenterWatch
http://www.centerwatch.com

COMMUNITY SERVICES

See also NURSING HOMES

Eldercare Locator
1112 16th Street, NW
Suite 100
Washington, DC 20036
(800) 677-1116 (toll-free)

This service of the National Association of Area Agencies on Aging provides information about and referrals to respite care and other home and community services offered by state and area agencies on aging.

Home Care and Hospice Agency Locator
http://www.nahc.org/Tango/HClocator/locator.html

A comprehensive database of more than 22,500 home care and hospice agencies to allow consumers to find all the agencies in any particular area of the country. Consumers can use the city and state or the first three digits of the zip code to get a range of companies.

Hospice Foundation of America
2001 S Street, NW, #300
Washington, DC 20009
(800) 854-3402 (toll-free)

Visiting Nurse Association of America
3801 East Florida Avenue
Suite 206
Denver, CO 80210
(800) 426-2547 (toll-free)

CREUTZFELDT-JAKOB DISEASE

Creutzfeldt-Jakob Disease Foundation
P.O. Box 611625
Miami, FL 33261-1626
http://www.cjdfoundation.org
crjakob@aol.com.
(954)-436-7591 (fax)

FAMILY SUPPORT

See also CAREGIVERS

Alzheimer's Family Relief Program
c/o American Health Assistance Foundation
15825 Shady Grove Road
Suite 140
Rockville, MD 20850
http://www.ahaf.org/afrp/afrp.htm

American Health Assistance Foundation (AHAF), The
http://www.ahaf.org/index.html

A nonprofit charitable organization with over 25 years dedicated to funding research on Alzheimer's disease and other health conditions, educating the public, and providing emergency financial assistance to Alzheimer's disease patients and their caregivers through the Alzheimer's Family Relief Program (see above). The group offers a range of free publications

Children of Aging Parents
1609 Woodbourne Road
Suite 302A
Levittown, PA 19057
(800) 227-7294 (toll-free)
http://www.caps4caregivers.org

Family Caregiver Alliance
690 Market Street
Suite 600
San Francisco, CA 94104
(415) 434 3388
http://www.caregiver.org

Interfaith Caregivers Alliance
112 West 9th
Suite 600
Kansas City, MO 64105
(816) 931-5442
http://www.interfaithcaregivers.org

National Family Caregivers Association
9223 Longbranch Parkway
Silver Spring, MD 20901
(301) 949-3638
http://www.nfcacares.org

GOVERNMENT ORGANIZATIONS

Alzheimer's Disease Education and Referral Center
P.O. Box 8250
Silver Spring, MD 20907-8250
(800) 438-4380 (toll-free)
adar@alzheimers.org
http://www.alzheimers.org/adear

ADEAR responds to requests from health professionals and the public. The center collects and disseminates information about Alzheimer's disease and related disorders and about recent research into the causes of and potential treatments for the disorder.

National Institute on Aging
Information Center
P.O. Box 8057
Gaithersburg, MD 20898-8057
(800) 222-2225 (toll-free) or (800) 222-4225 (TTY)
http://www.nih.gov/nia

National Institute on Aging Information Center
P.O. Box 8057
Gaithersburg, MD 20898
(800) 222-2225 (toll-free)

National Institute of Neurological Disorders and Stroke
Building 31, Room 8A06
9000 Rockville Pike
Bethesda, MD 20892
(301) 496-5751

HOSPICE

Foundation for Hospice and Home Care
519 C Street, NE
Washington, DC 20002
(202) 547-6586

Home Care and Hospice Agency Locator
http://www.nahc.org/Tango/HClocator/locator.html

A comprehensive database of more than 22,500 home care and hospice agencies to allow consumers to find all the agencies in any particular area of the country. Consumers can use the city and state or the first three digits of the zip code to get a range of companies.

Hospice Foundation of America
2001 S Street, NW, #300
Washington, DC 20009
(800) 854-3402 (toll-free)

HOUSING OPTIONS

American Association of Homes and Services for the Aging
2519 Connecticut Avenue NW
Washington, DC 20008-1520
(202) 783-2242
http://www.aahsa.org

Assisted Living Federation of America
11200 Waples Mill
Suite 150
Fairfax, VA 22030-7407
(703) 691-8100
http://www.alfa.org

National Association for Home Care
228 Seventh Street SE
Washington, DC 20003
(202) 547-7424
http://www.nahc.org

HUNTINGTON'S DISEASE

Huntington's Disease Society of America
158 W. 29th Street
7th Floor
New York, NY 10001-5300
http://www.hdsa.org/right.html
(212) 242-1968 (extension 10 for the receptionist) or
(800) 345-HDSA (toll-free)
(212) 239-3430 (fax)
hdsainfo@hdsa.org

Provides information on disease; referrals to physicians and support groups; answers questions on presymptomatic testing.

HYDROCEPHALUS

The Hydrocephalus Association
870 Market Street
Suite 705
San Francisco, CA 94102
(415) 732-7040 or (888) 598-3789 (toll-free)
http://www.hydroassoc.org

INCONTINENCE

Help for Incontinent People, Inc.
P.O. Box 544
Union, SC 29379
(800) BLADDER (toll-free)

INSURANCE

Health Insurance Association of America
1025 Connecticut Avenue, NW
Suite 1200
Washington, DC 20036
(202) 223-7780 or (800) 942-4242 (toll-free)

INTERNATIONAL ALZHEIMER'S GROUPS

Alzheimer's Disease International
45-46 Lower Marsh
London
SE1 7RG
44 20 7620 3011
info@alz.co.uk
http://www.alz.co.uk

Alzheimer Europe
http://www.alzheimer-europe.org/

Alzheimer Society of Canada
http://www.alzheimer.ca/

Federazione Alzheimer Italia
http://www.geocities.com/HotSprings/1420/

U.K. Alzheimer's Disease Society, Durham and Chester-le-Street Branch
http://www.users.zetnet.co.uk/durham.ads/

LEGAL AND FINANCIAL PLANNING

Center for Health Care Law
228 7th Street, SE
Washington, DC 20003
(202) 547-7424
chcl@nahc.org
http://www.nahc.org

Legal Services for the Elderly
130 W. 42nd Street
17th Floor
New York, NY 10036
(212) 391-0120

National Academy of Elder Law Attorneys, Inc.
National Academy of Elder Law Attorneys, Inc.
1604 North Country Club Road
Tucson, AZ 85716
(520) 881-4005
http://www.naela.org

National Senior Citizens Law Center
1101 14th Street, NW, Suite 400
Washington, DC 20005
(202) 289-6976
http://www.nsclc.org

NURSING HOMES/ASSISTED LIVING

The Alois Alzheimer Center
70 Damon Road
Cincinnati, OH 45218
(513) 605-1000

The American Association of Homes and Services for the Aging
901 E Street, NW
Suite 500
Washington, DC 20004-2011
(202) 783-2242
http://www.aahsa.org

American Health Care Association
7272 Greenville Avenue
Dallas, TX 75231
(800) 553-6321 (toll-free)

Assisted Living Federation of America
11200 Waples Mill Road
Suite 150
Fairfax, VA 22030
(703) 691-8100
http://www.alfa.org

Concerned Relatives of Nursing Home Patients
3130 Mayfield Road
Cleveland Heights, OH 44118
(216) 321-0403

The Health Care Financing Administration
(800) 638-6833 (toll-free)
http://www.hcfa.gov

HCFA publishes the *Guide to Choosing a Nursing Home* and the annual *Guide to Health Insurance for People with Medicare*. The nursing home guide includes a detailed checklist.

National Association of State Units on Aging
(202) 898-2578

Each state Office of the Long-Term Care Ombudsman visits nursing homes on a regular basis and handles complaints. Find a particular state ombudsman by calling the National Association of State Units on Aging. The association has publications about long-term care and can provide a list of facilities.

The National Citizens' Coalition for Nursing Home Reform
Suite 202
1424 16th Street, NW
Washington, DC 20036-2211
(202) 332-2275
http://www.nccnhr.org

Nursing Home Information Service
National Council of Senior Citizens
8403 Colesville Road
Suite 1200
Silver Spring, MD 20910
(301) 578-8938
http://www.ncscinc.org

This service has information on community services and offers a free guide on how to select a nursing home.

PARKINSON'S DISEASE

National Parkinson Foundation
Bob Hope Parkinson Research Center
1501 N.W. 9th Avenue
Bob Hope Road
Miami, FL 33136-1494
(305) 547-6666 or (800) 327-4545 (toll-free) or (800) 327-7872 (toll-free) or (800) 433-7022 (FL toll-free)
http://www.parkinson.org
mailbox@npf.med.miami.edu
Information, referrals, written material

PICK'S DISEASE

National Niemann-Pick Disease Foundation, Inc.
N1590 Fairview Lane
Ft. Atkinson, WI 53538
(877) CURE-NPC
http://www.nnpdf.org

PROFESSIONAL ORGANIZATIONS

American Academy of Neurology
1080 Montreal Avenue
St. Paul, MN 55116-2325
(651) 695-1940 or (800) 879-1960 (toll-free)
http://www.aan.com

American Association for Geriatric Psychiatry
7910 Woodmont Avenue
Bethesda, MD 20814-3004
(301) 654-7850
http://www.aagponline.org

American Geriatrics Society
The Empire State Building
350 Fifth Avenue
Suite 801
New York, NY 10118
(212) 308-1414
http://www.americangeriatrics.org/

Gerontological Society of America
1275 K Street, NW
Suite 350
Washington, DC 20005
(202) 842-1275
http://www.geron.org

National Association of Professional Geriatric Care Managers
(602) 881-8008

Society for Neuroscience
11 Dupont Circle, NW
Suite 500
Washington, DC 20036
(202) 462-6688
http://www.sfn.org

RESEARCH IN ALZHEIMER'S DISEASE

Alzheimer's Disease Cooperative Study
http://antimony.ucsd.edu/

American Health Assistance Foundation (AHAF), The
http://www.ahaf.org/index.html

A nonprofit charitable organization with over 25 years dedicated to funding research on Alzheimer's disease and other health conditions, educating the public, and providing emergency financial assistance to Alzheimer's disease patients and their caregivers through the Alzheimer's Family Relief Program. The group offers a range of free publications.

STROKE

National Institute of Neurological Disorders and Stroke
Public Inquiries
Building 31, Room 8A-16
Bethesda, MD 20892
(301) 496-5751

Part of the National Institutes of Health, NINDS conducts and sponsors research on neurological diseases.

APPENDIX II
ALZHEIMER'S DISEASE CENTERS

ALABAMA

University of Alabama at Birmingham
454 Sparks Center
1720 7th Avenue South
Birmingham, AL 35294-0017
(205) 934-2178
http://main.uab.edu/show.asp?durki=11627

ARIZONA

Arizona State University
Arizona Alzheimer's Disease Center
1111 East McDowell Road
Phoenix, AZ 85006
(602) 239-6999

ARKANSAS

University of Arkansas for Medical Sciences
Alzheimer's Disease Center
Donald W. Reynolds Department of Geriatrics
University of Arkansas for Medical Sciences
4301 W. Markham
Suite 811
Little Rock, AR 72205-7199
http://alzheimer.uams.edu
(501) 603-1294

CALIFORNIA

Stanford University
Alzheimer's Disease Center
Stanford University School of Medicine
Department of Psychiatry and Behavioral Science, C305
401 Quarry Road
Stanford, CA 94305-5717
(650) 852-3234
http://www.stanford.edu/~yesavage/ACRC.html

University of California, Davis
Alzheimer's Disease Center
Department of Neurology
University of California, Davis

4860 Y Street
Suite 3900
Sacramento, CA 95817
(916) 734-5496
http://alzheimer.ucdavis.edu/adc/

University of California, Irvine
Alzheimer's Disease Center
Institute for Brain Aging and Dementia
University of California, Irvine
1113 Gillespie Neuroscience Research Facility
Irvine, CA 92697
(949) 824-5847
http://www.alz.uci.edu/

University of California, Los Angeles
Alzheimer's Disease Center
Department of Neurology
University of California, Los Angeles
710 Westwood Plaza
Los Angeles, CA 90095-1769
(310) 206-5238
http://www.adc.ucla.edu

University of California, San Diego
Alzheimer's Disease Research Center
Department of Neurosciences
UCSD School of Medicine
9500 Gilman Drive
La Jolla, CA 92093-0624
(858) 622-5800
http://adrc.ucsd.edu/

University of Southern California
University of Southern California
Ethel Percy Andrus Gerontology Center
3715 McClintock Avenue
Los Angeles, CA 90089-0191
(213) 740-7777 (clinical core line for current studies
    and enrollment)
http://www.usc.edu/dept/gero/ADRC/

GEORGIA

Emory University
Emory Alzheimer's Disease Center
1841 Clifton Road, NE

Atlanta, GA 30329
(404) 728-6950
http://www.emory.edu/WHSC/MED/ADC

ILLINOIS

Northwestern University
Cognitive Neurology and Alzheimer's Disease Center
Northwestern University Medical School
320 East Superior Street
Searle 11-453
Chicago, IL 60611
(312) 908-9339
http://www.brain.nwu.edu

Rush-Presbyterian-St. Lukes Medical Center
Alzheimer's Disease Center
Rush-Presbyterian-St. Lukes Medical Center
Rush Institute for Healthy Aging
1645 West Jackson Boulevard
Suite 675
Chicago, IL 60612
(312) 942-4463
http://www.rush.edu/patients/radc/

INDIANA

Indiana University
Indiana Alzheimer's Disease Center
Indiana University School of Medicine
Department of Pathology and Laboratory Medicine
635 Barnhill Drive
MS-A142
Indianapolis, IN 46202-5120
(317) 278-2030
http://www.pathology.iupui.edu/ad/

KENTUCKY

University of Kentucky
Sanders-Brown Research Center on Aging
University of Kentucky
101 Sanders-Brown Building
Lexington, KY 40536-0230
(859) 323-6040
http://www.coa.uky.edu/

MARYLAND

The Johns Hopkins Medical Institutions
Alzheimer's Disease Center
Division of Neuropathology
The Johns Hopkins University School of Medicine
558 Ross Research Building
720 Rutland Avenue
Baltimore, MD 21205-2196

(410) 955-5632
http://www.alzresearch.org

MASSACHUSETTS

Boston University
Alzheimer's Disease Center
GRECC Program (182B)
Bedford VAMC
200 Springs Road
Bedford, MA 01730
(781) 687-2916
http://www.xfaux.com/Alzheimer/

Harvard Medical School/Massachusetts General Hospital
Massachusetts General Hospital
Department of Neurology
15 Parkman Street
Boston, MA 02114
(617) 726-1728
http://neuro-oas.mgh.harvard.edu/alzheimers

MICHIGAN

University of Michigan
Alzheimer's Disease Research Center
Department of Neurology
1500 E. Medical Center Drive
1914 Taubman Street
Ann Arbor, MI 48109-0316
(734) 764-2190
http://www.med.umich.edu/madrc/

MINNESOTA

Mayo Clinic
Department of Neurology
200 First Street, SW
Rochester, MN 55905
(507) 284-1324
http://www.mayo.edu/research/alzheimers_center/

MISSOURI

Washington University
Alzheimer's Disease Research Center
Washington University Medical Center
4488 Forest Park Avenue
Suite 130
St. Louis, MO 63108-2293
(314) 286-2881
http://www.adrc.wustl.edu/adrc

NEW YORK

Columbia University
Taub Institute for Research on Alzheimer's Disease and the Aging Brain
630 West 168th Street
P&S Box 16
New York, NY 10032
(212) 305-1818
http://www.alzheimercenter.org

Mount Sinai School of Medicine/Bronx VA Medical Center
Alzheimer's Disease Research Center
Department of Psychiatry
Box 1230
Mount Sinai School of Medicine
One Gustave L. Levy Place
New York, NY 10029-6574
(212) 241-8329
http://www.mssm.edu/psychiatry/adrc.shtml

New York University
New York University School of Medicine
Silberstein Aging and Dementia Research Center
Alzheimer's Disease Center
550 First Avenue
Room THN 312B
New York, NY 10016
(212) 263-5700
http://aging.med.nyu.edu/

University of Rochester
Alzheimer's Disease Center
Center for Aging and Developmental Biology
University of Rochester Medical Center
601 Elmwood Avenue
Box 645
Rochester, NY 14642
(716) 275-2581
http://www.urmc.rochester.edu/adc/index.html

NORTH CAROLINA

Duke University
Joseph and Kathleen Bryan Alzheimer's Disease Research Center
2200 West Main Street
Suite A-230
Durham, NC 27705
(919) 286-3228
http://adrc.mc.duke.edu/

OHIO

Case Western Reserve University
University Alzheimer Center
University Hospitals of Cleveland

Case Western Reserve University
12200 Fairhill Road
Cleveland, OH 44120-1013
(800) 252-5048
http://www.ohioalzcenter.org

OREGON

Oregon Health Sciences University
Alzheimer's Disease Center
Oregon Health Sciences University
3181 SW Sam Jackson Park Road
Department of Neurology, CR 131
Portland, OR 97201-3098
(503) 494-6976
http://www.ohsu.edu/som-alzheimers/

PENNSYLVANIA

University of Pennsylvania
Alzheimer's Disease Center
Center for Neurodegenerative Disease Research
University of Pennsylvania School of Medicine
3rd Floor Maloney Building
3600 Spruce Street
Philadelphia, PA 19104-4283
(215) 662-4708
http://www.med.upenn.edu/ADC

University of Pittsburgh
Alzheimer's Disease Research Center
University of Pittsburgh
4-West Montefiore University Hospital
200 Lothrop Street
Pittsburgh, PA 15213-2582
(412) 692-2700
http://www.adrc.pitt.edu/

TEXAS

Baylor College of Medicine
Alzheimer's Disease Research Center
Department of Neurology
Baylor College of Medicine
6550 Fannin Street, Smith Tower
Suite 1801
Houston, TX 77030
(713) 798-6660
http://www.bcm.tmc.edu/neurol/struct/adrc/adrc1.html

University of Texas, Southwestern Medical Center
Alzheimer's Disease Research Center
University of Texas Southwestern Medical Center
Southwestern Medical Center

5323 Harry Hines Boulevard
Dallas, TX 75390-9070
(214) 648-7444
http://www2.swmed.edu/alzheimer/

WASHINGTON

University of Washington
Alzheimer's Disease Center
VAPSHCS-GRECC 182B
1660 S. Columbian Way
Seattle, WA 98108
(206) 277-3491 or (800) 317-5382 (patient recruitment)
http://depts.washington.edu/adrcweb/

National Alzheimer's Coordinating Center (NACC)
4225 NE Roosevelt Way
Suite 301
Seattle, WA 98105
(206) 543-3121
naccmail@alz.washington.edu
http://www.alz.washington.edu

The NACC coordinates data collection and fosters collaborative research among the Alzheimer's Disease Centers.

APPENDIX III
AREA AGENCIES ON AGING

The Agency on Aging is responsible for coordinating and supporting special services for elderly Americans. There are branches in almost every local area in every state.

ALABAMA

Alabama Commission on Aging
RSA Plaza
Suite 470
770 Washington Ave.
Montgomery, AL 36130
(334) 242-5743

ALASKA

Alaska Commission on Aging
Division of Senior Services
Department of Administration
3601 C Street
#310
Juneau, AK
(907) 563-5654

ARIZONA

Aging and Adult Administration
Department of Economic Security
1789 W. Jefferson, 950 A Street
Phoenix, AZ 85007

ARKANSAS

Division Aging and Adult Services
Arkansas Department of Human Services
P.O. Box 1437
Slot 1412
1417 Donaghey Plaza South
Little Rock, AR 72203
(501) 682-2441

CALIFORNIA

California Department of Aging
1600 K Street
Sacramento, CA 95814
(916) 322-5290

COLORADO

Aging and Adult Services
Department of Social Services
110-16th Street
Suite 200
Denver, CO 80202
(303) 620-4147

CONNECTICUT

Community Services
Division of Elderly Services
25 Sigourney Street
Hartford, CT 06106
(203) 424-5281

DELAWARE

Delaware Department of Health and Social Services
Division of Services for Aging and Adults with Physical Disabilities
1901 N. DuPont Highway
New Castle, DE 19720
(302) 577-4791

DISTRICT OF COLUMBIA

District of Columbia Office on Aging
441 Fourth Street, NW
Suite 900 South
Washington, DC 20001
(202) 724-5622

FLORIDA

Department of Elder Affairs
4040 Esplanade Way
Tallahassee, FL 32399
(904) 414-2000

GEORGIA

Division of Aging Services
Department of Human Resources
2 Peachtree Street, NE
18th floor
Atlanta, GA 30303
(404) 657-5258

HAWAII

Hawaii Executive Office on Aging
335 Merchant Street
Room 241
Honolulu, HI 96813
(808) 586-0100

IDAHO

Idaho Commission on Aging
Room 108, Statehouse
Boise, ID 83720
(208) 334-3833

ILLINOIS

Illinois Department on Aging
421 East Capitol Avenue
Suite 100
Springfield, IL 62701
(217) 785-2870

INDIANA

Division of Disability, Aging and Rehabilitative Services
Family and Social Services Administration
Bureau of Aging and In-Home Services
402 W. Washington Street
Indianapolis, IN 46207

IOWA

Department of Elder Affairs
Jewett Building
Suite 236
914 Grand Avenue
Des Moines, IA 50319
(515) 281-4646

KANSAS

Department of Aging
Docking State Office Building
Room 150
915 S.W. Harrison
Topeka, KS 66612
(913) 296-0256

KENTUCKY

Kentucky Division of Aging Services
Department for Social Services
275 E. Main Street 6 West
Frankfort, KY 40621

LOUISIANA

Governor's Office of Elderly Affairs
P.O. Box 80374
Baton Rouge, LA 70898
(504) 925-1700

MAINE

Bureau of Elder and Adult Services
Department of Human Services
35 Anthony Avenue
State House, Station #11
Augusta, ME 04333

MARYLAND

Maryland Office on Aging
State Office Building
Room 1004
301 W. Preston Street
Baltimore, MD 21201

MASSACHUSETTS

Executive Office of Elder Affairs
One Ashburton Place, 5th floor
Boston, MA 02108
(617) 727-7750

MICHIGAN

Office of Services to the Aging
P.O. Box 30026
Lansing, MI 48909
(517) 373-8230

MINNESOTA

Board on Aging
444 Lafayette Road
St. Paul, MN 55155
(612) 296-2770

MISSISSIPPI

Division of Aging and Adult Services
750 State Street
Jackson, MS 39202
(601) 359-4925

MISSOURI

Division on Aging
Department of Social Services
P.O. Box 1357
615 Howerton Court
Jefferson City, MO 65102
(314) 751-3082

MONTANA

Senior and Long Term Care Division
Department of Public Health and Human Services
P.O. Box 4210
Helena, MT 59604
(406) 444-5900

NEBRASKA

Department of Health and Human Services
Division on Aging
P.O. Box 95044
301 Centennial Mall South
Lincoln, NE 68509
(402) 471-2306

NEVADA

Nevada Division for Aging Services
Department of Human Resources
340 North 11th Street
Suite 203
Las Vegas, NV 89101
(702) 486-3545

NEW HAMPSHIRE

Division of Elderly and Adult Services
State Office Park South
115 Pleasant Street

Annex Building #1
Concord, NH 03301
(603) 271-4680

NEW JERSEY

Department of Health and Senior Services
Division of Senior Affairs
101 South Broad Street, CN 807
Trenton, NJ 08625
(609) 292-3766

NEW MEXICO

State Agency on Aging
La Villa Rivera Building
Ground Floor
228 East Palace Avenue
Santa Fe, NM 87501
(505) 827-7640

NEW YORK

New York State Office for the Aging
2 Empire State Plaza
Albany, NY 12223
(800) 342-9871

NORTH CAROLINA

Division of Aging
CB 2953 1
693 Palmer Drive
Raleigh, NC 27626
(919) 733-3983

NORTH DAKOTA

Department of Human Services
Aging Services Division
600 South 2nd Street
Suite 1-C
Bismarck, ND 58504
(701) 328-2577

OHIO

Ohio Department of Aging
50 W. Broad Street
8th floor
Columbus, OH 43266
(614) 466-5500

OKLAHOMA

Services for the Aging
Department of Human Services
P.O. Box 25352
Oklahoma City, OK 73125
(405) 521-2281

OREGON

Senior and Disabled Services Division
500 Summer Street NE
2nd floor
Salem, OR 97310
(503) 945-5811

PENNSYLVANIA

Department of Aging
Commonwealth of Pennsylvania
400 Market Street
Harrisburg, PA 17101
(717) 783-1550

RHODE ISLAND

Department of Elderly Affairs
160 Pine Street
Providence, RI 02903
(401) 277-2858

SOUTH CAROLINA

Division on Aging
202 Arbor Lake Drive
Suite 301
Columbia, SC 29223
(803) 737-7500

SOUTH DAKOTA

Office of Adult Services and Aging
Richard F. Kneip Building
700 Governor's Drive
Pierre, SD 57501
(605) 773-3656

TENNESSEE

Commission on Aging
Andrew Jackson Building
9th floor

500 Deaderick Street
Nashville, TN 37243
(615) 741-2056

TEXAS

Texas Department on Aging
P.O. Box 12786
Capitol Station
Austin, TX 78711
(512) 444-2727

UTAH

Division of Aging and Adult Services
P.O. Box 45500
120 N. 200 West
Salt Lake City, UT 84145
(801) 538-3910

VERMONT

Department of Aging and Disabilities
Waterbury Complex
103 South Main Street
Waterbury, VT 05676
(802) 241-2400

VIRGINIA

Virginia Department for the Aging
700 E. Franklin Street 10th floor
Richmond, VA 23219

WASHINGTON

Aging and Adult Services Administration
Department of Social and Health Services
P.O. Box 45050
Olympia, WA
(360) 272-2300

WEST VIRGINIA

Commission on Aging
Holly Grove
State Capitol
1900 Kanawha Boulevard East
Charleston, WV 25305
(304) 558-3317

WISCONSIN

Bureau of Aging and Long Term Care Resources
Department of Health and Family Services
P.O. Box 7851
Madison, WI 53707
(608) 266-2536

WYOMING

Division on Aging
Department of Health
117 Hathaway Building
Room 139
Cheyenne, WY 82002
(307) 777-7986

APPENDIX IV
INTERNATIONAL ALZHEIMER'S DISEASE ASSOCIATIONS

ARGENTINA

Asociación de Lucha contra el Mal de Alzheimer
Lacarra No. 78
1407 Capital Federal, Buenos Aires
Argentina
+54 11 4671 1187
alma@satlink.com.ar
http://www.alma-alzheimer.org.ar

AUSTRALIA

Alzheimer's Association Australia
P.O. Box 108
Higgins
ACT 2615
Australia
+61 2 6254 4233
alzact@netspeed.com.au
www.alzheimers.org.au

AUSTRIA

Alzheimer Angehorige Austria
Obere Augartenstrasse 26-28
1020 Vienna, Austria
+43 1 332 5166
alzheimeraustria@via.at
www.alzheimer-selbsthilfe.at

BELGIUM

Ligue Alzheimer
Clinique Le Perî
4B Rue Montagne
Sainte Walburge
B-4000 Liège
+32 4 225 8793
henry.sabine@skynet.be
www.alzheimer.be

BRAZIL

FEBRAZ Federacao Brasileira de Associaçãoes de Alzheimer
Caixa Postal 3913
Sao Paulo - SP - Brazil
01160-970
+55 11 270 8791
abraz@abraz.com.br
www.abraz.com.br

CHILE

Corporación Chilena de la Enfermedad, de Alzheimer y Afecciones Similares
Desiderio Lemus 0143
Recoleta
Santiago, Chile
+56 2 236 0846
alzchile@mi.terra.cl

COLOMBIA

Asociacion Colombiana de Alzheimer y Desordenes Relacionados
Calle 69 A No. 10-16
Santa Fe de Bogotá, DC
Colombia
+57 1 348 1997
alzheimercolombia@hotmail.com

COSTA RICA

Alzheimer's Association of Costa Rica
Apartado 4755
San José 1000
Costa Rica
+506 290 28 44
ximajica@sol.racsa.co.cr

CUBA

Cuban Section of Alzheimer's Disease and Related Disorders
Calle 146 No. 2504 e/ 25 y 31
Cubanacan Playa
Ciudad de la Habana
Cuba
+537 220974
inmo@tleda.get.tur.cu

CYPRUS

Pancyprian Association of Alzheimer's Disease
31A Stadiou
6020 Larnaca
Cyprus
+357 4 627 104
alzhcyprus@yahoo.com

CZECH REPUBLIC

Ceska Alzheimerovska Spolecnost
Centre of Gerontology
Simunkova 1600
18200 Praha 8
Czech Republic
+420 2 88 36 76
Petr.Veleta@gerontocentrum.cz
www.gerontocentrum.cz

DENMARK

Alzheimerforeningen
Sankt Lukas Vej 6, 1
DK 2900 Hellerup
Denmark
+45 39 40 04 88
post@alzheimer.dk
www.alzheimer.dk

DOMINICAN REPUBLIC

Asociacion Dominicana de Alzheimer y Trastornos Relacionados
Apartado Postal #3321
Santo Domingo
Republica Dominicana
+1 809 544 1711
dr.pedro@codetel.net.do

ECUADOR

Alzheimer's Disease, Ecuador
Avenida de la Prensa #5204 y Avenida de Maestro
Quito
Ecuador
+593 2 594 997
alzheime@uio.satnet.net

EL SALVADOR

Asociacion de Familiares Alzheimer de El Salvador
Asilo Sara Zaldivar
Colonia Costa Rica
Avenida Irazu
San Salvador
El Salvador
+503 237 0787
ricardolopez@vianet.com.sv

FINLAND

Alzheimer Society of Finland
Luotsikatu 4E
00160 Helsinki
Finland
+358 9 6226 200
tarja.tapaninen@alzheimer.fi
www.alzheimer.fi

FRANCE

Association France Alzheimer
21 Boulevard Montmartre
75002 Paris, France
+33 1 42 97 52 41
www.maladie-alzheimer.com

GERMANY

Deutsche Alzheimer Gesellschaft
Friedrichstr. 236
10969 Berlin
Germany
+49 30 315 057 33
deutsche.alzheimer.ges@t-online.de
www.deutsche-alzheimer.de

GREECE

Greek Society of AD and Related Disorders
Charisio Old People's Home
Terma Dimitriou Charisi

Ano Toumba 543 52
Thessaloniki
+30 31 925802
alzhass@med.auth.gr
www.alzheimer-europe.org/Greece/

GUATEMALA

Asociación Grupo ERMITA
10a. Calle 11-63
Zona 1, Apto B
P.O. Box 2978
01901 Guatemala
+502 2 381122
alzguate@quetzal.net
www.alzheimer-guatemala.org.gt

HONG KONG

Hong Kong Alzheimer's Disease and Brain Failure Association
c/o GF Wang Lai House
Wang Tau Hom Estate
Kowloon, Hong Kong
+852 27943010
www.hkada.org.hk

ICELAND

FAAS
Austurbrún 31
104 Rejkjavik
Iceland
+354 533 1088
faas@isholf.is
www.obi.is/faas

INDIA

Alzheimer's & Related Disorders Society of India
P.O. Box 53
Kunnamkulam
Kerala 680 503
India
+91 488 523801
alzheimr@md2.vsnl.net.in
www.alzheimerindia.org

INDONESIA

IAzA Secretariat
c/o Wahyudi Nugroho
Sasana Tresna Werda "Yayasan Karya Bakti Ria Pembangunan"

jl. Pusdika RT 008 RW 07
KM 17 Cibubur, Jakarta 13720
Indonesia
+62 21 8730179
nasrun@indosat.net.id

IRELAND

The Alzheimer Society of Ireland
Alzheimer's House
43 Northumberland Avenue
Dunlaoghaire Co., Dublin
Ireland
+353 1 284 6616
alzheim@iol.ie
www.alzheimer.ie

ISRAEL

Alzheimer's Association of Israel
P.O. Box 8261
Ramat Gan
Israel 52181
+972 3 578 7660
a-a-i@zahav.net.il
medic.bgu.ac.il/aai

ITALY

Federazione Alzheimer Italia
Via Tommaso Marino 7
20121 Milano
Italy
+39 02 809767
alzit@tin.it
www.alzheimer.it

JAPAN

Alzheimer's Association Japan (Association of Family Caring for Demented Elderly Japan)
c/o Kyoto Social Welfare Hall
Horikawa-Marutamachi, Kamigyo-Ku, Kyoto, Japan
602-8143
+81 75 811 8195
afcdejpn@mbox.kyoto-inet.or.jp
www.alzheimer.or.jp

KOREA

Alzheimer's Association, Korea
#52, Machon 2-Dong
Songpa-ku

Seoul 138-122
Korea
+82 2 431 9963
afcde01@unitel.co.kr
www.alzza.or.kr

LUXEMBOURG

Alzheimer Europe
145, route de Thionville
L-2611 Luxembourg
+352 29 79 70
info@alzheimer-europe.org
http://www.alzheimer-europe.org

Association Luxembourg Alzheimer
45, rue Nicolas Hein
BP 5021
L 1050 Luxembourg
+352 421 676
info@alzheimer.lu
www.alzheimer.lu

MALAYSIA

Alzheimer's Disease Foundation, Malaysia
14 Lorong Utara A
46200 Petaling Jaya
Selangor
Malaysia
+603 758 1522
alzheimers@pd.jaring.my
www.adfm.org.my

MEXICO

AMAES
Insurgentes Sur No. 594 - 402
Col. Del Valle, Mexico 12
D.F. 03100 Mexico
+525 523 1526
amaes@data.net.mx
www.amaes.org.mx

NETHERLANDS

Alzheimer Nederland
Post Bus 183
3980 CD BUNNIK
The Netherlands
+31 30 659 6285

info@alzheimer-ned.nl
www.alzheimer-ned.nl

NEW ZEALAND

Alzheimer's Society, NZ
P.O. Box 2808
Christchurch
New Zealand
+64 3 365-1590
alzheimers@alzheimers.org.nz

NIGERIA

Alzheimer's Disease Association of Nigeria
c/o Department of Psychiatry
Nnamdi Azikiwe University Teaching Hospital
Nnewi
Anambra State
Nigeria
+234 046 463663
nauth@infoweb.abs.net

NORWAY

Nasjonalforeningen Demensforbundet
Oscarsgt 36 A, Postboks
7139 Majorstua
N 0307 Oslo
Norway
+47 23 12 00 00
post@nasjonalforeningen.no
www.nasjonalforeningen.no

PAKISTAN

Alzheimer's Pakistan
146/1 Shadman Jail Road
Lahore 54000
Pakistan
+92 42 759 6589
alzpak@hotmail.com

PERU

**Asociacion Peruana de Enfermedad
de Alzheimer y Otras Demencias**
Trinitarias 205
Surco

Lima 33
Perú
+511 275 8033
magasc@terra.com.pe

PHILIPPINES

ADAP
St. Luke's Medical Center
Medical Arts Building
Room 410
E. Rodriguez Sr. Avenue, Quezon City
Philippines
632 723 1039
mscmartinez@stluke.com.ph

POLAND

Polish Alzheimer's Association
ul. Hoza 54/1
00-682 Warszawa
Poland
+48 22 622 11 22
alzheimer_pl@hotmail.com
www.alzheimer.pl

PORTUGAL

Associaçäo Portuguesa de Familiares e Amigos de Doentes de Alzheimer
Rua Joäo de Menezes
16 - r/c - 1900-267
Lisboa
Portugal
+351 21 846 56 65
alzheimer@portugalnet.com
www.portugalnet.pt/ALZHEIMER

PUERTO RICO

Asociación de Alzheimer de P.R.
Apartado 362026
San Juan
Puerto Rico 00936-2026
+1 787 727 4151
alzheimerpr@alzheimerpr.org
www.alzheimerpr.org

ROMANIA

Romanian Alzheimer Society
Bd.Mihail Kogalniceanu 95A
Sc. A. Et. 1, Ap. 8, Sector 5

Bucharest
Romania 70603
+40 1 686 3470
alzsocro@fx.ro
www.alzheimer-europe.org

RUSSIA

Association for Support of Alzheimer's Disease Victims
34 Kashirskoye shosse
115522 Moscow
Russia
+7 095 324 9615
gavrilova@dionis.iasnet.ru

SCOTLAND

Alzheimer Scotland—Action on Dementia
22 Drumsheugh Gardens
Edinburgh
EH3 7RN
Scotland
+44 131 243 1453
alzheimer@alzscot.org
www.alzscot.org

SINGAPORE

Alzheimer's Disease Association
Block 157 Toa Payoh Lor 1 #01-1195
Singapore 310157
+65 353 8734
alzheimers.tp@pacific.net.sg

SLOVAK REPUBLIC

Slovak Alzheimer's Society
Dúbravaká 9
Bratislava 84246
Slovak Republic
+421 7 594 13353
nilunova@savba.sk

SOUTH AFRICA

Alzheimer's & Related Dementias Association
P.O. Box 81183
Parkhurst
Johannesburg 2120

South Africa
+27 11 478 2234/5/6
alzheimerssa@icon.co.za

SPAIN

Confederación Española de Familiares de Enfermos de Alzheimer
Avda Pio XII, 37
Entreplanta, Oficina 5
31008 Pamplona
Spain
+34 948 177 907
alzheimer@cin.es
www.ceafa.org

SWEDEN

Alzheimerforeningen I Sverig
Sunnanväg 14 S
222 26 Lund
Sweden
+46 46 14 73 18
alzheimf@algonet.se
www.alzheimerforeningen.nuDemensförbundet

Demensförbundet (The National Association for the Rights of the Demented)
Drakenbergsgatan 13 nb
117 41 Stockholm
08 658 52 22
rdr@demensforbundet.se
www.demensforbundet.se

SWITZERLAND

Association Alzheimer Suisse
8 Rue des Pêcheurs
CH-1400 Yverdon-les-Bains
Switzerland
+41 24 426 2000
alz@bluewin.ch
www.alz.ch

THAILAND

Alzheimer's and Related Disorders Association of Thailand
114 Pinakorn 4
Boramratchachunee Road
Talingchan
Bangkok 10170
Thailand
+66 2 880 8542/7539
c_sirintorn@hotmail.com
www.come.to/thaiAz

TRINIDAD AND TOBAGO

c/o Soroptimist International Port of Spain
15 Nepaul Street
St. James, Port of Spain
Republic of Trinidad and Tobago
+1 868 622 6134
klbtt@yahoo.com

TURKEY

Turkish Alzheimer Society

Siraci Sok
Baris Apt No: 24/8
Rumelihisari
Istanbul
Turkey
+90 212 2878581
ggurvit@alz.org.tr
www.medyatext.com/alzheimer/

UGANDA

Alzheimer's and Dementia Awareness Society
P.O. Box 361
Kabale
Uganda
+256 486 22290

UKRAINE

The Association for the Problems of Alzheimer's Disease
Institute of Gerontology
67 Vyshgorodskaya Street
04114 Kiev
Ukraine
+380 44 431 0526
direct@geront.freenet.kiev.ua

UNITED KINGDOM

Alzheimer's Disease International
45/46 Lower Marsh
London SE1 7RG
United Kingdom
+44 20 7620 3011
adi@alz.co.uk
http://www.alz.co.uk/

Alzheimer's Society
Gordon House
10 Greencoat Place
London

SW1P 1PH
United Kingdom
+44 20 7306 0606
info@alzheimers.org.uk
www.alzheimers.org.uk

URUGUAY

Asociación Uruguaya de Alzheimer y Similares
Casilla de Correo 5092
Montevideo, Uruguay

+598 2 400 8797
audasur@adinet.com.uy

VENEZUELA

Fundación Alzheimer de Venezuela
Av. El Limón, Qta. Mi Muñe—El Cafetal
Caracas
+58 2 9859546
alzven@cantv.net
www.mujereslegendarias.org.ve/alzheimer.htm

APPENDIX V
LEGAL/FINANCIAL ISSUES

Dealing with legal and financial issues is a crucial first step after a diagnosis of Alzheimer's disease. Prompt action, before the patient becomes incapacitated, will help the family understand the patient's wishes.

A. FINDING A PROFESSIONAL

The family of a patient with Alzheimer's may want to choose an attorney, accountant, or financial planner to help with planning of trusts, writing a will, dealing with Medicare and Medicaid, and financing long-term care. When going to the first meeting, the family should bring along information on:

- income
- bank accounts
- pensions
- trusts
- wills
- patient's birth certificate
- list of assets

B. LEGAL PROTECTION

When a person with Alzheimer's can no longer make decisions about money, health, or finances, it's important to have legal documents in place that name a person who can handle those situations. Every patient with Alzheimer's should have a will, a durable power of attorney, a living trust, a living will, and a medical power of attorney (health care proxy).

Will

A patient who is still mentally competent should prepare a will, if this has not already been com-

pleted. If the patient's mental state has deteriorated to the point where he or she is only sometimes lucid, a psychiatrist should examine the patient on the day the will is drawn to ensure competency. This is particularly important if there is any suspicion that the resulting will may be contested. A will can only be certified as valid if the following conditions are all true:

- the person understands what is being bequeathed
- the person can outline a sensible plan for the distribution of the property
- the person understands the relationship between the beneficiaries and himself or herself

Durable Power of Attorney

A patient with Alzheimer's disease should have a durable power of attorney, since the disease is progressive and this instrument gives a designated person the power to act on the patient's behalf. A nondurable power of attorney ceases when the patient needs it most. Most nondurable powers of attorney are used for limited transactions, such as when someone is briefly out of town and needs to have bills paid.

A durable power of attorney is permanent, and gives the appointed agent the right to take appropriate legal action on the patient's behalf without a court proceeding. A patient must be mentally competent when signing a power of attorney.

It is possible to restrict a power of attorney, giving power only over various accounts, for example, but if the integrity of the appointee is in question, another trusted individual should be named instead.

GENERAL POWER OF ATTORNEY

KNOW BY ALL THESE MEN PRESENT that I, _____ ,
of _____ (county) and _____ (state)
by these presents do constitute, make, and appoint _____
_____ and/or
_____ either
jointly or severally, my true and lawful attorney for me and in my stead:

1. to sign checks or other instruments of deposit, withdrawal, or instruction on my checking account or other banking account or bank deposit standing in my name;
2. to collect, demand, sue for, recover, and receive all such sums of money, debts, rents, goods, wares, accounts, and other demands whatsoever which are or shall be due, owing, payable, and belonging to me or detained from me in any manner whatsoever;
3. to execute and affirm or swear to all returns for the purposes of federal, state, or local taxation and all other papers in connection with my tax liability including claims for refunds of taxes;
4. to sell and assign all stocks and bonds belonging to me and to have access to any safety deposit box rented to or belonging to me;
5. to sell any real estate standing in my name and to make, execute, acknowledge, and deliver a deed for said real estate to the purchaser or purchasers and to satisfy mortgages;
6. to make gifts;
7. to create a trust for my benefit;
8. to make an addition to an existing trust for my benefit;
9. to claim an elective share of the estate of my deceased spouse;
10. to disclaim an interest in property;
11. to renounce fiduciary positions;
12. to withdraw and receive the income or corpus of a trust;
13. to authorize my admission to a medical, nursing, residential, or similar facility and to enter into agreement for my care;
14. to authorize medical and surgical procedures;
15. and generally to do and perform all matters and things, transact all business, make and execute and acknowledge all contracts, orders, writings, mortgages, bonds, U.S. Savings Bonds, assurances and instruments which may be requisite or proper to effectuate any matter or thing appertaining or belonging to me with the same powers, and to all intents and purposes with the same validity as I could, if personally present;
16. and to appoint one or more attorneys in fact under them for the purposes aforesaid, to make and constitute and again at pleasure to revoke such powers of attorney; hereby ratifying and confirming whatsoever my said attorney shall and may do by virtue heretofore; and hereby revoking any previous Power of Attorney signed by me. Notwithstanding the foregoing, this Power of Attorney shall apply not only to titles, documents, or assets standing in my name alone, but shall also apply to titles, documents, or assets standing in my name along with the name of another or others, such as joint tenancy, tenancy by the entirety, or tenancy in common, or tenancy in partnership.

This Power of Attorney shall not be affected by my disability or incompetency.
This Power of Attorney supersedes and replaces any prior Power of Attorney.

IN WITNESS THEREOF, I have hereunto set my hand and seal this _____ , day of _____ .
(date)   (month/year)

_____ (SEAL)

WITNESS

_____ , residing at _____

_____ , residing at _____

On this _____ day of _____ , 20_____ , before me, the undersigned officer, personally appeared _____ , known to me (or satisfactorily proven) to be the person whose name is subscribed to the within instrument and acknowledged that he or she executed the same for the purposes herein contained.
IN WITNESS THEREOF, I hereunto set my hand and official seal.

_____
Notary Public

Guardian

If the patient with Alzheimer's was not willing to assign a power of attorney and becomes mentally incompetent, a lawyer must then petition the court for a conservatorship (guardian of the property). It is up to the judge to decide if the patient is competent to handle personal affairs; if not, a guardian is assigned to care for the property, under court supervision. A guardian must file periodic reports to the court about the person's financial status.

A "guardian of the person" may be appointed by the court if the patient is not able to make decisions about medical or nursing home care, and the family members can't agree on what is to be done.

Living Trust

A living trust is a document into which a person transfers assets. The advantage of a living trust is that when the person dies, the assets pass directly to the beneficiaries, without having to go through probate. In a living trust, for example, a patient with Alzheimer's can name a trustee, who may be either a family member, friend, or bank (or combination of all three). In most cases, the spouse is usually named as a trustee. Trustees must follow the guidelines about how the assets are to be managed as written in the trust by the patient. Assets can be given away throughout the patient's lifetime, or preserved for distribution after death. While living trusts keep assets out of probate, they don't lessen the tax burden.

Living Will

This document allows a patient with Alzheimer's disease to outline what is to be done about specific health care decisions and whether life-sustaining treatment is to be carried out. Most states recognize living wills.

Health Care Proxy (Medical Power of Attorney)

A medical power of attorney/health care proxy allows a patient with Alzheimer's disease to authorize a spouse, parent, adult child, or other adult to make health care decisions on the patient's behalf once that person becomes incompetent. A medical POA can be used to make any type of medical decision. Having such a document can make difficult health care decisions easier, and can spare costly court proceedings that may be required without a proxy.

A health care proxy can be used only to make decisions regarding health care; it can't be used to make financial decisions for the patient.

Estate Planning

Estate planning with a competent financial planner can help provide for the patient with Alzheimer's disease in the event the person becomes mentally incapacitated.

C. PAYING FOR CARE

Paying for care for a patient with Alzheimer's may be taken care of by Medicare, Medicaid, or private insurance. While regulations vary from one state to the next, there are some basic provisions.

Medicare

A patient must be 65 or older, or disabled at any age, to qualify for Medicare coverage. Medicare does not cover chronic care, but if a patient with Alzheimer's gets sick, Medicare will probably cover the temporary illness. However, maximum coverage is just 150 days, and involves a copayment.

Medicaid

Medicaid may provide payment for nursing home care, adult day care, or at-home nursing care for patients with Alzheimer's if the person meets the financial need requirements. Medicaid also covers hospitalization, some medications, physical exams, and more. Patients usually become eligible for Medicaid only when their own money has been depleted to the point where they are below the federal poverty level. Eligibility is calculated not just on the patient's income, but also on the spouse's situation.

It is possible to transfer assets from the patient's name to another person (such as an adult child); however, this transfer must take place at least 30 months before the patient applies for Medicaid coverage. Each state has different Medicaid rules and regulations.

In some states, adult children and spouses are not legally required to spend their own money to support family members in nursing homes, but in

LIVING WILL

DECLARATION

I, _____, being of sound mind, willfully and voluntarily make this declaration to be followed if I become incompetent. This declaration reflects my firm and settled commitment to refuse life-sustaining treatment under the circumstances listed below.

I direct my attending physician to withhold or withdraw life-sustaining treatment that serves only to prolong the process of my dying, if I should be in a terminal condition or in a state of permanent unconsciousness.

In addition, if I am in the condition described above, I feel especially strong about the following forms of treatment:

I ( ) do ( ) do not want cardiac resuscitation.

I ( ) do ( ) do not want mechanical respiration.

I ( ) do ( ) do not want tube feeding or any other artificial or invasive form of nutrition or hydration.

I ( ) do ( ) do not want blood or blood products.

I ( ) do ( ) do not want any form of surgery or invasive diagnostic tests.

I ( ) do ( ) do not want kidney dialysis.

I ( ) do ( ) do not want antibiotics.

I realize that if I do not specifically indicate my preference regarding any of the forms of treatment listed above, I may receive that form of treatment.

Other instructions:

I ( ) do ( ) do not want to designate another person as my surrogate to make medical treatment decisions for me if I should be incompetent, in a terminal condition, or in a state of permanent unconsciousness.

Name and address of surrogate: _____
_____
_____

Name and address of alternate surrogate: _____
_____
_____

I make this declaration on the _____ day of _____, 20_____.

Declarant's signature _____

Declarant's address _____
_____

The declarant knowingly and voluntarily signed this writing by signature or marked in my presence:

Witness' signature _____

Witness' address _____
_____

Witness' signature _____

Witness' address _____
_____

ADVANCE DIRECTIVE FOR HEALTH CARE DECLARATION

I [print your name] _____

Being of sound mind, willfully and voluntarily make this declaration to be followed if I become incompetent. This declaration reflects my firm and settled commitment to refuse life-sustaining treatment under the circumstances listed below.

I direct my attending physician to withhold or withdraw life-sustaining treatment that serves only to prolong the process of my death, if I should be in a terminal condition or in a state of permanent unconsciousness.

I direct that treatment be limited to measures to keep me comfortable and to relieve pain, including any pain that might occur by withholding or withdrawing life-sustaining treatment.

In addition, if I am in the condition described above, I feel especially strong about the following forms of treatment:

I ( ) do ( ) do not want cardiac resuscitation.

I ( ) do ( ) do not want mechanical respiration.

I ( ) do ( ) do not want tube feeding or any other artificial or invasive form of nutrition or hydration.

I ( ) do ( ) do not want blood or blood products.

I ( ) do ( ) do not want any form of surgery or invasive diagnostic tests.

I ( ) do ( ) do not want kidney dialysis.

I ( ) do ( ) do not want antibiotics.

I realize that if I do not specifically indicate my preference regarding any of the forms of treatment listed above, and I do not name a surrogate to make medical treatment decisions for me, I may receive that form of treatment.
Other instructions:

I ( ) do ( ) do not want to designate another person as my surrogate to make medical treatment decisions for me if I should be incompetent, in a terminal condition, or in a state of permanent unconsciousness. I authorize my surrogate to make decisions regarding any of the medical treatments listed above as to which I do not specifically indicate my preference, and any other form of treatment not listed in this declaration.

Name and address of surrogate: _____
_____
_____

Name and address of alternate surrogate: _____
_____
_____

I do _____ do not _____ want to make an anatomical gift of all or any of my body, subject to the following limitations, if any:
_____
_____

I make this declaration on the _____ day of _____, 20_____.

Declarant's signature _____
Declarant's address _____

If this declaration was signed by another person on behalf of and at the direction of the declarant, please explain the circumstances:

The declarant, or the person on behalf of and at the direction of the declarant, knowingly and voluntarily signed this writing by signature or marked in my presence:

Witness' signature _____

Witness' address _____

Witness' signature _____

Witness' address _____

PLEASE NOTE: This declaration is based on the model form set forth in the Pennsylvania Advance Directive for Health Care Act at 20 Pa. CSA 5454 (b). This form may not be best suited for every patient. If you have questions, consult your attorney.

other states relative responsibility laws require family to support the patient financially.

Private Insurance

Long-term care insurance may pay for nursing home costs, but the policies differ a great deal in their coverage, deductibles, waiting periods, and so on. Such a long-term policy must have been purchased before the patient was diagnosed with Alzheimer's, however, because after such a diagnosis it would be almost impossible to buy such a policy. Some companies will add a long-term care rider to a life insurance policy to provide a monthly stipend that equals a fixed percentage of the death benefit. Experts suggest the best time to buy long-term care insurance is when patients are in their late 50s to early 60s; after this, the cost becomes prohibitive.

A long-term care policy should include:

- custodial care
- intermediate care
- skilled nursing care
- respite care/home health care/home nursing care provision
- no exemptions for certain illnesses or diseases
- physician's statement to trigger benefits (not hospitalization)

APPENDIX VI
READ MORE ABOUT IT

Carly, R. Hellen. *Alzheimer's Disease: Activity Focused Care.* Woburn, Mass.: Butterworth-Heinemann Medical, 1998.

Castleman, Michael, et al. *There's Still a Person in There: The Complete Guide to Treating and Coping with Alzheimer's.* New York: Putnam, 2000.

Davidson, Ann. *Alzheimer's: A Love Story: One Year in My Husband's Journey.* Palo Alto, Calif.: Birch Lane Press, 1997.

Davies, Helen, and Michael Jensen. *Alzheimer's: The Answers You Need.* Forest Knolls, Calif.: Elder Books, 1998.

Dowling, James R., and Nancy Mace. *Keeping Busy: A Handbook of Activities for Persons With Dementia.* Baltimore: Johns Hopkins University Press, 1995.

Feil, Naomi. *Validation Breakthrough: Simple Techniques for Communicating with People with Alzheimer's-Type Dementia.* Baltimore: Health Professions Press, 1993.

Gray-Davidson, Freena. *The Alzheimer's Sourcebook for Caregivers.* New York: McGraw Hill, 1999.

Gruetzner, Howard. *A Caregiver's Guide and Sourcebook* (3rd ed.). New York: John Wiley & Sons, 2001.

Haisman, Pam. *Alzheimer's Disease: Caregivers Speak Out.* Fort Myers, Fla.: Chippendale House, 1998.

Harper, M.A. *The Worst Day of My Life, So Far.* Athens, Ga.: Hill Street Press, 2001.

Henderson, Cary. *Partial View: An Alzheimer's Journal.* Dallas, Tex.: Southern Methodist University Press, 1998.

Hodgson, Harriet. *Alzheimer's—Finding the Words: A Communication Guide for Those Who Care.* New York: Wiley, 1995.

Kuhn, David, and David Bennett. *Alzheimer's Early Stages: First Steps in Caring and Treatment.* New York: Hunter House, 1999.

Leviton, Richard. *Brain Builders!: A Lifelong Guide to Sharper Thinking, Better Memory, and an Ageproof Mind.* Upper Saddle River, N.J.: Prentice Hall, 1995.

Mace, Nancy L., and Peter V. Rabins. *The 36-Hour Day (revised).* New York: Warner Books, 2001.

Marcell, Jacqueline. *Elder Rage or Take My Father . . . Please!: How to Survive Caring for Aging Parents.* Irvine, Calif.: Impressive Press, 2001.

Molloy, William, and Paul Caldwell. *Alzheimer's Disease: Everything You Need to Know.* Westport, Conn.: Firefly Books, 1998.

Newman, Diane Kaschak, and Mary Dzvirnko. *The Urinary Incontinence Sourcebook.* Los Angeles: Lowell House, 1997.

Shanks, Lela Knox. *Your Name Is Hughes Hannibal Shanks: A Caregiver's Guide to Alzheimer's.* New York: The Penguin Group, 1999.

Shenk, David. *The Forgetting: Alzheimer's: Portrait of an Epidemic.* New York: Doubleday, 2001.

Snyder, Lisa. *Speaking Our Minds: Personal Reflections from Individuals With Alzheimer's Disease.* New York: W. H. Freeman, 2000.

Tanzi, Rudolph, and Ann Parson. *Decoding Darkness: The Search for the Genetic Causes of Alzheimer's Disease.* New York: Perseus Press, 2001.

Volicer, Vladimir. *Hospice Care for Patients with Advanced Progressive Dementia.* New York: Springer Publishing Co., 1998.

APPENDIX VII
ALZHEIMER'S DISEASE CLINICAL TRIALS

TOLERABILITY AND PRIMARY EFFICACY OF CX516 IN ALZHEIMER'S DISEASE AND RELATED DISORDERS

This double-blind, placebo-controlled outpatient study will determine the safety and effectiveness of experimental medication CX516 (Ampalex) to improve mental function in patients with Alzheimer's disease. Patients who volunteer for this study will either receive CX516 or will receive a harmless, inactive pill called a placebo. Neither the volunteers nor the physicians will know which type of pill a patient receives.

Ampalex stimulates certain glutamate receptors and has been shown to improve memory in animal and normal volunteer studies. Patients must be generally healthy and have mild-to-moderate dementia. There must be a patient caregiver who can watch for side effects, ensure that the patient takes the study pills on schedule, and accept legal responsibility for the patient during the study.

Patients will undergo weekly neuropsychological tests as well as laboratory evaluations, and will be seen in the National Institutes of Health Clinical Center outpatient clinic once a week for nine weeks with one follow-up visit. Each visit will last approximately six hours.

IA0005

Contact information: http://clinicalstudies.info.nih.gov/detail/A_1997-N-0049.html

TREATMENT OF BEHAVIORAL SYMPTOMS IN ALZHEIMER'S DISEASE

This study focuses on treating behavioral symptoms in Alzheimer's disease with haloperidol and whether long-term treatment is necessary. Alzheimer's patients with behavioral problems, such as sleep disturbance or agitation, and/or severe psychiatric symptoms, such as hallucinations or delusions, are often treated with antipsychotic medications such as haloperidol, a widely prescribed medication for Alzheimer's patients with such problems.

The study is conducted in two phases: First, for five months the medication is given in adjusted doses to manage behavioral problems or psychosis.

In phase two, those patients who respond and remain stable on the medication are randomized, double-blind, to continue taking haloperidol or placebo for 24 weeks. Researchers will examine whether it is necessary for them to stay on this medicine. To accomplish this, patients continue for another five to six months on either a placebo pill (pill containing an inactive substance) or continuation on active haloperidol, while the researchers continue to monitor behavioral symptoms. After completing the study, patients continue to receive treatment for behavioral problems and/or psychosis if required.

IA0013

Contact: Gregory Pelton, MD, 722 West 168th Street Unit 126, New York, NY 10032; (212)543-5957, e-mail: ghp4@columbia.edu

ANTI-INFLAMMATORY TREATMENT FOR AGE-ASSOCIATED MEMORY IMPAIRMENT: A DOUBLE-BLIND PLACEBO-CONTROLLED TRIAL

This project is designed to study whether nonsteroidal anti-inflammatory drugs (NSAID) such as Celecoxib may delay age-related mental decline and whether genetic risk and brain structure can predict mental decline. Several epidemiological studies indicate that anti-inflammatory treatments prevent the symptoms of Alzheimer's disease (AD). Neuropathological studies also support inflammatory or immune mechanisms in AD. Because such evidence is circumstantial, controlled, randomized drug trials are needed to determine efficacy.

A total of 135 subjects with age-associated memory impairment (AAMI) (mild memory complaints, decreased performance in selected memory tests) between 65 and 90 years of age will be randomly assigned to treatment groups, receiving either an inactive substance (placebo) or Celecoxib (400 mg/day). The subjects will receive a magnetic resonance imaging (MRI) scan, routine laboratory blood tests, electrocardiogram, and cognitive tests. The study will continue for about two years, with follow-up testing at specific intervals. Measures of brain structure will be derived from baseline MRI scans, and blood will be drawn and tested to determine which genotypes (apolipoprotein E [apoE] or human leukocyte antigen [HLA]) the patient has. The study will explore how deep white matter disease, hippocampal asymmetry, and atrophy and genetic risk for AD onset influence decline rates and treatment outcome.

Subjects receiving Celecoxib (400 mg/day) are expected to show less evidence of cognitive decline than those receiving placebo. The proposed project builds upon earlier work on early detection of AD using brain imaging, genetic risk, and neuropsychological assessments. This project also is a logical follow-up to recent observational studies of a promising early intervention and will represent one of the first controlled, anti-inflammatory treatment trials for persons at high risk for age-related cognitive decline and the eventual development of AD. Subjects will be followed closely to ensure that medication is safely used, without side effects.
ID # IA0015
Contact person: Andrea Kaplan, 760 Westwood Plaza, Los Angeles, CA 90024; (310) 206-7392, e-mail: akaplan@mednet.ucla.edu

THE EFFECTS OF SEX HORMONES ON COGNITION AND MOOD IN OLDER ADULTS

This double-blind, placebo-controlled, crossover study will investigate the effects of estrogen and testosterone replacement on memory, mental abilities, and mood in older adults aged 65 to 90. During the study, men will take testosterone for three months and women will take estrogen for three months. At four points during the study (once every three months), participants will complete a test battery and have blood drawn.

Women who have not had a hysterectomy will be given Prempro (estrogen with progesterone to protect the uterine lining); women who have had a hysterectomy will be given Premarin (estrogen only).

While taking estrogen, some women experience vaginal bleeding, breast tenderness, headache, mood changes, nausea, bloating, weight changes, changes in sleeping patterns, fatigue, or change in sex drive. With only three months of estrogen replacement, women are not thought to be at increased risk for uterine or breast cancer. While taking testosterone, some men experience problems urinating, swelling or tenderness in the chest, behavioral changes, or elevated hematocrit levels.
ID # IA0016
CONTACT: Kristen Mordecai, Gerontology Research Center 5600 Nathan Shock Drive, Baltimore, MD 21224; (410) 558-8536; e-mail mordecai@lpc.grc.nia.nih.gov

ALZHEIMER'S DISEASE PREVENTION TRIAL

This is a multi-center, randomized, double-blind, placebo controlled trial of estrogen (or estrogen and progesterone) to see whether they can prevent or delay Alzheimer's disease and loss of memory in elderly women with a family history of the disease.

While taking estrogen some women experience vaginal bleeding, breast tenderness, headache, mood changes, nausea, bloating, weight changes, changes in sleep.
ID # IA0018
Contact Person: Alba Raghnauth, 630 West 168 Street P&S Box 16, New York, NY 10032; (877) DELAY-AD, E-mail: alba@delay-ad.org

ESTROGEN EFFECTS ON MEMORY FUNCTIONING IN POST-MENOPAUSAL WOMEN AND PATIENTS WITH ALZHEIMER'S DISEASE

The primary goal of this study is to examine whether three months of estrogen administered to postmenopausal women and women with mild to moderate Alzheimer's disease who are concurrently treated with standard therapy (generally Aricept) will enhance the system in the brain involving memory and learning. Estrogen may have significant benefits in preserving cognitive functioning in normal aging after menopause and in decreasing the incidence of Alzheimer's disease. Subjects will be blindly placed on estrogen or placebo for three months each. After each three-month period, they will be cognitively assessed after receiving single doses of the cholinergic antagonists scopolamine and mecamylamine. These results will have direct implications for the use of estrogen in postmenopausal women as well as interactive treatment with cholinergic drugs for AD.

Possible side effects in taking estrogen or progesterone include breast tenderness and breakthrough spotting. Rare side effects include nausea, cramps, bloating, headaches. Scopolamine (administered during one study visit day) may temporarily cause drowsiness, decreased salivation, or memory impairment. Mecamylamine (administered during one study visit day) may temporarily cause low blood pressure or decreased salivation. Aricept side effects include nausea, diarrhea, trouble sleeping, vomiting, muscle cramps, fatigue, and decreased appetite. Aricept treatment has also rarely been associated with headache, pain, accidents, difficulty thinking, bruising, weight loss, arthritis, depression, nightmares, drowsiness, and urinary frequency.
ID #A0023
Contact Person: Katie Hancur, UHC Campus, Arnold 6 1 South Prospect St, Burlington, VT 05401; (802) 847-8596, E-mail: Catherine.Hancur@vtmednet.org

ALZHEIMER'S DISEASE ANTI-INFLAMMATORY PREVENTION TRIAL (ADAPT)

ADAPT is a randomized trial that will test the ability of the nonsteroidal anti-inflammatory drugs (NSAIDs) naproxen and celecoxib to delay or prevent the onset of Alzheimer's disease (AD) and age-related cognitive decline. This long-term trial will run for five to seven years.

Considerable evidence suggests that inflammation may play a role in the neurodegenerative

process of Alzheimer's disease (AD), and the use of NSAIDs may be associated with reduced occurrence of AD.

The study is sponsored by the National Institute on Aging and is being conducted at the University of South Florida in Tampa, the Veterans Affairs Puget Sound Health Care System with the University of Washington in Seattle, Boston University School of Medicine, the Johns Hopkins Medical Institutions in Baltimore, Sun Health Research Institute in Phoenix, and the University of Rochester. At each of these sites, the goal is to enroll approximately 2,625 men and women 70 years of age or older, with a parent, brother, or sister who has had serious age-related memory loss, senility, dementia, or Alzheimer's disease.

Participants will be asked to take an anti-inflammatory medication or placebo (inactive pill) twice daily. Before enrolling in the trial, participants will be asked to go to a study site for two medical evaluations. Once enrolled, they will need to go to a study site for a medical evaluation every six months and to participate in a telephone interview twice a year for an average of up to 7 years of follow-up.
ID # IA0026
Contact Person: Janette Negele, Veterans Administration (VA) Puget Sound Health Care System 1660 S. Columbian Way, Seattle, WA 98108 (206) 277-6548, e-mail: jnegele@u.washington.edu

A NUTRITIONAL BRAIN METABOLIC ENHANCER FOR ALZHEIMER'S DISEASE

This double-blind, placebo-controlled, parallel-group trial followed by an open-label period will investigate a nutritional supplement designed to improve brain metabolism and function in patients with Alzheimer's disease (AD). The design of the nutritional supplement is based on observations of abnormalities in mitochondria in AD. The constituents of the nutritional supplement are components of the normal American diet and are classified by the Food and Drug Administration as GRAS (generally regarded as safe).

The ability of the brain to use glucose is reduced in patients with Alzheimer's disease. A nutritional supplement has been developed to improve the function of the brain affected by Alzheimer's by increasing its ability to use sugar effectively. The ingredients of the supplement are natural products and are found in the normal American diet. Results have been encouraging in open trials where the patients knew they were taking the active medicine. Patients are now being invited to participate in a placebo-controlled trial, followed by an open-label trial where all patients will receive the active preparation.

During the placebo-controlled portion of the trial, half of the participants will receive the active preparation and half a sugar pill. During this first phase, neither the patients nor those testing them will know who is taking active medicine and who is taking placebo. The active supplement or placebo are taken as one tablespoon twice a day, between meals. If desired, the supplement or placebo can be stirred into, or washed down with, water, coffee or tea without milk or sugar, or the soft drink TAB. Patient visits to the Burke Medical Research Institute will be once a month, after the screening and baseline visits.

Results with the supplement have been favorable in preliminary open trials. The supplement is taken as one tablespoon of a fluid, between meals. Since other sugars or citrate can be expected to interfere with the actions of the supplements, food or drinks containing sugar or citrate and diet drinks containing citrate are to be avoided for one and one-half hours before and one and one-half hours after taking the supplement. Water, coffee or tea without sugar or milk, or the diet drink TAB are permitted. (TAB contains neither sugar nor citrate.)

No significant adverse events have been associated with this supplement. However, standard precautions for patient safety are being taken, including medical examination and clinical laboratory tests at screening and at the completion of the double-blind and open-label phases.

ID # IA0027

Contact Person: Mireya Montalvan-Panzer, 785 Mamaroneck Avenue, White Plains, NY 10605; (914) 597-2596; E-mail: mmontalv@burke.org

CATIE ALZHEIMER'S DISEASE TRIAL

The CATIE Alzheimer's Disease Trial is part of the Clinical Antipsychotic Trials of Intervention Effectiveness (CATIE) Project and is designed for people with Alzheimer's disease who are having trouble with their thinking or behavior. In particular, this study is trying to find out the best treatment for people who have hallucinations, delusions, or agitation. The design of the trial helps to increase the chance that participants in the study receive a medication that helps them.

The study uses three atypical antipsychotic medications (olanzapine, quetiapine, and risperidone), which are the newest medications that are currently available for treating these problems. Participants may also receive an antidepressant (citalopram). Participants are given a thorough evaluation at no cost to ensure that this study is appropriate, and the caregiver, family member, or friend who comes with the participant will be offered an educational program about Alzheimer's disease. There are four phases to the study.

During Phase I (the initial treatment phase), participants will be assigned randomly to one of the three atypical antipsychotics or placebo groups. After two weeks, the patient can move to the next phase because of lack of efficacy or tolerability. At week 12, the investigator can decide whether the current medication is sufficiently optimal or if it would be more beneficial to try another randomized medication.

Phase 2 starts when the patient is randomized to a second medication (olanzapine, quetiapine, risperidone, or citalopram). Patients will be randomized from an antipsychotic treatment to another antipsychotic treatment or citalopram, or from placebo to an antipsychotic treatment or citalopram. Therefore, half of patients who took placebo in Phase 1 will be randomized to an antipsychotic in Phase 2, and half will be randomized to citalopram in Phase 2. After the initial two weeks in Phase 2, the investigator can move the patient to the next phase, due to lack of efficacy or tolerability. After the patient has been on the Phase 2 study drug for approximately 12 weeks, the investigator can decide whether the current medication is sufficiently optimal or whether it would be more beneficial to try another randomized medication.

Phase 3 is a randomized open-label treatment of one of the medications not previously received (olanzapine, quetiapine, risperidone, or citalopram). Treatment failures to the second treatment can be switched to a third open-label treatment. During Phase 3, patients will be maintained on their treatments openly and managed clinically until week 36.

If the investigator determines that the participant's response is not sufficiently optimal to the randomized open-label medication, then after the first two weeks of Phase 3, the investigator can prescribe another medication (of the investigator's choice) to the patient. If this occurs then patients are classed as being in the Open-Choice Phase.

Open-Choice Phase can begin at any time during the 36-week study and directly from any of the three phases. There are four reasons a patient can enter the open choice phase:

- withdrawal from Phase 1 or Phase 2 with the participant or patient's decision-maker refusing to proceed to the next randomized phase
- withdrawal from Phase 3
- withdrawal from current study drug from any of the three previous phases because antipsychotic medication is no longer required
- withdrawal due to concomitant treatment with an exclusionary medication.

The Open-Choice Phase is designed to keep patients monitored in the trial for the 36-week duration.
ID #IA0028
Contact Person: Karen Dagerman, (323) 442-3715, e-Mail dagerman@hsc.usc.edu

A PHASE I STUDY OF EX VIVO NERVE GROWTH FACTOR GENE THERAPY FOR ALZHEIMER'S DISEASE

This Phase I clinical trial is the first step in testing gene therapy and is considered to be a safety/toxicity study. It will determine whether the experimental protocol is safe for humans, whether the study procedure causes side effects in humans, and also may provide a preliminary sense of whether this will be effective in combating Alzheimer's disease (AD) in humans. The study investigators are proceeding with this human clinical trial because the identical procedure in nonhuman primates has been safe and has not produced negative side effects at the cell doses that are planned for this study. However, animals do not suffer from Alzheimer's, so this experimental procedure has not been tested in this disease.

The eventual goal of this clinical program will be to determine whether growth factor gene therapy will be useful in Alzheimer's disease. This approach has prevented cell loss in animal models that mimic some aspects of the cell loss that occurs in Alzheimer's, but it has not been tested in this disease.

Not all of the cells in the brain that are affected by Alzheimer's are expected to respond to growth factor gene therapy. One class of cell in particular (a basal forebrain cholinergic neuron) is expected to respond. This type of cell undergoes extensive loss in AD; preventing loss of this cell type could help to slow down intellectual decline. Nonetheless, animals in which this gene therapy approach has been tested do not have AD, and it remains to be established whether this procedure will be effective in humans with AD.

This study will involve brain surgery. Each person's own cells will be genetically modified to produce a natural substance called nerve growth factor (NGF). A person's cells (fibroblasts) will be obtained from skin biopsies and then genetically modified in the test tube; they will then be implanted into either five or 10 locations in the person's brain. The eventual goal of this research effort will be to determine whether NGF produced by the cells implanted into the brain can prevent the death of some nerve cells that are affected in AD and enhance the function of some remaining brain cells. However, the primary goal of this first study will be to determine whether this gene therapy procedure is safe.

In animal studies, fibroblasts genetically modified to produce NGF have been shown to prevent the death of certain nerve cells in the brain. This effectiveness has been shown in both the rat brain and the monkey brain. The genetically modified cells prevent cell death after injury, as well as cell atrophy that is a natural consequence of aging in primates.

Although the precise pathogenesis of AD is unknown, certain pathological features accompany the disease. These pathological features include the abnormal accumulation of amyloid, the formation of neurofibrillary tangles, synapse loss, and cellular degeneration. Cellular degeneration occurs in several neuronal populations in the central nervous system, but it is especially severe in the basal forebrain cholinergic neurons. Loss of cholinergic neurons in AD correlates best with severity of dementia, the density of amyloid plaques in the brain, and the amount of synapse. To date, the only Food and Drug Administration-approved therapies for AD focus on augmenting the function of degenerating cholinergic neurons. The present trial will move beyond compensating for cholinergic neuronal degeneration by attempting to protect cholinergic neurons from degeneration, and augment the function of remaining cholinergic neurons by directly elevating choline acetyltransferase (ChAT) function in neurons. These two therapeutic interventions will be brought about by the delivery of human NGF to the brain.

NGF has been shown to prevent both lesion-induced and spontaneous, age-related degeneration of basal forebrain cholinergic neurons. Further, NGF infusions reversed both lesion-induced memory loss and spontaneous, age-related memory loss in rodents. Based on these findings, NGF administration offers significant potential as a neuroprotective strategy in AD. Grafts of primary fibroblasts transduced to express human NGF have been shown to sustain NGF in vivo gene expression for at least 18 months in the rodent central nervous system. In addition, these grafts sustain NGF messenger RNA production for at least 14 months in vivo. In primate systems, ex vivo NGF gene therapy has been demonstrated to sustain NGF protein production in the brain in the rhesus monkey for at least one year. Thus, the available data suggests that ex vivo NGF gene therapy is an effective means of preventing loss of basal forebrain cholinergic neurons and of augmenting cholinergic function in the primate brain. In animals, this procedure is safe and well tolerated. Based on these data, clinical trials of ex vivo NGF gene therapy in AD has begun.

There are four main hypothetical risks of this study that any person should seriously consider before agreeing to participate:

- **Risk of bleeding into the brain (hemorrhage):** Since cells will be surgically implanted into five or ten locations in the brain, there is an estimated risk of bleeding of one to five percent. If bleeding occurred, it could result in death or permanent disability in addition to that which would result from Alzheimer's disease.

- **Risk of tumor formation:** It is possible that the implanted cells could become cancerous. If this happened, it could be extremely difficult to treat. Although tumors have not formed in any monkeys that have undergone this procedure (approximately 30 monkeys to date that have received more than 200 implants), tumor formation remains a hypothetical possibility. Individuals considering enrollment in this experimental trial should carefully reflect on this possibility before volunteering.

- **Risk of a chronic pain syndrome:** A pain syndrome has never been known to occur in any monkey or rat that has undergone the gene therapy procedure planned in this clinical trial, but in past animal experiments, NGF has been pumped into the fluid space that surrounds and cushions the brain and spinal cord, causing pain. Three humans in Sweden have also undergone NGF pumping into the brain fluid space and experienced pain. It is believed that this side effect occurred because NGF "flooded" the fluid space that surrounds the brain, causing growth of pain fibers into the fluid space. This gene therapy trial is not expected to cause this side effect because much lower doses of NGF are being delivered directly into the brain. NGF is not expected to leak into the fluid space, and pain is not expected to occur as a complication of this procedure. Nonetheless, the development of a chronic pain syndrome remains a hypothetical possibility, and it would be difficult to effectively treat this complication if it developed. Individuals considering enrollment in this experimental trial should carefully reflect on this possibility before volunteering.

- **Risk of weight loss:** Substantial weight loss has not occurred in monkeys that have undergone the gene therapy procedure planned in this clinical trial, but in past experiments, animals lost weight when NGF was pumped into the fluid space of the brain and spinal cord. Three humans in Sweden have also lost weight after undergoing NGF pumping into the brain fluid space. It is believed that this side effect occurred because NGF "flooded" the fluid space that surrounds the brain, suppressing appetite centers in the brain. This gene therapy trial is not expected to cause this side effect because much lower doses of NGF are being delivered directly into the brain. While monkeys have not shown signs of substantial weight loss from the procedure, the development of weight loss remains a hypothetical possibility, and it would be difficult to effectively treat this complication if it developed. Individuals considering enrollment in this experimental trial should carefully reflect on this possibility before volunteering.

ID# IA0029
Contact: Stephanie McKinney, 8950 Villa La Jolla Suite 1200, La Jolla, CA 92037, (858) 622-5800, e-mail: smckinney@ucsd.edu

EFFECT OF THE HMG-COA REDUCTASE INHIBITOR ATORVASTATIN CALCIUM, LIPITOR, IN THE TREATMENT OF ALZHEIMER'S DISEASE

This clinical trial is designed to assess the benefit of a cholesterol-lowering drug (Lipitor) compared to placebo in the treatment of Alzheimer's disease.
ID# IA0031
Contact Person: David Lawrence Sparks, 10515 West Santa Fe Drive Sun City, AZ 85351, (623) 876-5463, e-mail: Larry.Sparks@SunHealth.org

PREVENTION OF ALZHEIMER'S DISEASE BY VITAMIN E AND SELENIUM (PREADVISE)

The Prevention of Alzheimer's Disease with Vitamin E and Selenium (PREADVISE) trial is an important addition to the Selenium and Vitamin E Cancer Prevention Trial (SELECT). As a prevention trial, PREADVISE is trying to find out if taking selenium and/or vitamin E supplements can help to prevent memory loss and dementia such as Alzheimer's disease. Studies have suggested that these supplements may increase antioxidant defenses in the brain, so they are being evaluated

for their potential to protect against AD. Men over the age of 62, or 60 if African-American or Hispanic, enrolled or enrolling in SELECT are eligible for PREADVISE. This involves annual checkups that take less than 15 minutes.

Participants accepted into the study will be given vitamin E and selenium supplements alone or in combination, or a placebo plus a multivitamin, visiting the study site every six months for seven to 12 years. A short memory test will be administered on an annual basis to detect memory changes.
ID# IA0033
Contact Person: Cecil R. Runyons, 800 South Limestone St., Lexington, KY 40536, toll-free (800) 333-8874 or tollfree (866) 846-1412, e-mail: preadvise@lsv.uky.edu

TREATMENT OF AGITATION/PSYCHOSIS IN DEMENTIA/PARKINSONISM (TAP/DAP)

This multicenter, randomized, double-blind, placebo-controlled trial is investigating the efficacy and tolerability of quetiapine (QUET) and donepezil (DONEP), used alone or in combination, for psychosis and/or agitation in patients with a primary dementia (probable Alzheimer's disease or dementia with Lewy bodies) complicated by coexistent parkinsonism, or patients with Parkinson's disease with dementia.

Psychosis and agitation often occur in the course of dementia and are a major source of patient disability and caregiver stress. For the common situation in which extrapyramidal (parkinsonian) motor dysfunction accompanies dementia, there is a therapeutic dilemma since the most frequently used drugs to treat the behavioral problems, neuroleptic antipsychotics, can worsen parkinsonism and have been associated with severe extrapyramidal reactions in some types of dementia. To date, the efficacy and tolerability of the most promising alternative medications to treat psychosis and agitation (atypical antipsychotics and cholinesterase inhibitors) have not been tested in patients with a primary dementia selected for coexisting parkinsonism. Furthermore, no study has examined the possible additive benefits or risks of these two drug classes when used in combination.

1. In this study, subjects will be randomized to one of four treatment groups: quetiapine (QUET; an atypical antipsychotic with a favorable extrapyramidal side effect profile)
2. donepezil (a cholinesterase inhibitor)
3. the combination of QUET + DONEP
4. placebo.

Each subject participates in the trial for 10 weeks; systematic ratings of behavior, motor function, cognition, adverse events, and other outcomes occur at baseline and after six and 10 weeks of assigned treatment.
ID# IA0034
Contact Person: Cheryl Deeley, (585) 341-7515 University of Rochester Medical Center, Department of Neurology 919 Westfall Road, Building C, Suite 220, Rochester, NY 14618, (585) 3411-7500, e-mail: cdeeley@mct.rochester.edu

NEUROTRANSMITTER RECEPTOR MEASUREMENTS IN AGING AND IN ALZHEIMER'S DISEASE

This study is designed to help researchers better devise ways to study how brain cells work in Alzheimer's disease.

The brain communicates among its brain cells using chemicals called neurotransmitters that are secreted from the cell and bind to specific sites on other cells called neurotransmitter receptors. In order for normal communication to occur between brain cells, there has to be adequate amounts of neurotransmitter and receptors.

One specific neurotransmitter is acetylcholine (ACh), which binds to acetylcholine receptors. Acetylcholine receptors are affected by the aging process and by Alzheimer's disease (AD). In both aging and AD, the number of neurons secreting ACh decreases, and the function of some acetylcholine receptors is changed. The effect of AD is much more severe than the effect of aging.

Researchers want to study the effects of aging and AD on a specific type of acetylcholine receptor (muscarinic type 2 [M2]). In order to do this, researchers will use a PET scan to investigate the functional activity of the brain. The PET technique allows doc-

tors to study the normal biochemical and metabolic processes of the central nervous system of normal individuals and patients with neurologic illnesses without physical/structural damage to the brain.

In this study, patients will be given a radioactive tracer, which will bind to acetylcholine receptors and allow researchers to see them under PET scan.

The goal of this study is to provide information about how well the tracer binds to acetylcholine receptors in young and old healthy volunteers and patients with AD. This information can be used later in other studies to design experiments to improve the understanding of the effects of aging and AD on the nervous (cholinergic) system.
ID# IA0036
Contact Person: NIMH Patient Recruitment and Public Liaison Office, Bethesda, MD 20892, (800) 411-1222, e-mail: prpl@mail.cc.nih.gov

PILOT STUDY OF IMMUNOMODULATORY ANTI-INFLAMMATORY THERAPY IN ALZHEIMER'S DISEASE

This randomized, placebo-controlled trial is designed to study the immune and inflammatory reactions in Alzheimer's disease (AD) and the possibility that blocking the inflammatory response may alter the course of the illness. The specific plan is to evaluate the biologic and clinical effects of two doses of cyclophosphamide (CY) immunotherapy in AD patients compared to placebo. Two doses of CY or placebo will be compared over a six-month period. Those subjects who receive placebo over the first six months will have the option of receiving CY for a second six months.

Three times during the study candidates will have a physical examination, cognitive testing for memory and thought processes, functional evaluation, blood tests, electrocardiogram, and spinal tap to monitor their health, side effects of medication, and effects of the medication on disease progression. These tests will be done before starting medication, at three months (in the middle of the study), and at six months (the end of the study). Patients will have DNA testing of a blood sample to study the genetic influences on Alzheimer's Disease and magnetic resonance imaging (MRI) of the brain.

While the primary outcome measures will be safety and immunologic data, cognitive and other behavioral measures will also be collected. The biological outcome measures will include measures of brain volume (assessed by magnetic resonance imaging) and cerebrospinal fluid biomarkers of neurodegeneration, neuroinflammation, and neuroimmune activation. In addition, peripheral lymphocyte subsets and peripheral markers of inflammation will be assessed. This design is meant to provide dose-finding data to help design a more definitive efficacy trial with CY if the safety/tolerability parameters are acceptable in this pilot study.

Inflammation and immunologic response appear to contribute significantly to neurodegeneration in Alzheimer's. In a pathological process called gliosis, the brain's immune cells (microglia and astroglia) undergo chronic activation and possible proliferation, promoting neuronal injury and death by several means. Activated microglia and astroglia produce compounds that are directly cytotoxic to neurons, and they express molecules that greatly amplify immune and inflammatory processes in the brain. Excessive glial activation and proliferation are thought to be pivotal events hastening the demise of synapses and neurons in AD. Conversely, the growing understanding of immune and inflammatory pathology in AD has provided new opportunities for designing disease-altering treatments for AD.

Preliminary clinical trails of anti-inflammatory drugs in AD patients, epidemiologic studies of anti-inflammatory drug use, and experimental models linking neurodegeneration with neuroimmune/neuroinflammatory processes suggest strongly that medications such as nonsteroidal-anti-inflammatory drugs (NSAIDs) and immunomodulatory agents may have an important role in altering the course of AD. CY is a potent anti-inflammatory and immunomodulatory drug that acts primarily by inhibiting proliferation of immune cells. Moreover, as immune-cell proliferation appears to be an important aspect of AD pathophysiology and disease progression, an exploratory, dose-finding trial of a cytotoxic/ cytostatic drug such as CY is appropriate, especially since CY is already widely used for the treatment of other immune-mediated illnesses. Furthermore, a preliminary European trial of CY in AD patients has already demonstrated an improvement in cognitive function that correlated highly with the degree of immunomodulation achieved.

ID# IA0037

Contact Person: Patient Recruitment and Public Liaison Office, (800) 411-1222, e-mail: prpl@mail.cc.nih.gov

CHOLESTEROL LOWERING AGENT TO SLOW PROGRESSION (CLASP) OF ALZHEIMER'S DISEASE STUDY

This research study will investigate the safety and effectiveness of simvastatin (a cholesterol lowering drug, or statin) to slow the progression of Alzheimer's disease (AD). Statins are commonly used to treat high cholesterol levels, which increase the risk of heart disease and stroke.

The clinical trial will include the treatment of patients with mild to moderate AD, evaluating the safety and efficacy of simvastatin to slow the progression of AD, as measured by the cognitive portion of the AD Assessment Scale. Measures of clinical global change (ADCS-CGIC), mental status, functional ability, behavioral disturbances, quality of life, and economic indicators also will be made. The study is a randomized, double-blind, placebo-controlled, parallel group design with equal randomization to drug and placebo.

During the study, 20 mg of simvastatin or matching placebo will be given for six weeks, followed by 40 mg of simvastatin or matching placebo for the remainder of the 18-month study period. Participants will be instructed to take the medication once a day in the evening. Safety parameters to be checked will include adverse events, symptom checklists, vital signs, physical and neurological examinations, and laboratory tests.

This medication is well tolerated, but there may be side effects, the most common being constipation, diarrhea, dizziness, gas, headache, heartburn, nausea, skin rash, and stomach pain. Less common or rare side effects are fever, muscle aches or cramps, severe stomach pain, unusual tiredness or weakness, or liver problems. Rare side effects include decreased sexual ability, progression of cataracts, or trouble sleeping. Doctor should check progress of participant at regular visits to see if medication is working properly. Do not stop taking medication without first checking with doctor, and check with doctor before any surgery.

ID# IA0038

Principal Investigator: Dr. Mary Sano, Mount Sinai School of Medicine, Alzheimer Disease Research Center, Department of Psychiatry, Box 1230, New York, NY 10029-6574

GLOSSARY

adrenergic Term that means "associated with catecholamines."

adverse reaction An unexpected effect of drug treatment that may range from trivial to serious or life-threatening, such as an allergic reaction.

agnosia A perceptual impairment characterized by an inability to recognize familiar objects or associate an object with its use.

agonist A molecule that stimulates receptors to produce a desired reaction, increasing the effect of a neurotransmitter.

allele One of two or more alternative forms of a gene; for example, one allele of the gene for eye color may code for blue eyes, while another allele may code for brown eyes.

amino acids The basic building blocks of proteins. Genes contain the code for the production of the 20 amino acids necessary for human growth and function.

antagonist A chemical that blocks the action of a neurotransmitter receptor. Antagonists inhibit the effects of agonists.

anterior In medicine, a directional term meaning "toward the front."

antibodies Specialized proteins produced by the cells of the immune system that counteract a specific foreign substance. The production of antibodies is the first line of defense in the body's immune response.

assay The evaluation or testing of a substance for toxicity, impurities, or other variables.

atherosclerosis A condition caused by fatty deposits along the inner lining of blood vessels that narrow the vessel and restrict blood flow.

atrophy Shrinking of size; often used to describe the loss of brain mass seen in Alzheimer's disease during autopsy.

axon The arm of a nerve cell that normally transmits outgoing signals from one cell body to another. Each nerve cell has one axon, which can be relatively short in the brain but can be up to three feet long in other parts of the body.

blood-brain barrier The selective barrier that controls the entry of substances from the blood into the brain.

caudal In medicine, a directional term that means "toward the tail end."

cell The fundamental unit of all organisms; the smallest structural unit capable of independent functioning.

cell body Also called the soma, this is the part of the cell that contains the nucleus.

cell membrane The outer boundary of the cell. The cell membrane helps control what substances enter or exit the cell.

cerebral cortex The outermost layer of the cerebral hemispheres of the brain, responsible for conscious experience, including perception, emotion, thought, and planning.

cholinergic system The system of nerve cells that uses acetylcholine as its neurotransmitter.

chromosome An H-shaped structure inside the cell nucleus made up of tightly coiled strands of genes. Each chromosome is numbered (in humans, 1 through 46). Genes on chromosomes 1, 14, 19, and 21 are associated with Alzheimer's disease.

circadian rhythm A cycle of behavior or physiological change lasting approximately 24 hours.

cortisol A hormone manufactured by the adrenal cortex. In humans, it is secreted in highest amounts before dawn, readying the body for the daily activities.

dendrites Branched extensions of the nerve cell body that receive signals from other nerve cells. Each nerve cell usually has many dendrites.

diuretic A type of medication that washes out salt from the body and helps to reduce swelling and high blood pressure.

edema   Swelling due to excess fluid in tissue spaces.

enzyme   A protein produced by living organisms that promotes or otherwise influences chemical reactions.

fatty acids   Acids within the body derived from the breakdown of fats.

gene   The basic unit of heredity; a section of DNA coding for a particular trait. Each gene is located at a specific spot on a particular chromosome, and is made up of a string of chemicals arranged in a certain sequence along the DNA molecule.

genome   All the genes of an organism.

glutamate   An amino acid neurotransmitter that excites neurons (including receptors involved in learning and memory).

hippocampus   A structure located within the brain and considered to be an important part of the limbic system. It functions in learning, memory, and emotion.

hormones   Chemical messengers secreted by endocrine glands to regulate the activity of target cells that play a role in sexual development, calcium and bone metabolism, growth, and many other activities.

hypothalamus   A brain structure composed of many nuclei with different functions, including regulation of activities of internal organs, monitoring information from the autonomic nervous system, and controlling the pituitary gland.

immediate memory   A phase of memory that is extremely short-lived, with information stored for a few seconds. Also known as short-term and working memory.

incontinence   Involuntary discharge of feces or urine.

limbic system   A group of brain structures including the amygdala, hippocampus, septum, and basal ganglia, that regulate emotions, memory, and certain aspects of movement.

melatonin   Produced from serotonin, melatonin is released by the pineal gland into the bloodstream and affects physiological changes related to time and light cycles.

nerve   A bundle of axons through which signals pass to and from the brain.

nerve cell (neuron)   The basic working unit of the nervous system. The nerve cell is typically composed of a cell body containing the nucleus, several short branches (dendrites), and one long arm (the axon) with short branches along its length and at its end. Nerve cells send signals that control the actions of other cells in the body, such as other nerve cells and muscle cells.

nerve fiber   Structures of a neuron, aside from the cell body; nerve fibers include such things as dendrites and axons.

neurofibrillary tangle   A buildup of twisted fibers in the nerve cells of the cerebral cortex that is believed to play a role in the development of Alzheimer's disease.

neuron   The cellular unit of the central and peripheral nervous systems.

neurotransmitter   A chemical released by neurons at a synapse for the purpose of relaying information via receptors.

plaque   An abnormal protein deposit in the brain of a person with Alzheimer's disease. Plaques and neurofibrillary tangles in the brain are the hallmark of the disease.

pressure sore   Skin breakdown as a result of pressure on one area of the skin, usually from sitting or lying in one position for too long. Pressure sores are also called bedsores or decubitus ulcers.

receptor   A site on a nerve cell that receives a specific neurotransmitter; the message receiver.

synapse   The tiny gap between two nerve cells. Messages are transmitted across this gap from one nerve cell to another, usually by a neurotransmitter.

BIBLIOGRAPHY

Alzheimer's Association. "General Statistics/Demographics." Available on-line. URL: http://www.alz.org/hc/overview/stats.htm. Downloaded March 29, 2000.

Alzheimer's Association. "Progress in Alzheimer Research and Care." *Alzheimer's Association Newsletter* 19, no. 4 (Winter 2000): 3, 11.

American Psychiatric Association. "Practice Guideline for the Treatment of Patients with Alzheimer's Disease and Other Dementias of Late Life." *American Journal of Psychiatry* 154 (1997): 1–39.

Anand, R., J. Messina, and R. Hartman. "Dose-Response Effect of Rivastigmine in the Treatment of Alzheimer's Disease." *Internal Journal of Geriatric Psychopharmacology* 2 (2000): 68–72.

Arkin, Sharon. "Elder Rehab: A Student-Supervised Exercise Program for Alzheimer's Patients." *The Gerontologist* 39, no. 6 (1999): 729–735.

Aronstein, Zelda, Richard Olsen, and Ellen Schulman. "Nursing Assistants' Use of Recreational Interventions for Behavioral Management of Residents with Alzheimer's Disease." *American Journal of Alzheimer's Disease* 11, no. 3 (May/June 1996): 26–31.

Artiga, M. J., et al. A. Goate, and F. Valdivieso. "Risk for Alzheimer's Disease Correlates with Transcriptional Activity of the APOE Gene." *Human Molecular Genetics* 7 (1998): 1,887–1,892.

Auriacombe, S., J. J. Pere, Y. Loria-Kanza, and B. Vellas. "Efficacy and Safety of Rivastigmine in Patients with Alzheimer's Disease Who Failed to Benefit From Treatment With Donepezil." *Current Medical Research and Opinion* 18, no. 3 (2002): 129–138.

Axelsson, S. "The Basic Reality of Mind and Spongiform Diseases." *Medical Hypotheses* 57, no. 5 (November 2001): 549–554.

Balasubramanian, A. S. "Amyloid Beta Peptide Processing, Insulin Degrading Enzyme, and Butyrylcholinesterase." *Neurochemical Research* 26 (2001): 453–536.

Ballard, C., M. Johnson, M. Piggott, R. Perry, J. O'Brien, E. Rowan, E. Perry, P. Lantos, N. Cairns, and C. Holmes. "A Positive Association Between 5HT Reuptake Binding Sites and Depression in Dementia with Lewy Bodies." *Journal of Affective Disorders* 69, no. 1–3 (May 2002): 219–223.

Barber, R., A. Panikkar, and I. G. McKeith. "Dementia with Lewy bodies: Diagnosis and Management." *International Journal of Geriatric Psychiatry* 16, Supp 1, (December 2001): S12–S18.

Barker, W., D. Harwood, R. Duara, M. Mullan, D. Fallin, P. S. Hyslop, E. Rogaeva, and Y. Song. "The APOE-epsilon4 Allele and Alzheimer Disease Among African Americans, Hispanics, and Whites [letter]." *Journal of the American Medical Association* 280 (1998): 1,661–1,662.

Batson, K., B. McCabe, and M. M. Baun. "Effects of a Therapy Dog on Socialization and Physiologic Indicators of Stress in Persons Diagnosed with Alzheimer's Disease." In *Companion Animals in Human Health*, edited by C. C. Wilson and D. C. Turner. Thousand Oaks, Calif.: Sage, 1998.

Beal, M. F. "Energy, Oxidative Damage, and Alzheimer's Disease: Clues to the Underlying Puzzle." *Neurobiology of Aging* 15 Suppl. 2 (1994): S171–S174.

Beyersdorfer, P. S., and D. M. Birkenhauer. "The Therapeutic Use of Pets on an Alzheimer's Unit." *American Journal of Alzheimer's Care and Related Disorders and Research* 5, no. 1 (1990): 13–17.

Behl, C., and B. Moosmann. "Antioxidant Neuroprotection in Alzheimer's Disease as Preventive and Therapeutic Approach(2)." *Free Radical Biology and Medicine* 15, no. 332 (July 2002): 182–191.

Bhagat, Y. A., A. Obenaus, J. S. Richardson, and E. J. Kendall. "Evolution of Beta-Amyloid Induced Neuropathology: Magnetic Resonance Imaging and Anatomical Comparisons in the Rodent Hippocampus." *MAGMA* 14, no. 3 (June 2002): 223–232.

Bi, X., C. M. Gall, J. Zhou, and G. Lynch. "Uptake and Pathogenic Effects of Amyloid Beta Peptide 1-42 Are Enhanced by Integrin Antagonists and Blocked by NMDA Receptor Antagonists." *Neuroscience* 112, no. 4 (2002): 827–840.

Blacker, D., and R. E. Tanzi. "The Genetics of Alzheimer Disease: Current Status and Future Prospects." *Archives of Neurology* 55 (1998): 294–296.

Blass, J. P. "Brain Metabolism and Brain Disease: Is Metabolic Deficiency the Proximate Cause of Alzheimer Dementia?" *Journal of Neuroscience Research* 66, no. 5 (December 1, 2001): 851–856.

Blessed, G., B. Tomlinson, and M. Roth. "The Association Between Quantitative Measures of Dementia and of Senile Change in the Cerebral Gray Matter of Elderly Subjects." *British Journal of Psychiatry* 114 (1968): 797–811.

Bliwise, D. L., D. B. Rye, B. Dihenia, and P. Gurecki. "Greater Daytime Sleepiness in Subcortical Stroke Relative to Parkinson's Disease and Alzheimer's Disease." *Journal of Geriatric Psychiatry and Neurology* 15, no. 2 (Summer 2002): 61–67.

Blount, P. J., C. D. Nguyen, and J. T. McDeavitt. "Clinical Use of Cholinomimetic Agents: A Review," *Journal of Head Trauma and Rehabilitation* 17, no. 4 (August 2002): 314–321.

Bobinski, M., M. de Leon, A. Convit, et al. "MRI of Entorhinal Cortex in Mild Alzheimer's Disease." *Lancet* 353 (1999): 38–39.

Bonner, A. P., and S. O. Cousins. "Exercise and Alzheimer's Disease: Benefits and Barriers." *Activities, Adaptation and Aging* 20, no. 4 (1996): 21–34.

Brayne, C., C. R. Harrington, C. M. Wischik, F. A. Huppert, L. Y. Chi, J. H. Xuereb, D. W. O'Connor, and E. S. Paykel. "Apolipoprotein E genotype in the Prediction of Cognitive Decline and Dementia in a Prospectively Studied Elderly Population." *Dementia* 7 (1996): 169–174.

Brill, P. A., A. M. Drimmer, L. A. Morgan, et al. "The Feasibility of Conducting Strength and Flexibility Programs for Elderly Nursing Home Residents with Dementia." *Gerontologist* 35, no. 2 (1995): 263–266.

Burton, T., B. Liang, A. Dibrov, and F. Amara. "Transcriptional Activation and Increase in Expression of Alzheimer's Beta-Amyloid Precursor Protein Gene Is Mediated by TGF-beta in Normal Human Astrocytes." *Biochemical and Biophysical Research Communications* 295, no. 3 (July 2002): 702–12.

Burton, T., B. Liang, A. Dibrov, and F. Amara. "Transforming Growth Factor-Beta-Induced Transcription of the Alzheimer's Beta-Amyloid Precursor Protein Gene Involves Interaction Between the CTCF-complex and Smads." *Biochemical and Biophysical Research Communications* 295, no. 3 (July 2002): 713–23.

Butterfield, D. A., J. Drake, C. Pocernich, and A. Castegna. "Evidence of Oxidative Damage in Alzheimer's Disease Brain: Central Role for Amyloid Beta Peptide." *Trends in Molecular Medicine* 7, no. 12 (December 2001): 548–54.

Calhoun, M. E., K. H. Wiederhold, D. Abramowski, A. L. Phinney, A. Probst, C. Sturchler-Pierrat, M. Staufenbiel, B. Sommer, and M. Jucker. "Neuron Loss in APP Transgenic Mice [letter]." *Nature* 395 (1998): 755–756.

Campion, D., C. Dumanchin, D. Hannequin, B. Dubois, S. Belliard, M. Puel, C. Thomas-Anterion, A. Michon, C. Martin, F. Charbonnier, G. Raux, A. Camuzat, C. Penet, V. Mesnage, M. Martinez, F. Clerget-Darpoux, A. Brice, and T. Frebourg. "Early-onset Autosomal Dominant Alzheimer Disease: Prevalence, Genetic Heterogeneity, and Mutation Spectrum." *American Journal of Human Genetics* 65 (1999): 664–670.

Canadian Study of Health and Aging, "Risk Factors for Alzheimer's Disease in Canada." *Neurology* 44, no. 11 (1994): 2073–80.

Carr, J. "Long-term Outcome for People with Down's Syndrome." *Journal of Child Psychology & Psychiatry & Allied Disciplines* 35, no. 3 (March 1994): 425–439.

Carta, M. G., P. Serra, A. Ghiani, E. Manca, M. C. Hardoy, G. S. Del Giacco, G. Diaz, B. Carpiniello, and P. E. Manconi. "Chemokines and Pro-inflammatory Cytokines in Down's Syndrome: An Early Marker for Alzheimer-type Dementia?" *Psychotherapy and Psychosomatics* 71, no. 4 (July–August 2002): 233–236.

Cassel, C. K. "Genetic Testing and Alzheimer Disease: Ethical Issues for Providers and Families." *Alzheimer Disease and Associated Disorders* 12, Suppl. 3 (1998): S16–S20.

Castleman, M., et al. *There's Still a Person in There: The Complete Guide to Treating and Coping with Alzheimer's.* New York: Putnam, 2000.

Chan, C., A. Dharmarajan, C. S. Atwood, et al. "Anti-apoptotic Action of Alzheimer Ab." *Alzheimer's Reports* 2, no. 2 (1999): 113–119.

Chen, Q., H. Kimura, and D. Schubert. "A Novel Mechanism for the Regulation of Amyloid Precursor Protein Metabolism." *Journal of Cellular Biology* 158, no. 1 (July 8, 2002): 79–89.

Chui, D. H., T. Tabira, S. Izumi, G. Koya, and J. Ogata. "Decreased Beta Amyloid and Increased Abnormal Tau Deposition in the Brain of Aged Patients with Leprosy." *American Journal of Pathology* 145, no. 4 (October 1994): 771–775.

Churchill, M., J. Safaoui, B. W. McCabe, and M. M. Baun. "Effects of a Therapy Dog in Alleviating the Agitation Behavior of Sundown Syndrome and in Increasing Socialization for Persons with Alzheimer's Disease." *Journal of Psychosocial Nursing and Mental Health Services* 37, no. 4 (1999): 16–22.

Cohen, C. I., K. Hyland, and C. Magai. "Interracial and Intraracial Differences in Neuropsychiatric Symptoms, Sociodemography, and Treatment Among Nursing Home Patients with Dementia." *Gerontologist* 38, no. 3 (June 1998): 353–361.

Cohen, C. I., and C. Magai. "Racial Differences in Neuropsychiatric Symptoms Among Dementia Outpatients." *American Journal of Geriatric Psychiatry* 7, no. 1 (Winter 1999): 57–63.

Compton, J., T. van Amelsvoort, and D. Murphy. "HRT and Its Effect on Normal Aging of the Brain and Dementia." *British Journal of Clinical Pharmacology* 52, no. 6 (December 2001): 647–653.

Coon, D. W., H. Davies, C. McKibben, and D. Gallagher-Thompson. "The Psychological Impact of Genetic Testing for Alzheimer Disease." *Genetics Testing* 3 (1999): 121–131.

Copple, P. "Movement Is Life." *Geriatric Nursing Home Care* 7, no. 10 (1987): 20–22.

Corder, E., L. Lannfelt, and M. Mulder. "Apolipoprotein E and Herpes Simplex Virus 1 in Alzheimer's Disease." *Lancet* 352 (1998): 1,312–1,313.

Corder, E. H., K. Robertson, L. Lannfelt, N. Bogdanovic, G. Eggertsen, J. Wilkins, and C. Hall. "HIV-Infected Subjects with the E4 Allele for APOE Have Excess Dementia and Peripheral Neuropathy." *Nature Medicine* 4 (1998): 1,182–1,184.

Corder, E. H., L. Lannfelt, N. Bogdanovic, L. Fratiglioni, and H. Mori. "The Role of APOE Polymorphisms in Late-Onset Dementias." *Cellular and Molecular Life Sciences* 54 (1998): 928–934.

Corder, E., L. Lannfelt, and M. Mulder. "Apolipoprotein E and Herpes Simplex Virus 1 in Alzheimer's Disease [letter]." *Lancet* 352 (1998): 1,312–1,313.

Corey-Bloom, J., L. J. Thal, D. Galasko, et al. "Diagnosis and Evaluation of Dementia." *Neurology* 45 (1995): 211–218.

Corey-Bloom, J., D. Galasko, and L. J. Thai. "Is It Alzheimer's? A Strategy for Diagnosis." *Internal Medicine* 16 (1995): 28–37.

Corey-Bloom, J., R. Anand, J. Veach, et al. "A Randomized Trial Evaluating the Efficacy and Safety of ENA 713 (Rivastigmine Tartrate), a New Acetylcholinesterase Inhibitor, in Patients with Mild to Moderately Severe Alzheimer's Disease." *International Journal of Geriatric Psychopharmacology* 1 (1998): 55–65.

Cotton, P. "Constellation of Risks and Processes Seen in Search for Alzheimer's Clues." *Journal of the American Medical Association* 271 (1994): 89–91.

Craddock, N. and C. Lendon. "New Susceptibility Gene for Alzheimer's Disease on Chromosome 12?" *Lancet* 352 (1998): 1,720–1,721.

Crawford, F., T. Town, M. Freeman, J. Schinka, M. Gold, R. Duara, and M. Mullan. "The Alpha-2 Macroglobulin Gene Is Not Associated with Alzheimer's Disease in a Case-control Sample." *Neuroscience Letters* 270 (1999): 133–136.

Crawford, F., M. Freeman, T. Town, D. Fallin, M. Gold, R. Duara, and M. Mullan. "No Genetic Association Between Polymorphisms in the Tau Gene and Alzheimer's Disease in Clinic or Population Based Samples." *Neuroscience Letters* 266 (1999): 193–196.

Crawford, F., L. Abdullah, J. Schinka, Z. Suo, M. Gold, R. Duara, and M. Mullan. "Gender-Specific Association of the Angiotensin Converting Enzyme Gene with Alzheimer's Disease." *Neuroscience Letters* 280 (2000): 215–219.

Cummings, J., M. Mega, K. Gray. et al. "The Neuropsychiatric Inventory: Comprehensive Assessment of Psychopathology in Dementia." *Neurology* 44 (1994): 2,308–2,314.

Cummings, J. L. "The Neuropsychiatric Inventory: Assessing Psychopathology in Dementia Patients." *Neurology* 48, Suppl. 6 (1997): S10–S16.

Cummings, J. L., J. C. Frank, D. Cherry, N. D. Kohatsu, B. Kemp, L. Hewett, and B. Mittman. "Guidelines for Managing Alzheimer's Disease: Part II. Treatment." *American Family Physician* 65, no. 12 (June 15, 2002): 2,525–2,534.

Cutter, K. "Alzheimer's Disease." *Wellbeing Magazine* 60 (1995): 14–19.

Czech, C., G. Tremp, and L. Pradier. "Presenilins and Alzheimer's Disease: Biological Functions and Pathogenic Mechanisms." *Progress in Neurobiology* 60 (2000): 363–384.

Dahiyat, M., A. Cumming, C. Harrington, C. Wischik, J. Xuereb, F. Corrigan, G. Breen, D. Shaw, and D. St Clair. "Association Between Alzheimer's Disease and the NOS3 Gene." *Annals of Neurology* 46 (1999): 664–667.

Daly, M. J. "Untangling the Genetics of a Complex Disease [editorial; comment]." *Journal of the American Medical Association* 280 (1998): 652–653.

Danet, S., T. Brousseau, F. Richard, P. Amouyel, and C. Berr. "Risk of Dementia in Parents of Probands with and without the Apolipoprotein E4 Allele. The EVA Study." *Journal of Epidemiology & Community Health* 53 (1999): 393–398.

Davidson, Ann. *Alzheimer's: A Love Story: One Year in My Husband's Journey.* Palo Alto, Calif: Birch Lane Press, 1997.

Davies, Helen, and Michael Jensen. *Alzheimer's: The Answers You Need.* Forest Knolls, Calif: Elder Books, 1998.

Davis, C. M. "The Role of the Physical and Occupational Therapist in Caring for the Victim of Alzheimer's Disease." *Physical and Occupational Therapy in Geriatrics* 4, no. 3 (Spring 1986): 15–28.

Daw, E. W., H. Payami, E. J. Nemens, D. Nochlin, T. D. Bird, G. D. Schellenberg, and E. M. Wijsman. "The Number of Trait Loci in Late-onset Alzheimer Disease." *American Journal of Human Genetics* 66 (2000): 196–204.

Deb, S., and M. Janicki. "International Colloquium on Mental Retardation and Alzheimer's Disease: Conference Report." *Journal of Intellectual Disability Research* 39 (pt 2) (April 1995): 149–150.

de Knijff, P., and C. M. van Duijn. "Role of APOE in Dementia: A Critical Reappraisal." *Haemostasis* 28 (1998): 195–201.

Dekroon, R. M., and P. J. Armati. "The Effects of Oxidative Stress and Altered Intracellular Calcium Levels on Vesicular Transport of ApoE-egfp." *Cellular Biology International* 26, no. 5 (2002): 407–420.

Devanand, D. P., et al. "Olfactory Deficits in Patients with Mild Cognitive Impairment Predict Alzheimer's Disease at Follow-up." *American Journal of Psychiatry* 157 (September 2000): 1,399.

Dilworth-Anderson, P. "Family Issues and the Care of Persons with Alzheimer's Disease." *Aging Mental Health* 5, Suppl. 1(2) (May 2001): 49–51.

Dobson, C. B., and R. F. Itzhaki. "Herpes Simplex Virus Type 1 and Alzheimer's Disease." *The Neurobiology of Aging* 20 (1999): 457–465.

Doraiswamy, M., R. Hartman, and S. Graham. "Early Intervention with a Cholinesterase Inhibitor Produces Long-term Beneficial Effects in Moderately Severe AD Patients." *Neurobiology of Aging* 21, Suppl. 1 (2000): S275.

Dow, D. J., N. Lindsey, N. J. Cairns, C. Brayne, D. Robinson, F. A. Huppert, E. S. Paykel, J. Xuereb, G. Wilcock, J. L. Whittaker, and D. C. Rubinsztein. "Alpha-2 Macroglobulin Polymorphism and Alzheimer Disease Risk in the UK." *Nature Genetics* 22 (1999): 16–17.

Dowling, James R., and Nancy Mace. *Keeping Busy : A Handbook of Activities for Persons With Dementia.* Baltimore: Johns Hopkins University Press, 1995.

Drachman, D. A. "The Treatment of Alzheimer's Disease: Where Have We Been, and Where Are We Going?" *American Journal of Alzheimer's Disease and Other Dementias* 17, no. 3 (May–June 2002): 133–134.

Eaton, M. L. "Surrogate Decision Making for Genetic Testing for Alzheimer's Disease." *Genetics Testing* 3, (1999): 93–97.

Edwardson, J., and C. Morris. "The Genetics of Alzheimer's Disease." *British Medical Journal* 317 (1998): 361–362.

Engelhart, M. J., M. I. Geerlings, A. Ruitenberg, J. C. van Swieten, A. Hofman, J. C. Witteman, and M. M. Breteler. "Dietary Intake of Antioxidants and Risk of Alzheimer's Disease." *Journal of the American Medical Association* 287, no. 24 (June 26, 2002): 3,223–3,229.

Endoh, M., T. Kunishita, and T. Tabira. "No Effect of Anti-Leprosy Drugs in the Prevention of Alzheimer's Disease and Beta-Amyloid Neurotoxicity." *Journal of Neurological Science* 165, no. 1 (May 1, 1999): 28–30.

Espiritu, D. A., H. Rashid, B. T. Mast, J. Fitzgerald, J. Steinberg, and P. A. Lichtenberg. "Depression, Cognitive Impairment and Function in Alzheimer's Disease." *International Journal of Geriatric Psychiatry* 16, no. 11 (November 2001): 1,098–1,103.

Evans, D. A., L. A. Beckett, T. S. Field, L. Feng, M. S. Albert, D. A. Bennett, B. Tycko, and R. Mayeux. "Apolipoprotein E epsilon4 and Incidence of Alzheimer Disease in a Community Population of Older Persons." *Journal of the American Medical Association* 277 (1997): 822–824.

Evenhuis, H. M. "Natural History of Dementia in Down's Syndrome." *Archives of Neurology* 47, no. 3 (March 1990): 263–267.

Farkas, B. L. "The APOE-epsilon4 Allele and Alzheimer Disease Among African Americans, Hispanics, and Whites." *Journal of the American Medical Association* 280 (1998): 1,662.

Farlow, M. R. "Etiology and Pathogenesis of Alzheimer's Disease." *American Journal of Health-System Pharmacy* 55, Supp. 21 (1998): 5s–10s.

Farrer, L. A., L. A. Cupples, J. L. Haines, B. Hyman, W. A. Kukull, R. Mayeux, R. H. Myers, M. A. Pericak-Vance, N. Risch, and C. M. van Duijn. "Effects of Age, Sex, and Ethnicity on the Association Between Apolipoprotein E Genotype and Alzheimer Disease. A Meta-Analysis." *Journal of the American Medical Association* 278 (1997): 1,349–1,356.

Farrer, M., K. Gwinn-Hardy, M. Hutton, and J. Hardy. "The Genetics of Disorders with Synuclein Pathology and Parkinsonism." *Human Molecular Genetics* 8, (1999): 1,901–1,905.

Feil, Naomi. *Validation Breakthrough: Simple Techniques for Communicating with People with Alzheimer's-Type Dementia.* Baltimore: Health Professions Press, 1993.

Fine, R. E. "The Biochemistry of Alzheimer Disease." *Alzheimer Disease Association Disorders* 13, Suppl. 1 (1999): S82–S87.

Fogarty, M. "Genetic Testing, Alzheimer Disease, and Long-term Care Insurance." *Genetics Testing* 3 (1999): 133–137.

Folstein, M. F., S. E. Folstein, and P. R. McHugh. "Mini-Mental State: A practical method for grading the cognitive state of patients for the clinician." *Journal of Psychiatric Research* 12 (1975): 189–198.

Francis, P. T., A. M. Palmer, M. Snape, and G. K. Wilcock. "The Cholinergic Hypothesis of Alzheimer's Disease: a Review of Progress." *The Journal of Neurology and Neurosurgical Psychiatry* 66, no. 2 (February 1999): 137–47.

Fraser, M., and E. H. Snyder, Jr. "The Economic Benefits of Delaying Progression in Alzheimer's Disease Using Cholinesterase Inhibitors." *Clinical Geriatrics* 8 (2000): 72–93.

Fratiglioni, L., D. De Ronchi, and H. Aguero-Torres. "Worldwide Prevalence and Incidence of Dementia." *Drugs and Aging* 15 (1999): 365–375.

Fritz, C. L., B. F. Thomas, P. H. Kass, and Lynette Hart. "Association with Companion Animals and the Expression of Noncognitive Symptoms in Alzheimer's Patients." *Journal of Nervous and Mental Disease* 183, no. 7 (1995): 459–463.

Fruton, J. S. "A History of Pepsin and Related Enzymes." *Quarterly Review of Biology* 77, no. 2 (June 2002): 127–47.

Gasparini, L., W. J. Netzer, P. Greengard, and H. Xu. "Does Insulin Dysfunction Play a Role in Alzheimer's Disease?" *Trends in Pharmacological Sciences* 23, no. 6 (June 2002): 288–93.

Gatz, M., B. Lowe, and S. Berg, et al. "Dementia: Not Just a Search for the Gene." *Gerontologist* 34, no. 2 (1994): 251–255.

Gauthier, S., ed. *Clinical Diagnosis and Management of Alzheimer's Disease.* London: Martin Dunitz, 1999.

Geldmacher, D. S., and P. J. Whitehouse, Jr. "Differential Diagnosis of Alzheimer's Disease." *Neurology* 48, Suppl. 6 (1997): S2–S9.

Gelernther, J., H. Kranzler, and J. Lacobelle. "Population Studies of Polymorphisms at Loci of Neuropsychiatric Interest (Tryptophan Hydroxylase (TPH), Dopamine Transporter Protein (SLC6A3), D3 Dopamine Receptor (DRD3), Apolipoprotein E (APOE), Mu Opioid Receptor (OPRM1), and Ciliary Neurotrophic Factor (CNTF))." *Genomics* 52 (1998): 289–297.

Geller, L. N., and H. Potter. "Chromosome Missegregation and Trisomy 21 Mosaicism in Alzheimer's Disease." *Neurobiological Disease* 6 (1999): 167–179.

Gervais, F. G., D. Xu, G. S. Robertson, J. P. Vaillancourt, Y. Zhu, J. Huang, A. LeBlanc, D. Smith, M. Rigby, M. S. Shearman, E. E. Clarke, H. Zheng, L. H. Van Der Ploeg, S. C. Ruffolo, N. A. Thornberry, S. Xanthoudakis, R. J. Zamboni, S. Roy, and D. W. Nicholson. "Involvement of Caspases in Proteolytic Cleavage of Alzheimer's Amyloid-Beta Precursor Protein and Amyloidogenic A Beta Peptide Formation." *Cell* 97 (1999): 395–406.

Giacobini, E. "Cholinesterase Inhibitors Stabilize Alzheimer Disease." *Neurochemical Research* 25 (2000): 1,185–1,190.

Gluck, M. R., R. G. Thomas, K. L. Davis, and V. Haroutunian. "Implications for Altered Glutamate and GABA Metabolism in the Dorsolateral Prefontal Cortex of Aged Schizophrenic Patients." *American Journal of Psychiatry* 159, no. 7 (July 2002): 1165–73.

Goate, A., et al. "Susceptibility Locus for Alzheimer's Disease on Chromosome 10." *Science* 290 (2000): 2,304–2,305.

Goldsmith, S. M., B. Hoeffer, and J. Rader. "Problematic Wandering Behavior in the Cognitively Impaired Elderly." *Journal of Psychosocial Nursing & Mental Health Services* 33, no. 2 (February 1995): 6–12.

Goto, M., T. Kimura, S. Hagio, K. Ueda, S. Kitajima, H. Tokunaga, and E. Sato. "Neuropathological Analysis of Dementia in a Japanese Leprosarium." *Dementia* 6, no. 3 (May–June 1995): 157–61.

Grant, W. B. "The APOE-epsilon4 Allele and Alzheimer Disease Among African Americans, Hispanics, and Whites [letter]." *Journal of the American Medical Association* 280 (1998): 1,662–1,663.

Grant, William B. "Dietary Links to Alzheimer's Disease." The online journal *Alzheimer's Disease Review.* Posted on 19 June 1997. http://www.mc.uky.edu/adreview/Vol2-97.htm

Gray-Davidson, Freena. *The Alzheimer's Sourcebook for Caregivers.* New York: McGraw Hill, 1999.

Greely, H. T. "Special Issues in Genetic Testing for Alzheimer Disease." *Genetic Testing* 3 (1999): 115–119.

Grootendorst, J., E. R. de Kloet, S. Dalm, M. S. Oitzl. "Reversal of Cognitive Deficit of Apolipoprotein E Knockout Mice After Repeated Exposure to a Common Environmental Experience." *Neuroscience* 10; 108, no. 2 (December 2001): 237–247.

Grossbergm, G. T., H. B. Stahelinm, J. C. Messina, et al. "Lack of Adverse Pharmacodynamic Drug Interactions with Rivastigmine and Twenty-two Classes of Medications." *International Journal of Geriatric Psychiatry* 15 (2000): 242–247.

Gruetzner, Howard. *A Caregiver's Guide and Sourcebook* (3rd ed.). New York: John Wiley & Sons, 2001.

Guillozet, A. L., J. F. Smiley, D. C. Mash, et al. "Butyrylcholinesterase in the Life Cycle of Amyloid Plaques." *Annals of Neurology* 42 (1997): 909–918.

Gwyther, Lisa, and Peter Rabins. "Practical Approaches for Treating Behavioral Symptoms of People with Mild to Moderate Alzheimer's Disease." *Primary Psychiatry* 3, no. 12 (December 1996): 27, 79.

Haisman, Pam. *Alzheimer's Disease: Caregivers Speak Out.* Fort Myers, Fla.: Chippendale House, 1998.

Haraguchi, T., H. Ishizu, Y. Takehisa, et al. "Lead Content of Brain Tissue in Diffuse Neurofibrillary Tangles with Calcification (DNTC): the Possibility of Lead Neurotoxicity." *Neuroreport* 12, no. 18 (December 2001): 3,887–3,890.

Hardin, S., and B. Schooley. "A Story of Pick's Disease: A Rare Form of Dementia." *Journal of Neuroscience Nursing* 34 no. 3 (June 2002): 117–122.

Hardy, J., and K. Gwinn-Hardy. "Genetic Classification of Primary Neurodegenerative Disease." *Science* 282 (1998): 1,075–1,079.

Hardy, J., K. Duff, K. Gwinn Hardy, J. Perez-Tur, and M. Hutton. "Genetic Dissection of Alzheimer's Disease and Related Dementias: Amyloid and Its Relationship to Tau." *Nature Neuroscience* 1 (1998): 355–358.

Hardy, J., and A. Israel. "In Search of Gamma-Secretase." *Nature* 398 (1999): 466–467.

Harris, C. M., M. W. Dysken, P. Fovall, et al. "Effect of Lecithin on Memory in Normal Adults." *American Journal of Psychiatry* 140 (1983): 1,010–1,012.

Harvey, P. D. "Cognitive Impairment in Elderly Patients with Schizophrenia: Age Related Changes." *International Journal of Geriatric Psychiatry* 16, Suppl 1. (December 2001): S78–S85.

Hauss-Wegrzyniak, B., P. Dobrzanski, J. D. Stoehr, L. G. Wenk. "Chronic Neuroinflammation in Rats Reproduces Components of the Neurobiology of Alzheimer's Disease." *Brain Research* 780 (1997): 294–303.

Heiss, W. D., J. Kessler, R. Mielke, et al. "Long-term Effects of Phosphatidylserine, Pyritinol, and Cognitive Training in Alzheimer's Disease. A Neuropsychological, EEG, and PET Investigation." *Dementia* 5 (1994): 88–98.

Henderson, Cary. *Partial View: An Alzheimer's Journal.* Dallas: Southern Methodist University Press, 1998.

Henderson, A. S., S. Easteal, A. F. Jorm, A. J. Mackinnon, A. E. Korten, H. Christensen, L. Croft, and P. A. Jacomb. "Apolipoprotein E Allele Epsilon 4, Dementia, and Cognitive Decline in a Population Sample." *Lancet* 346 (1995): 1,387–1,390.

Henderson, V. W., A. Paganini-Hill, B. L. Miller, and et al. "Estrogen for Alzheimer's Disease in Women: Randomized, Double-blind, Placebo-Controlled Trial." *Neurology* 54 (2000): 295–301.

Hodgson, Harriet. *Alzheimer's—Finding the Words: A Communication Guide for Those Who Care.* New York: Wiley, 1995.

Ho, L. W., L. J. Cook, and D. C. Rubinsztein. "Decoding Darkness—The Search for the Genetic Causes of Alzheimer's Disease." *Journal of Medical Genetics* 38, no. 12 (December 2001): 894.

Hofman, A., A. Ott, M. M. Breteler, M. L. Bots, A. J. Slooter, F. van Harskamp, C. N. van Duijn, C. van Broeckhoven, and D. E. Grobbee. "Atherosclerosis, Apolipoprotein E, and Prevalence of Dementia and Alzheimer's Disease in the Rotterdam Study." *Lancet* 349 (1997): 151–154.

Hogervorst, E., M. Combrinck, P. Lapuerta, J. Rue, K. Swales, and M. Budge. "The Hopkins Verbal Learning Test and Screening for Dementia." *Dementia Geriatric Cognitive Disorders* 13, no. 1 (January–February 2002): 13–20.

Holmberg, S. K. "Evaluation of a Clinical Intervention for Wanderers on a Geriatric Nursing Unit." *Archives of Psychiatric Nursing* 11 no. 1 (February 1997): 21–28.

Holmes, C., M. J. Arranz, J. F. Powell, D. A. Collier, and S. Lovestone. "5-HT2A and 5-HT2C Receptor Polymorphisms and Psychopathology in Late Onset Alzheimer's Disease." *Human Molecular Genetics* 7 (1998): 1,507–1,509.

Holtzman, S., E. Ozanne, B. Carone, M. K. Goldstein, G. Steinke, and J. Timbs. "Decision Analysis and Alzheimer Disease: Three Case Studies." *Genetic Testing* 3 (1999): 71–83.

Hope, T., K. M. Tilling, K. Gedling, et al. "The Structure of Wandering in Dementia." *International Journal of Geriatric Psychiatry* 9, no. 2 (February 1994): 149–155.

Hoyer S. "Cholesterol and Alzheimer's Disease." *Neurology* 9, no. 59 (July 2002): 150–151.

Hu, Q., W. A. Kukull, S. L. Bressler, M. D. Gray, J. A. Cam, E. B. Larson, G. M. Martin, and S. S. Deeb. "The Human FE65 Gene: Genomic Structure and an Intronic Biallelic Polymorphism Associated with Sporadic Dementia of the Alzheimer Type." *Human Genetics* 103 (1998): 295–303.

Hughes, C., L. Berg, and W. Danzinger. "A New Clinical Scale for the Staging of Dementia." *British Journal of Psychiatry* 140 (1982): 566–572.

Hutton, M., et al. "Linkage of Plasma Ab42 to a Quantitative Locus on Chromosome 10 in Late-onset Alzheimer's Disease Pedigrees." *Science* 290 (2000): 2,303–2,304.

Hutton, M., J. Perez-Tur, and J. Hardy. "Genetics of Alzheimer's Disease." *Essays in Biochemistry* 33 (1998): 117–131.

Hyman, B. T., and R. Tanzi. "Molecular Epidemiology of Alzheimer's Disease." *New England Journal of Medicine* 333 (1995): 1,283–1,284.

Ihl, R., J. Brinkmeyer, M. Janner, M. S. Kerdar. "A Comparison of ADAS and EEG in the Discrimination of Patients with Dementia of the Alzheimer Type from Healthy Controls." *Neuropsychobiology* 41, no. 2 (January 2000): 102–107.

Ishihara, Takeshi, Ming Hong, Bin Zhang, Yasushi Nakagawa, Michael K. Lee, John Q. Trojanowski, and Virginia M.-Y Lee. "Age-dependent Emergence and Progression of a Tauopathy in Transgenic Mice Overexpress the Shortest Human Tau Isoform." *Neuron* 24, no. 1 (November 1999): 751–762.

Itzhaki, R. F., et al. "Herpes Simplex Virus 1 in Brain & Risk of Alzheimer's Disease." *Lancet* 349 (1997): 241–244.

Jann, M. W. "Rivastigmine, a New-Generation Cholinesterase Inhibitor for the Treatment of Alzheimer's Disease." *Pharmacotherapy* 20 (2000): 1–12.

Josefson, D. "Foods Rich in Antioxidants May Reduce Risk of Alzheimer's Disease." *British Medical Journal* 325, no. 7354 (6 July 2002): 7.

Joseph, J. A., B. Shukitt-Hale, N. A. Denisova, D. Bielinksi, A. Martin, J. J. McEwen, and P. C. Bickford. "Reversals of Age-Related Declines in Neuronal Signal Transduction, Cognitive, and Motor Behavioral Deficits with Blueberry, Spinach, or Strawberry Dietary Supplementation." *Journal of Neuroscience* 19, no. 18 (15 September 1999): 8,114–8,121.

Jost, B. C., G. T. Grossberg. "The Evolution of Psychiatric Symptoms in Alzheimer's Disease: A Natural History Study." *Journal of the American Geriatric Society* 44 (1996): 1,078–1,081.

Kaplan, H. I., B. J. Sadock, eds. *Kaplan & Sadock's Synopsis of Psychiatry: Behavioral Sciences/Clinical Psychiatry,* 8th ed. Baltimore: Williams & Wilkins, 1998.

Karlawish, J. H., D. Casarett, K. J. Propert, B. D. James, and C. M. Clark. "Relationship Between Alzheimer's Disease Severity and Patient Participation in Decisions About Their Medical Care." *Journal of Geriatric Psychiatry and Neurology* 15, no. 2 (Summer 2002): 68–72.

Kawas, C., S. Resnick, A. Morrison, R. Brookmeyer, M. Corrada, A. Zonderman, C. Bacal, and E. Metter. "A Prospective Study of Estrogen Replacement Therapy and the Risk of Developing Alzheimer's Disease." *Neurology* 48 (1997): 1,517–1,521.

Kennedy, G. J. "Advances in the Epidemiology of Alzheimer's Disease: Will Empiricism Improve the Public's Health?" *International Journal of Geriatric Psychiatry* 16, no. 11 (November 2001): 1028–1029.

Khachaturian, Z. S. "Calcium Hypothesis of Alzheimer's Disease and Brain Aging." *Annals of the New York Academy of Sciences* (1994): 7,471–7,481.

Kilpatrick, G. J., and G. S. Tilbrook. "Memantine." *Current Opinions in Investigative Drugs* 3, no. 5 (May 2002): 798–806.

Klegeris, A., E. A. Singh, and P. L. McGeer. "Effects of C-reactive Protein and Pentosan Polysulphate on Human Complement Activation." *Immunology* 106 no. 3 (July 2002): 381–388.

Klepper, H., and M. Rorty. "Personal Identity, Advance Directives, and Genetic Testing for Alzheimer Disease." *Genetic Testing* 3 (1999): 99–106.

Knapp, M. J., D. S. Knopman, P. R. Solomon, and et al. "A 30-week Randomized Controlled Trial of High-Dose Tacrine in Patients with Alzheimer's Disease." *Journal of the American Medical Association* 271 (1994): 985–991.

Knopman, D., M. Knapp, S. Gracon, and et al. "The Clinician Interview-based Impression (CIBI)—A Clinician Global Change Rating Scale in Alzheimer's Disease." *Neurology* 44 (1994): 2,315–2,321.

Knopman, D., L. Schneider, K. Davis, and et al. "Long-Term Tacrine (Cognex) Treatment: Effects on Nursing Home Placement and Mortality." *Neurology* 47 (1996): 166–177.

Koenig, B. A., and H. L. Silverberg. "Understanding Probabilistic Risk in Predisposition Genetic Testing for Alzheimer Disease." *Genetic Testing* 3 (1999): 55–63.

Koistinaho, M., M. I. Kettunen, D. M. Holtzman, R. A. Kauppinen, L. S. Higgins, and J. Koistinaho. "Expression of Human Apolipoprotein E Downregulates Amyloid Precursor Protein-induced Ischemic Susceptibility." *Stroke* 33, no. 7 (July 2002): 1905–10.

Kongable, L., K. Buckwalter, and J. Stolley. "The Effects of Pet Therapy on the Social Behavior of Institutionalized Alzheimer's Clients." *Archives of Psychiatric Nursing* 3, no. 4 (1989): 191–198.

Korovaitseva, G. I., A. Bukina, L. A. Farrer, and E. I. Rogaev. "Presenilin Polymorphisms in Alzheimer's Disease." *Lancet* 350 (1997): 959.

Korovaitseva, G. I., S. Premkumar, A. Grigorenko, Y. Molyaka, V. Galimbet, N. Selezneva, S. I. Gavrilova, L. A. Farrer, and E. I. Rogaev. "Alpha-2 Macroglobulin Gene in Early- and Late-Onset Alzheimer Disease. *Neuroscience Letters* 271 (1999): 129–131.

Kosik, K. S. "A Partnership that Delivers." *Natural Medicine* 5 (1999): 149–150.

Kovacs, D. M., and R. E. Tanzi. "Monogenic Determinants of Familial Alzheimer's Disease: Presenilin-1 Mutations." *Cellular and Molecular Life Sciences* 54 (1998): 902–909.

Kremer, B., P. Goldberg, S. E. Andrew, J. Theilmann, H. Telenius, J. Zeisler, F. Squitieri, B. Lin, A. Bassett, and E. Almqvist. "A Worldwide Study of the Huntington's Disease Mutation. The Sensitivity and Specificity of Measuring CAG Repeats." *New England Journal of Medicine* 330 (1994): 1,401–1,406.

Kruger, R., A. M. Vieira-Saecker, W. Kuhn, D. Berg, T. Muller, N. Kuhnl, G. A. Fuchs, A. Storch, M. Hungs, D. Woitalla, H. Przuntek, J. T. Epplen, L. Schols, and O. Riess. "Increased Susceptibility to Sporadic Parkinson's Disease by a Certain Combined Alpha-Synuclein/apolipoprotein E Genotype." *Annals of Neurology* 45 (1999): 611–617.

Kruman, I., T. S. Kumaravel, A. Lohani, W. Pedersen, R. G. Cutler, Y. Kruman, N. Haughey, J. Lee, M. Evans, and M. P. Mattson. "Folic Acid Deficiency and Homocysteine Impair DNA Repair in Hippocampal Neurons and Sensitize Them to Amyloid Toxicity in Experimental Models of Alzheimer's Disease." *Journal of Neuroscience* 22, no. 5 (1 March 2002): 1,752–1,762.

Kuhn, David, and David Bennett. *Alzheimer's Early Stages: First Steps in Caring and Treatment.* New York: Hunter House, 1999.

Kumari, V., M. T. Mitterschiffthaler, and T. Sharma. "Neuroimaging to Predict Preclinical Alzheimer's Disease." *Hosp Medicine* 63, no. 6 (June 2002): 341–345.

Lahiri, D. K., C. Nall, D. Chen, M. Zaphiriou, C. Morgan, and J. I. Nurnberger, Sr. "Developmental Expression of the Beta-Amyloid Precursor Protein and Heat-Shock Protein 70 in the Cerebral Hemisphere Region of the Rat Brain." *Annals of the New York Academy of Science* 965 (June 2002): 324–333.

Lahiri, D. K., T. Utsuki, D. Chen, M. R. Farlow, M. Shoaib, D. K. Ingram, and N. H. Greig. "Nicotine Reduces the Secretion of Alzheimer's Beta-Amyloid Precursor Protein Containing Beta-Amyloid Peptide in the Rat Without Altering Synaptic Proteins." *Annals of the New York Academy of Science* 965 (June 2002): 364–372.

Lai, F., E. Kammann, G. W. Rebeck, A. Anderson, Y. Chen, and R. A. Nixon. "APOE Genotype and Gender Effects on Alzheimer Disease in 100 Adults With Down Syndrome." *Neurology* 53 (1999): 331–336.

Lambert, J. C., C. Berr, F. Pasquier, A. Delacourte, B. Frigard, D. Cottel, J. Rez-Tur, V. Mouroux, M. Mohr, D. Cyre, D. Galasko, C. Lendon, J. Poirier, J. Hardy, D. Mann, P. Amouyel, and M. C. Chartier-Harlin. "Pronounced Impact of Th1/E47cs Mutation Compared with -491 AT Mutation on Neural APOE Gene Expression and Risk of Developing Alzheimer's Disease." *Human Molecular Genetics* 7 (1998): 1,511–1,516.

Lambert, J. C., T. Brousseau, V. Defosse, A. Evans, D. Arveiler, J. B. Ruidavets, B. Haas, J. P. Cambou, G. Luc, P. Ducimeti, F. Cambien, M. C. Chartier-Harlin, and P. Amouyel. "Independent Association of an APOE Gene Promoter Polymorphism with Increased Risk of Myocardial Infarction and Decreased APOE Plasma Concentrations—the ECTIM Study." *Human Molecular Genetics* 9 (2000): 57–61.

Lambert, J. C., L. Araria-Goumidi, L. Myllykangas, C. Ellis, J. C. Wang, M. J. Bullido, J. M. Harris, M. J. Artiga, D. Hernandez, J. M. Kwon, B. Frigard, R. C. Petersen, A. M. Cumming, F. Pasquier, I. Sastre, P. J. Tienari, A. Frank, R. Sulkava, J. C. Morris, D. St. Clair, D. M. Mann, F. Wavrant-DeVrieze, M. Ezquerra-Trabalon, P. Amouyel, J. Hardy, M. Haltia, F. Valdivieso, A. M. Goate, J. Perez-Tur, C. L. Lendon, and M. C. Chartier-Harlin. "Contribution of APOE Promoter Polymorphisms to Alzheimer's Disease Risk." *Neurology* 9, no. 59 (1 July 2002): 59–66.

Lapalio, L. R., and S. S. Sakla. "Distinguishing Lewy Body Dementia." *Hospital Practice* 33 (1998): 93–102, 107.

Lauderback, C. M., J. Kanski, J. M. Hackett, N. Maeda, M. S. Kindy, and D. A. Butterfield. "Apolipoprotein E modulates Alzheimer's Abeta(1-42)-induced Oxidative Damage to Synaptosomes in an Allele-Specific Manner." *Brain Research* 924, no. 1 (4 January 2002): 90–97.

Laws, S. M., K. Taddei, G. Martins, et al. "The -491AA Polymorphism in the APOE Gene Is Associated with Increased Plasma ApoE Levels in Alzheimer's Disease." *NeuroReport* 10 (1999): 879–882.

Lawton, M., and E. Brody. "Assessment of Older People: Self Maintaining and Instrumental Activities of Daily Living." *The Gerontologist* 9 (1969): 179–86.

Le Bars, P. J., et al. "A Placebo-Controlled, Double-Blind, Randomized Trial of an Extract of Ginkgo Bilboa for Dementia." *Journal of the American Medical Association* 278 (1997): 1,327–1,332.

LeBlanc, A. "Estrogen and Alzheimer's Disease." *Current Opinions in Investigative Drugs* 3 no. 5 (May 2002): 768–773.

Lehmann, D. J., J. Williams, J. Mcbroom, and A. D. Smith. "Using Meta-analysis to Explain the Diversity of Results in Genetic Studies of Late-onset Alzheimer's Disease and to Identify High-risk Subgroups." *Neuroscience* 108 no. 4 (December 2001): 541–554.

LeMaire, D., and R. Lacy. "Patience Is a Virtue." *Caring* 13 no. 8 (August 1994): 60–62.

Levy-Lahad, E., D. Tsuang, and T. D. Bird. "Recent Advances in the Genetics of Alzheimer's Disease." *Journal of Geriatric Psychiatry and Neurology* 11 (1998): 42–54.

Lewis, C., and J. Bottomly. *Geriatric Physical Therapy: A Clinical Approach.* East Norwalk, Conn.: Appleton & Lange, 1994.

Li, G., J. M. Silverman, L. D. Altstiel, V. Haroutunian, D. P. Perl, D. Purohit, S. Birstein, M. Lantz, R. C. Mohs, and K. L. Davis. "Apolipoprotein E-epsilon 4 Allele and Familial Risk in Alzheimer's Disease." *Genet Epidemiol* 13 (1996): 285–298.

Liao, A., R. M. Nitsch, S. M. Greenberg, U. Finckh, D. Blacker, M. Albert, G. W. Rebeck, T. Gomez-Isla, A. Clatworthy, G. Binetti, C. Hock, T. Mueller-Thomsen, U. Mann, K. Zuchowski, U. Beisiegel, H. Staehelin, J. H. Growdon, R. E. Tanzi, and B. T. Hyman. "Genetic Association of an Alpha2-macroglobulin (Val1000lle) Polymorphism and Alzheimer's Disease." *Human Molecular Genetics* 7 (1998): 1,953–1,956.

Licastro, F., S. Pedrini, M. Govoni, A. Pession, C. Ferri, G. Annoni, V. Casadei, F. Veglia, S. Bertolini, and L. M. Grimaldi. "Apolipoprotein E and Alpha-1-Antichymotrypsin Allele Polymorphism in Sporadic and Familial Alzheimer's Disease." *Neuroscience Letters* 270 (1999): 129–132.

Lilius, L., F. S. Froelich, H. Basun, C. Forsell, K. Axelman, K. Mattila, A. Andreadis, M. Viitanen, B. Winblad, L. Fratiglioni, and L. Lannfelt. "Tau Gene Polymorphisms and Apolipoprotein E Epsilon4 May Interact to Increase Risk for Alzheimer's Disease." *Neuroscience Letters* 277 (1999): 29–32.

Lindenmuth, G. F., and E. B. Lindenmuth. "Effects of a Three-Year Exercise Therapy Program on Cognitive Functioning." *American Journal of Alzheimer's Care and Related Disorders & Research*. 9, no. 1 (January/February 1994): 20–24.

Lovestone, S. "Early Diagnosis and the Clinical Genetics of Alzheimer's Disease." *Journal of Neurology* 246 (1999): 69–72.

Lucca, U. "Nonsteroidal Anti-inflammatory Drugs and Alzheimer's Disease." *CNS Drugs* 11 (1999): 207–224.

Lukiw, W. J., and N. G. Bazan. "Neuroinflammatory Signaling Upregulation in Alzheimer's Disease." *Neurochemical Research* 25 (2000): 1,173–1,184.

Lyketsos, C. G., J. M. Sheppard, M. Steinberg, J. A. Tschanz, M. C. Norton, D. C. Steffens, and J. C. Breitner. "Neuropsychiatric Disturbance in Alzheimer's Disease Clusters into Three Groups: the Cache County Study." *International Journal of Geriatric Psychiatry* 16, no. 11 (November 2001): 1,043–1,053.

Mace, Nancy L., and Peter V. Rabins. *The 36-Hour Day* (revised). New York: Warner Books, 2001.

Mahoney, D. F., B. J. Tarlow, R. N. Jones, and J. Sandaire. "Effects of a Multimedia Project on Users' Knowledge about Normal Forgetting and Serious Memory Loss." *Journal of the American Medical Information Association* 9, no. 4 (July–August 2000): 383–394.

Maiorini, A. F., M. J. Gaunt, T. M. Jacobsen, A. E. McKay, L. D. Waldman, and R. B. Raffa. "Potential Novel Targets for Alzheimer Pharmacotherapy: I. Secretases." *Journal of Clinical Pharmacy and Therapeutics* 27, no. 3 (June 2002): 169–83.

Manor, W. "Alzheimer's Patients and Their Caregivers: The Role of the Human-Animal Bond." *Holistic Nursing Practice* 5, no. 2 (1991): 32–37.

Marcell, Jacqueline. *Elder Rage or Take My Father . . . Please! : How to Survive Caring for Aging Parents*. Irvine, Calif.: Impressive Press, 2001.

Marshall, E. "The Alzheimer's Gene Puzzle." *Science* 280 (1998): 1002.

Marx, J. "New Gene Tied to Common Form of Alzheimer's." *Science* 281 (1998): 508–509.

Masters, C. L., and K. Beyreuther. "Alzheimer's Disease." *British Medical Journal* 316 (1998): 446–448.

Matteson, M. A., and A. Linton. "Wandering Behaviors in Institutionalized Persons with Dementia." *Journal of Gerontological Nursing* 22, no. 9 (September 1996): 39–46.

Mattson, M. P., S. L. Chan, and W. Duan. "Modification of Brain Aging and Neurodegenerative Disorders by Genes, Diet, and Behavior." *Physiological Reviews* 82, no. 3 (July 2002): 637–672.

Mayeux, Richard, et al. "The APOE-~4 Allele and the Risk of Alzheimer Disease Among African Americans, Whites and Hispanics." *Journal of the American Medical Association* (11 March 1998).

Mayeux, R., A. M. Saunders, S. Shea, S. Mirra, D. Evans, A. D. Roses, B. Hyman, B. Crain, M. X. Tang, and C. Phelps. "Utility of the Apolipoprotein E Genotype in the Diagnosis of Alzheimer Disease." *New England Journal of Medicine* 338 (1998): 506–511.

Mayeux, R., and R. Ottman. "Alzheimer's Disease Genetics: Home Runs and Strikeouts." *Annals of Neurology* 44 (1998): 716–719.

McConnell, L. M., B. A. Koenig, H. T. Greely, and T. A. Raffin. "Genetic Testing and Alzheimer Disease: Has the Time Come?" *Nature Medicine* 4 (1998): 757–759.

McConnell, L. M., G. D. Sanders, and D. K. Owens. "Evaluation of Genetic Tests: APOE Genotyping for the Diagnosis of Alzheimer Disease." *Genetics Testing* 3 (1999): 47–53.

McConnell, L. M., B. A. Koenig, H. T. Greely, and T. A. Raffin. "Genetic Testing and Alzheimer Disease: Recommendations of the Stanford Program in Genomics, Ethics, and Society." *Genetics Testing* 3 (1999): 3–12.

McKeith, I. G., D. Galasko, K. Kosaka, et al. "Consensus Guidelines for the Clinical and Pathologic Diagnosis of Dementia with Lewy Bodies (DLB): Report of the Consortium on DLB International Workshop." *Neurology* 47 (1996): 1,113–1,124.

McKeith, I., T. Del Ser, R. Anand, et al. "Rivastigmine Provides Symptomatic Benefit in Dementia with Lewy Bodies: Findings From a Placebo-Controlled International Multicenter Study." *Neurology* 54, Suppl. 3 (2000): A450.

McKeith, I., T. Del Ser, and P. Spano. "Effectiveness of Rivastigmine in Dementia With Lewy Bodies: a Randomised, Double-Blind, Placebo-Controlled International Study." *Lancet* 356 (2000): 2031–2036.

Mesulam, M. M., and C. Geula. "Butyrylcholinesterase Reactivity Differentiates the Amyloid Plaques of Aging From Those of Dementia." *Annals of Neurology* 36 (1994): 722–727.

Miklossy, J., K. Taddei, R. N. Martins. et. al. "Alzheimer Disease: Curly Fibers and Tangles in Organs Other than Brain." *Journal of Neuropathology and Experimental Neurology* 58/8 (1999): 803–814.

Molloy, William, and Paul Caldwell. *Alzheimer's Disease: Everything You Need to Know.* Westport, Conn.: Firefly Books, 1998.

Morris, J. C. "Differential Diagnosis of Alzheimer's Disease." *Clinical Geriatric Medicine* 10 (1994): 257–276.

Multhaup, G., S. Scheuermann, A. Schlicksupp, A. Simons, M. Strauss, A. Kemmling, C. Oehler, R. Cappai, R. Pipkorn, and T. A. Bayer. "Possible Mechanisms of APP-mediated Oxidative Stress in Alzheimer's Disease(1,2)." *Free Radical Biology and Medicine* 1 no. 33 (1 July 2002): 45–51.

Musha, T., T. Asada, F. Yamashita, T. Kinoshita, Z. Chen, H. Matsuda, M. Uno, and W. R. Shankle. "A New EEG Method for Estimating Cortical Neuronal Impairment That Is Sensitive to Early Stage Alzheimer's Disease." *Clinical Neurophysiology* 113, no. 7 (July 2002): 1,052–1,058.

Myers, D. L. "Remedies Beyond Counting Sheep." *Provider* 22, no. 2 (February 1996): 62–4.

Myers, C. E., A. Kluger, J. Golomb, S. Ferris, M. J. de Leon, G. Schnirman, and M. A. Gluck. "Hippocampal Atrophy Disrupts Transfer Generalization in Nondemented Elderly." *Journal of Geriatric Psychiatry and Neurology* 15, no. 2 (Summer 2002): 82–90.

Mendez, H. A. "The APOE-epsilon4 Allele and Alzheimer Disease Among African Americans, Hispanics, and Whites." *Journal of the American Medical Association* 280 (1998): 1663.

Mez-Isla, G., W. B. Growdon, M. J. McNamara, D. Nochlin, T. D. Bird, J. C. Arango, F. Lopera, K. S. Kosik, P. L. Lantos, N. J. Cairns, and B. T. Hyman. "The Impact of Different Presenilin 1 and Presenilin 2 Mutations on Amyloid Deposition, Neurofibrillary Changes and Neuronal Loss in the Familial Alzheimer's Disease Brain: Evidence for Other Phenotype-Modifying Factors." *Brain* 122 (1999): 1,709–1,719.

Morrison-Bogorad, M., C. Phelps, and N. Buckholtz. "Alzheimer Disease Research Comes of Age." *Journal of the American Medical Association* 277 (1997): 837–840.

Mullan, M., P. Scibelli, R. Duara, D. Fallin, M. Gold, J. Schinka, J. Hoyne, A. Osborne, S. Sevush, and F. Crawford. "Familial and Population-Based Studies of Apolipoprotein E and Alzheimer's Disease." *Annals of the New York Academy of Science* 802 (1996): 16–26.

Myllykangas, L., T. Polvikoski, R. Sulkava, A. Verkkoniemi, R. Crook, P. J. Tienari, A. K. Pusa, L. Niinisto, P. O'Brien, K. Kontula, J. Hardy, M. Haltia, and J. Perez-Tur. "Genetic Association of Alpha2-macroglobulin With Alzheimer's Disease in a Finnish Elderly Population." *Annals of Neurology* 46 (1999): 382–390.

Newman, Diane Kaschak, and Mary Dzvirnko. *The Urinary Incontinence Sourcebook.* Los Angeles: Lowell House, 1997.

Nichols, M., and D. Hwaleshka. "Studies Suggest that Aluminum May Play a Role in Alzheimer's Disease." *Maclean's* (10 April 1995): 45.

Nitsch, R. M., M. Deng, M. Tennis, D. Schoenfeld, and J. H. Growdon. "The Selective Muscarinic M1 Agonist AF102B Decreases Levels of Total A[beta] in Cerebrospinal Fluid of Patients With Alzheimer's Disease." *Annals of Neurology* 48 (2000): 913–918.

Nordberg, A., and A. L. Svensson. "Cholinesterase Inhibitors in the Treatment of Alzheimer's Disease: A Comparison of Tolerability and Pharmacology." *Drug Safety* 19 (1998): 465–480.

Ott, A., A. J. C. Slooter, A. Hofman, F. van Harskamp, J. C. M. Witteman, C. van Broeckhoven, and C. M. van Duijn. "Smoking and Risk of Dementia and Alzheimer's Disease in a Population-Based Cohort Study: the Rotterdam Study." *Lancet* 351 (1998): 1,840–1,843.

Panza, F., V. Solfrizzi, F. Torres, F. Mastroianni, A. Del Parigi, A. M. Colacicco, A. M. Basile, C. Capurso, R. Noya, and A. Capurso. "Decreased Frequency of Apolipoprotein E Epsilon4 Allele From Northern to Southern Europe in Alzheimer's Disease Patients and Centenarians." *Neuroscience Letters* 277, no. 1 (17 December 1999): 49–52.

Papassotiropoulos, A., M. Bagli, F. Jessen, T. A. Bayer, W. Maier, M. L. Rao, and R. Heun. "A Genetic Variation of the Inflammatory Cytokine Interleukin-6 Delays the Initial Onset and Reduces the Risk for Sporadic Alzheimer's Disease." *Annals of Neurology* 45 (1999): 666–668.

Papassotiropoulos, A., M. Bagli, O. Feder, F. Jessen, W. Maier, M. L. Rao, M. Ludwig, S. G. Schwab, and R. Heun, "Genetic Polymorphism of Cathepsin D Is Strongly Associated with the Risk for Developing Sporadic Alzheimer's Disease." *Neuroscience Letters* 262 (1999): 171–174.

Pappolla, M. A., M. A. Smith, T. Bryant-Thomas, N. Bazan, S. Petanceska, G. Perry, L. J. Thal, M. Sano, and L. M. Refolo. "Cholesterol, Oxidative Stress, and Alzheimer's Disease: Expanding the Horizons of Pathogenesis (1)." *Free Radical Biological Medicine* 15, no. 33 (2 July 2002): 173–181.

Payami, H., G. D. Schellenberg, S. Zareparsi, J. Kaye, G. J. Sexton, M. A. Head, S. S. Matsuyama, L. F. Jarvik, B. Miller, D. Q. McManus, T. D. Bird, R. Katzman, L. Heston, D. Norman, and G. W. Small. "Evidence for Association of HLA-A2 Allele With Onset Age of Alzheimer's Disease." *Neurology* 49 (1997): 512–518.

Pericak-Vance, M. A., C. C. Johnson, J. B. Rimmler, A. M. Saunders, L. C. Robinson, E. G. D'Hondt, C. E. Jackson, and J. L. Haines. "Alzheimer's Disease and Apolipoprotein E-4 Allele in an Amish Population." *Annals of Neurology* 39 (1996): 700–704.

Perry, E. K., A. T. Pickering, W. W. Wang, P. J. Houghton, and N. S. Perry. "Medicinal Plants and Alzheimer's Disease: From Ethnobotany to Phytotherapy." *Journal of Pharmacology* 51, no. 5 (May 1999): 527–34.

Petronis, A. "Alzheimer's Disease and Down Syndrome: From Meiosis to Dementia." *Experimental Neurology* 158 (1999): 403–413.

Pettegrew, J. W., K. Panchalingam, R. L. Hamilton, and R. J. McClure. "Brain Membrane Phospholipid Alterations in Alzheimer's Disease." *Neurochemical Research* 26 (2001): 771–82.

Petit-Turcotte, C., S. M. Stohl, U. Beffert, J. S. Cohn, N. Aumont, M. Tremblay, D. Dea, L. Yang, J. Poirier, and N. S. Shachter. "Apolipoprotein C-I Expression in the Brain in Alzheimer's Disease." *Neurobiological Disease* 8, no. 6 (December 2001): 953–963.

Pfeffer, R., T. Kurosaki, C. Harrah, and et al. "Measurement of Functional Activities of Older Adults in the Community." *Journal of Gerontology* 37 (1982): 323–329.

Poeggeler, B., L. Miravalle, M. G. Zagorski, T. Wisniewski, Y. J. Chyan, Y. Zhang, H. Shao, T. Bryant-Thomas, R. Vidal, B. Frangione, J. Ghiso, and M. A. Pappolla. "Melatonin Reverses the Profibrillogenic Activity of Apolipoprotein E4 on the Alzheimer Amyloid A-beta Peptide." *Biochemistry* 40, no. 49 (11 December 2001): 14995–5001.

Poirier, J. "Apolipoprotein E: A Pharmacogenetic Target for the Treatment of Alzheimer's Disease." *Molecular Diagnosis* 4 (1999): 335–341.

Poirier, J., J. Davignon, D. Bouthillier, S. Kogan, P. Bertrand, and S. Gauthier. "Apolipoprotein E Polymorphism and Alzheimer's Disease." *Lancet* 342 (1993): 697–699.

Polinsky, R. J. "Clinical Pharmacology of Rivastigmine: A New-Generation Acetylcholinesterase Inhibitor for the Treatment of Alzheimer's Disease." *Clinical Therapy* 20 (1998): 634–647.

Polvikoski, T., R. Sulkava, M. Haltia, K. Kainulainen, A. Vuorio, A. Verkkoniemi, L. Niinisto, P. Halonen, and K. Kontula. "Apolipoprotein E, Dementia, and Cortical Deposition of Beta-amyloid Protein." *New England Journal of Medicine* 333 (1995): 1,242–1,247.

Post, S. G., P. J. Whitehouse, R. H. Binstock, T. D. Bird, S. K. Eckert, L. A. Farrer, L. M. Fleck, A. D. Gaines, E. T. Juengst, H. Karlinsky, S. Miles, T. H. Murray, K. A. Quaid, N. R. Relkin, A. D. Roses, P. H. St. George-Hys-lop, G. A. Sachs, B. Steinbock, E. F. Truschke, and A. B. Zinn. "The Clinical Introduction of Genetic Testing for Alzheimer Disease. An Ethical Perspective." *Journal of the American Medical Association* 277 (1997): 832–836.

Post, S. G. "Future Scenarios for the Prevention and Delay of Alzheimer's Disease Onset in High-Risk Groups." *American Journal of Preventive Medicine* 16 (1999): 105–110.

Prasher, V. P., and V. H. R. Krishnan. "Age of Onset and Duration of Dementia in People with Down Syndrome: Integration of 98 Reported Cases in the Literature." *International Journal of Geriatric Psychiatry* 8, no. 11 (November 1993): 915–922.

Price, D. L., S. S. Sisodia, and D. R. Borchelt. "Genetic Neurodegenerative Diseases: the Human Illness and Transgenic Models." *Science* 282 (1998): 1,079–1,083.

Pulst, S. M. "Genetic Linkage Analysis." *Archives of Neurology* 56 (1999): 667–672.

Ramassamy, C., D. Averill, U. Beffert, S. Bastianetto, L. Theroux, S. Lussier-Cacan, J. S. Cohn, Y. Christen, J. Davignon, R. Quirion, and J. Poirier. "Oxidative Damage and Protection by Antioxidants in the Frontal Cortex of Alzheimer's Disease Is Related to the Apolipoprotein E Genotype." *Free Radical Biological Medicine* 27 (1999): 544–553.

Ramassamy, C., D. Averill, U. Beffert, L. Theroux, S. Lussier-Cacan, J. S. Cohn, Y. Christen, A. Schoofs, J. Davignon, and J. Poirier. "Oxidative Insults Are Associated With Apolipoprotein E Genotype in Alzheimer's Disease Brain." *Neurobiology of Disease* 7 (2000): 23–37.

Raskind, M. A., C. H. Sadowsky, W. R. Sigmund, P. J. Beitler, and S. B. Auster. "Effect of Tacrine on Language, Praxis, and Noncognitive Behavioral Problems in Alzheimer's Disease." *Archives of Neurology* 54 (1997): 836–840.

Raskind, M. A., E. R. Peskind, T. Wessel, and et al. "Galantamine in AD: A 6-Month Randomized, Placebo-controlled Trial with a 6-month Extension." *Neurology* 54 (2000): 2,261–2,268.

Rasmussen, D. E., and D. Sobsey. "Age, Adaptive Behavior, and Alzheimer Disease in Down Syndrome: Cross-sectional and Longitudinal Analyses." *American Journal of Mental Retardation* 99, no. 2 (September 1994): 151–165.

Rebeck, G. W., B. S. Cheung, W. B. Growdon, A. Deng, P. Akuthota, J. Locascio, S. M. Greenberg, and B. T. Hyman. "Lack of Independent Associations of Apolipoprotein E Promoter and Intron 1 Polymorphisms with Alzheimer's Disease." *Neuroscience Letters* 272 (1999): 155–158.

Reichman, W. E., and A. Negron. "Negative Symptoms in the Elderly Patient With Dementia." *International Journal of Geriatric Psychiatry* 16, Suppl. 1 (December 2001): S7–S11.

Reiman, E. M., R. J. Caselli, L. S. Yun, K. Chen, D. Bandy, S. Minoshima, S. N. Thibodeau, and D. Osborne. "Preclinical Evidence of Alzheimer's Disease in Persons Homozygous for the Epsilon 4 Allele for Apolipoprotein E." *New England Journal of Medicine* 334 (1996): 752–758.

Reisberg, B., J. Borenstein, S. Salob, and et al. "Behavioral Symptoms in Alzheimer's Disease: Phenomenology and Treatment." *Journal of Clinical Psychiatry* 48 (1987): s9–s15.

Relkin, N. R. "Promise and Peril: New Genetic Discoveries and Alzheimer Disease." *Alzheimer Disease and Associated Disorders* 12, Suppl. 3 (1998): S1–S2.

Renbaum, P., and E. Levy-Lahad. "Monogenic Determinants of Familial Alzheimer's Disease: Presenilin-2 Mutations." *Cellular Molecular Life Science* 54 (1998): 910–919.

Richard, F., N. Helbecque, E. Neuman, D. Guez, R. Levy, and P. Amouyel. "APOE Genotyping and Response to Drug Treatment in Alzheimer's Disease." *Lancet* 349 (1997): 539.

Riley, K., D. Snowdon, and W. Markesbery. "Alzheimer's Neurofibrillary Pathology and the Spectrum of Cognitive Function: Findings from the Nun Study." *Annals of Neurology* 51 (2002): 567–577.

Ritchie, K., and A. M. Dupuy. "The Current Status of Apo E4 as a Risk Factor for Alzheimer's Disease: An Epidemiological Perspective." *International Journal of Geriatric Psychiatry* 14 (1999): 695–700.

Robbins, T. W., M. James, A. M. Owen, B. J. Sahakian, L. McInnes, and P. Rabbitt. "Cambridge Neuropsychological Test Automated Battery (CANTAB): A Factor Analytic Study of a Large Sample of Normal Elderly Volunteers." *Dementia* 5, no. 5 (September/October 1994): 266–281.

Roberts, C. "The Management of Wandering in Older People With Dementia." *Journal of Psychiatric & Mental Health Nursing* 3, no. 2 (April 1996): 138–139.

Robertson, T., et al. "Early Deposition of B-Amyloid Protein in Brains of ApoE Deficient Mice." *Neuroscience* 82, no. 1 (1998): 171–180.

Rocha, L., C. Garcia, A. de Mendonca, J. P. Gil, D. T. Bishop, and M. C. Lechner. "N-Acetyltransferase (NAT2) Genotype and Susceptibility of Sporadic Alzheimer's Disease." *Pharmacogenetics* 9 (1999): 9–15.

Rogaeva, E., S. Premkumar, Y. Song, S. Sorbi, N. Brindle, A. Paterson, R. Duara, G. Levesque, G. Yu, M. Nishimura, M. Ikeda, C. O'Toole, T. Kawarai, R. Jorge, D. Vilarino, A. C. Bruni, L. A. Farrer, and P. H. St. George-Hyslop. "Evidence for an Alzheimer Disease Susceptibility Locus on Chromosome 12 and for Further Locus Heterogeneity." *Journal of the American Medical Association* 280 (1998): 614–618.

Rogaeva, E. A., S. Premkumar, J. Grubber, L. Serneels, W. K. Scott, T. Kawarai, Y. Song, D. L. Hill, S. M. Abou-Donia, E. R. Martin, J. J. Vance, G. Yu, A. Orlacchio, Y. Pei, M. Nishimura, A. Supala, B. Roberge, A. M. Saunders, A. D. Roses, D. Schmechel, A. Crane-Gatherum, S. Sorbi, A. Bruni, G. W. Small, and M. A. Pericak-Vance. "An Alpha-2-Macroglobulin Insertion-deletion Polymorphism in Alzheimer Disease [letter]." *Nature Genetics* 22 (1999): 19–22.

Rogers, J., L. C. Kirby, S. R. Hempelman, and et al. "Clinical Trial of Indomethacin in Alzheimer's Disease." *Neurology* 43 (1993): 1,609–1,611.

Rogers, S. L., M. R. Farlow, R. S. Doody, and et al. "A 24-week, Double-Blind, Placebo-Controlled Trial of Donepezil in Patients with Alzheimer's Disease." *Neurology* 50 (1998): 136–145.

Rohn, T. T., E. Head, W. H. Nesse, C. W. Cotman, and D. H. Cribbs. "Activation of Caspase-8 in the Alzheimer's Disease Brain." *Neurobiological Disease* 8 no. 6 (December 2001): 1,006–1,016.

Romas, S. N., M. X. Tang, L. Berglund, and R. Mayeux. "APOE Genotype, Plasma Lipids, Lipoproteins, and AD in Community Elderly." *Neurology* 53 (1999): 517–521.

Rosenberg, R. N. "Molecular Neurogenetics: the Genome Is Settling the Issue [editorial comment]." *Journal of the American Medical Association* 278 (1997): 1,282–1,283.

Rosen, W. G., R. D. Terry, P. A. Fuld, et al. "Pathological Verification of Ischemic Score in Differentiation of Dementias." *Annals of Neurology* 7 (1980): 486–488.

Rosen, W., R. Mohs, and K. Davis. "A New Rating Scale for Alzheimer's Disease." *American Journal of Psychiatry* 14 (1984): 1,356–1,364.

Rosler, M., R. Anand, A. Cicin-Sain, et al. "Efficacy and Safety of Rivastigmine in Patients with Alzheimer's Disease: International Randomised Controlled Trial." *British Medical Journal* 318 (1999): 633–638.

Rubinsztein, D. C., J. Hon, F. Stevens, I. Pyrah, C. Tysoe, F. A. Huppert, D. F. Easton, and A. J. Holland. "Apo E Genotypes and Risk of Dementia in Down Syndrome." *American Journal of Medical Genetics* 88 (1999): 344–347.

Rubinsztein, D. C., and D. F. Easton. "Apolipoprotein E Genetic Variation and Alzheimer's Disease, a Meta-analysis." *Dementia and Geriatric Cognitive Disorders* 10 (1999): 199–209.

Rudrasingham, V., V. F. Wavrant-De, J. C. Lambert, S. Chakraverty, P. Kehoe, R. Crook, P. Amouyel, W. Wu, F. Rice, J. Perez-Tur, B. Frigard, J. C. Morris, S. Carty, R. Petersen, D. Cottel, N. Tunstall, P. Holmans, S. Lovestone, M. C. Chartier-Harlin, A. Goate, J. Hardy, M. J. Owen, and J. Williams. "Alpha-2 Macroglobulin Gene and Alzheimer Disease." *Nature Genetics* 22 (1999): 17–19.

Ryan, J. P., J. McGown, N. McCaffrey, et al. "Graphomotor Perseveration and Wandering in Alzheimer's Disease." *Journal of Geriatric Psychiatry & Neurology* 8, no. 4 (October 1995): 209–12.

Sano, M., C. Ernesto, R. G. Thomas, et al. "A Controlled Trial of Selegiline, Alpha-Tocopherol, or Both as Treatment for Alzheimer's Disease." *New England Journal of Medicine* 336 (1997): 1,216–1,222.

Saunders, A. M., O. Hulette, K. A. Welsh-Bohmer, D. E. Schmechel, B. Crain, J. R. Burke, M. J. Alberts, W. J. Strittmatter, J. C. Breitner, and C. Rosenberg. "Specificity, Sensitivity, and Predictive Value of Apolipoprotein-E Genotyping for Sporadic Alzheimer's Disease." *Lancet* 348 (1996): 90–93.

Saunders, A. M., K. Schmader, J. C. Breitner, M. D. Benson, W. T. Brown, L. Goldfarb, D. Goldgaber, M. G. Manwaring, M. H. Szymanski, and N. McCown. "Apolipoprotein E Epsilon 4 Allele Distributions in Late-onset Alzheimer's Disease and in Other Amyloid-Forming Diseases." *Lancet* 342 (1993): 710–711.

Schaub, R. T., D. Anders, G. Golz, K. Gohringer, and R. Hellweg. "Serum Nerve Growth Factor Concentration and Its Role in the Preclinical Stage of Dementia." *American Journal of Psychiatry* 159 (7 July 2002): 1,227–1,229.

Schneider, L. S., M. R. Farlow, V. W. Henderson, and et al. "Effects of Estrogen Replacement Therapy on Response to Tacrine in Patients With Alzheimer's Disease." *Neurology* 46 (1996): 1,580–1,584.

Schneider, L. S. "An Overview of Rating Scales Used in Dementia Research." *Alzheimer Insights* 2 (1996): 1–7.

Schorderet, M. "Alzheimer's Disease: Fundamental and Therapeutic Aspects," *Experientia* 51 (1995): 99–105.

Schutte, D. L. "Genetic Testing in Alzheimer's Disease. Benefits Risks and Public Policy." *Journal of Gerontological Nursing* 24 (1998): 17–23.

Scott, J. "Apolipoprotein E and Alzheimer's Disease." *Lancet* 342 (1993): 696.

Scott, W. K., J. M. Grubber, S. M. Abou-Donia, T. D. Church, A. M. Saunders, A. D. Roses, M. A. Pericak-Vance, P. M. Conneally, G. W. Small, and J. L. Haines. "Further Evidence Linking Late-Onset Alzheimer Disease With Chromosome 12." *Journal of the American Medical Association* 281 (1999): 513–514.

Selkoe, D. J. "Translating Cell Biology into Therapeutic Advances in Alzheimer's Disease." *Nature* 399 (1999): A23–A31.

Shadlen, M. F., and E. B. Larson. "What's New in Alzheimer's Disease Treatment? Reasons for Optimism About Future Pharmacologic Options." *Postgraduate Medicine* 105 (1999): 109–118.

Shanks, Lela Knox. *Your Name Is Hughes Hannibal Shanks: A Caregiver's Guide to Alzheimer's.* New York: The Penguin Group, 1999.

Shapira, J. "Research Trends in Alzheimer's Disease." *Journal of Gerontological Nursing* 20, no. 4 (1994): 4–10.

Sheikh, J. I., and J. A. Yesavage. "Geriatric Depression Scale (GDS): Recent Evidence and Development of a Shorter Version." *Clinical Gerontology* 5 (1986): 165–173.

Shenk, David. *The Forgetting: Alzheimer's: Portrait of an Epidemic.* New York: Doubleday, 2001.

Sherrard, D. J. "Aluminum—Much Ado About Something." *The New England Journal of Medicine* 324, no. 8 (1991): 558–60.

Shibata, N., T. Ohnuma, T. Takahashi, E. Ohtsuka, A. Ueki, and H. Arai. "Genetic Association Between Alpha-2 Macroglobulin and Japanese Sporadic Alzheimer's Disease." *Neuroscience Letters* 271 (1999): 132–134.

Siegler, I. C., L. A. Bastian, D. C. Steffens, H. B. Bosworth, and P. T. Costa. "Behavioral Medicine and Aging." *Journal of Consulting and Clinical Psychology* 70 (3 June 2002): 843–51.

Sigurdsson, E. M., D. R. Brown, M. Daniels, R. J. Kascsak, R. Kascsak, R. Carp, H. C. Meeker, B. Frangione, and T. Wisniewski. "Immunization Delays the Onset of Prion Disease in Mice." *American Journal of Pathology* 161 (1 July 2002): 13–17.

Silverman, J. M., C. J. Smith, D. B. Marin, S. Birstein, M. Mare, R. C. Mohs, and K. L. Davis. "Identifying Families with Likely Genetic Protective Factors Against Alzheimer Disease." *American Journal of Human Genetics* 64 (1999): 832–838.

Singleton, A. B., A. M. Gibson, A. L. Atkinson, A. Daly, and C. M. Morris. "Presenilin Polymorphisms in Alzheimer's Disease." *Lancet* 350 (1997): 958–959.

Sjogren, M., M. Blomberg, M. Jonsson, L. O. Wahlund, L. Rosengren, K. Blennow, and A. Wallin. "Neurofilament Protein in Cerebrospinal Fluid: A Marker of White Matter Changes." *Journal of Neuroscience Research* 66, no. 3 (1 November 2001): 510–516.

Skoog, I., J. Marcusson, and K. Blennow. "Dementia: It's Getting Better All the Time." *Lancet* 352, Suppl. 4 (1998): SIV4.

Sloane, Philip. "Advances in the Treatment of Alzheimer's Disease." *American Family Physician* 58 no. 6 (1 November 1998): 1,577–1,586.

Slooter, A. J., M. Cruts, S. Kalmijn, A. Hofman, M. M. Breteler, C. van Broeckhoven, and C. M. van Duijn. "Risk Estimates of Dementia by Apolipoprotein E Genotypes from a Population-Based Incidence Study." *Archives of Neurology* 55 (1998): 964–968.

Slooter, A. J. C., and C. M. van Duijn. "Genetic Epidemiology of Alzheimer Disease." *Epidemiological Review* 19 (1997): 107–119.

Small, G. W., P. V. Rabins, P. P. Barry, et al. "Diagnosis and Treatment of Alzheimer Disease and Related Disorders: Consensus Statement of the American Association for Geriatric Psychiatry, the Alzheimer's Association, and the American Geriatrics Society." *Journal of the American Medical Association* 278 (1997): 1,363–1,371.

Small, G. W. "Treatment of Alzheimer's Disease: Current Approaches and Promising Developments." *American Journal of Medicine* 104, Suppl. 4A (1998): 32S–38S.

Small, G. W., S. T. Chen, S. Komo, et al. "Memory Self-appraisal and Depressive Symptoms in People at Genetic Risk for Alzheimer's Disease." *International Journal of Geriatric Psychiatry* 16, no. 11 (November 2001): 1,071–1,077.

Small, G. W., S. T. Chen, S. Komo, L. Ercoli, S. Bookheimer, K. Miller, H. Lavretsky, S. Saxena, A. Kaplan, D. Dorsey, W. K. Scott, A. M. Saunders, J. L. Haines, A. D. Roses, and M. A. Pericak-Vance. "Memory Self-Appraisal in Middle-Aged and Older Adults With the Apolipoprotein E-4 Allele." *American Journal of Psychiatry* 156 (1999): 1,035–1,038.

Small, G. W., W. K. Scott, S. Komo, L. H. Yamaoka, L. A. Farrer, S. H. Auerbach, A. M. Saunders, A. D. Roses, J. L. Haines, and M. A. Pericak-Vance. "No Association between the HLA-A2 Allele and Alzheimer Disease." *Neurogenetics* 2 (1999): 177–182.

Snowdon, D. *Aging with Grace: What the Nun Study Teaches Us About Leading Longer, Healthier, and More Meaningful Lives.* New York: Bantam Books, 2001.

Sobel, E., M. Dunn, Z. Davanipour, Z. Qian, and H. C. Chui. "Elevated Risk of Alzheimer's Disease Among Workers With Likely Electromagnetic Field Exposure." *MD NEUROLOGY* 47 (December 1996): 1,477–1,481.

Sodeyama, N., M. Yamada, Y. Itoh, N. Suematsu, M. Matsushita, E. Otomo, and H. Mizusawa. "Lack of Genetic Associations of Alpha-1-Antichymotrypsin Polymorphism With Alzheimer-type Neuropathological Changes or Sporadic Alzheimer's Disease." *Dementia and Geriatric Cognitive Disorders* 10 (1999): 221–225.

Sodeyama, N., M. Yamada, Y. Itoh, N. Suematsu, M. Matsushita, E. Otomo, and H. Mizusawa. "No Association of Paraoxonase Gene Polymorphism with Atheroscle-

rosis or Alzheimer's Disease." *Neurology* 53 (1999): 1,146–1,148.

Solfrizzi, V., F. Panza, F. Torres, C. Capurso, A. D'Introno, A. M. Colacicco, and A. Capurso. "Selective Attention Skills in Differentiating Between Alzheimer's Disease and Normal Aging." *Journal of Geriatric Psychiatry and Neurology* 15, no. 2 (Summer 2002): 99–109.

Spillantini, M. G., R. A. Crowther, R. Jakes, M. Hasegawa, and M. Goedert. "Alpha-Synuclein in Filamentous Inclusions of Lewy Bodies From Parkinson's Disease and Dementia With Lewy Bodies." *Proceedings of the National Academy of Science* 95 (1998): 6,469–6,473.

Squire, L., and E. Kandel. *Memory: From Mind to Molecules.* New York: Scientific American Library, 2000.

Sramek, J., and N. Cutler. "Recent Developments in the Drug Treatment of Alzheimer's Disease." *Drugs and Aging* 14, no. 5 (May 1999): 359–373.

St. George-Hyslop, P. H. "Molecular Genetics of Alzheimer's Disease." *Biological Psychiatry* 47 (2000): 183–199.

Steiner, H., A. Capell, U. Leimer, and C. Haass. "Genes and Mechanisms Involved in Beta-Amyloid Generation and Alzheimer's Disease." *European Archives of Psychiatry and Clinical Neuroscience* 249 (1999): 266–270.

Stern, R. G., R. C. Mohs, M. Davidson, et al. "A Longitudinal Study of Alzheimer's Disease: Measurement, Rate, and Predictors of Cognitive Deterioration." *American Journal of Psychiatry* 151 (1994): 390–396.

Stewart, W. F., C. Kawas, M. Corrada, and E. J. Metter. "Risk of Alzheimer's Disease and Duration of NSAID use." *Neurology* 48 (1997): 627–631.

Stockdale, A. "Public Understanding of Genetics and Alzheimer Disease." *Genetics Testing* 3 (1999): 139–145.

Stone, R. I. "Alzheimer's Disease and Related Dementias: Important Policy Issues." *Aging Mental Health* 5, Suppl. 1, no. 2 (May 2001): 146–148.

Stoppe, G., H. Sandholzer, J. Staedt, et al. "Sleep Disturbances in the Demented Elderly: Treatment in Ambulatory Care." *Sleep* 18, no. 10 (December 1995): 844–848.

Swanberg, M. M., and J. L. Cummings. "Benefit-risk Considerations in the Treatment of Dementia With Lewy Bodies." *Drug Safety* 25, no. 7 (2002): 511–523.

Swartz, R. H., S. E. Black, and P. St. George-Hyslop. "ApolipoproteinE and Alzheimer's Disease: A Genetic, Molecular and Neuroimaging Review." *Canadian Journal of Neurological Science* 26 (1999): 77–88.

Taddei, K., D. Yang, C. Fisher, et al. "No Association of Presenilin-1 Intronic Polymorphism and Alzheimer's

Disease in Australia." *Neuroscience Letters* 246 (1998): 178–180.

Taddei, K., J. B. J. Kwok, J. J. Kril, et al. "Two Novel Presenilin-1 Mutations (Ser169Leu and Pro436Gln) Associated With Very Early Onset Alzheimer's Disease." *NeuroReport* 9, no. 14 (1998): 3,335–3,339.

Takehashi, M., S. Tanaka, E. Masliah, and K. Ueda. "Association of Monoamine Oxidase A Gene Polymorphism With Alzheimer's Disease and Lewy Body Variant." *Neuroscience Letters* 19 no. 327 (2 July 2002): 79–82.

Tanzi, R., and A. Parson. *Decoding Darkness: The Search for the Genetic Causes of Alzheimer's Disease.* New York: Perseus Press, 2001.

Tanzi, R. E. "A Genetic Dichotomy Model for the Inheritance of Alzheimer's Disease and Common Age-Related Disorders." *Journal of Clinical Investigations* 104 (1999): 1,175–1,179.

Tanzi, R., et al. "Evidence for Genetic Linkage of Alzheimer's Disease to Chromosome 10q." *Science* 290 (2000): 2,302–2,303.

Tariot, P. N., P. R. Solomon, J. C. Morris, and et al. "A 5-month, Randomized, Placebo-controlled Trial of Galantamine in AD." *Neurology* 54 (2000): 2,269–2,276.

Taylor, G. S., I. B. Vipond, I. D. Paul, S. Matthews, G. K. Wilcock, and E. O. Caul. "Failure to Correlate C. Pneumoniae With Late Onset Alzheimer's Disease." *Neurology* 9, no. 59 (1 July 2002): 142–143.

Teri, L., et.al. "Treatment of Agitation in Alzheimer's Disease: A Randomized, Placebo-Controlled Clinical Trial." *Neurology* 55, no. 9 (14 November 2000): 1,271–1,278.

Terry, R. D., R. Katzman, K. L. Bick, eds. *Alzheimer Disease.* New York: Raven Press, 1994.

Theuns, J., J. Del-Favero, B. Dermaut, C. M. Duijn, H. Backhovens, M. V. Broeck, S. Serneels, E. Corsmit, C. V. Broeckhoven, and M. Cruts. "Genetic Variability in the Regulatory Region of Presenilin 1 Associated With Risk for Alzheimer's Disease and Variable Expression." *Human Molecular Genetics* 9 (2000): 325–331.

Thomas, D. "Wandering: A Proposed Definition." *Journal of Gerontological Nursing* 21, no. 9 (September 1995): 35–41.

Tilley, L., K. Morgan, and N. Kalsheker. "Genetic Risk Factors in Alzheimer's Disease." *Molecular Pathology* 51 (1998): 293–304.

Tobin, S. L., N. Chun, T. M. Powell, and L. M. McConnell. "The Genetics of Alzheimer Disease and the Application of Molecular Tests." *Genetics Testing* 3 (1999): 37–45.

Tractenberg, R. E., M. F. Weiner, M. B. Patterson, A. Gamst, and L. J. Thal. "Emergent Psychopathology in Alzheimer's Disease Patients Over 12 Months Associated With Functional, Not Cognitive, Changes." *Journal of Geriatric Psychiatry and Neurology* 15, no. 2 (Summer 2002): 110–117.

Tsolaki, M., V. Iakovidou, E. Papadopoulou, M. Aminta, E. Nakopoulou, T. Pantazi, and A. Kazis. "Greek Validation of the Seven-Minute Screening Battery for Alzheimer's Disease in the Elderly." *American Journal of Alzheimer's Disease and Other Dementias* 17, no. 3 (May–June 2002): 139–148.

Tsuang, D., E. B. Larson, J. Bowen, W. McCormick, L. Teri, D. Nochlin, J. B. Leverenz, E. R. Peskind, A. Lim, M. A. Raskind, M. L. Thompson, S. S. Mirra, M. Gearing, G. D. Schellenberg, and W. Kukull. "The Utility of Apolipoprotein E Genotyping in the Diagnosis of Alzheimer Disease in a Community-Based Case Series." *Archives of Neurology* 56 (1999): 1,489–1,495.

Tunstall, N., and S. Lovestone. "UK Alzheimer's Disease Genetics Consortium." *International Journal of Geriatric Psychiatry* 14 (1999): 789–791.

Turner, R. T., III, J. A. Loy, C. Nguyen, T. Devasamudram, A. K. Ghosh, G. Koelsch, and J. Tang. "Specificity of Memapsin 1 and Its Implications on the Design of Memapsin 2 (beta-secretase) Inhibitor Selectivity." *Biochemistry* 9, no. 41 (27 July 2002): 8,742–8,746.

VanDenBerg, C., Y. Kazmi, and M. Jann. "Cholinesterase Inhibitors for the Treatment of Alzheimer's Disease in the Elderly." *Drugs and Aging* 16, no. 2 (February 2000): 123–138.

van Allen, M. I., J. Fung, and S. B. Jurenka. "Health Care Concerns and Guidelines for Adults with Down Syndrome." *American Journal of Medical Genetics* 89 (1999): 100–110.

van Duijn, C. M., L. Hendriks, L. A. Farrer, H. Backhovens, M. Cruts, A. Wehnert, A. Hofman, and C. Van Broeckhoven. "A Population-Based Study of Familial Alzheimer Disease: Linkage to Chromosomes 14, 19, and 21." *American Journal of Human Genetics* 55 (1994): 714–727.

Vladeck, B. C. "Genetic Testing for Alzheimer Disease: A View from Washington." *Alzheimer Diseases and Associated Disorders* 12, Suppl. 3 (1998): S29–S32.

Vellas, B., F. Inglis, S. Potkin, et al. "Interim Results from an International Clinical Trial With Rivastigmine Evaluating a 2-week Titration Rate in Mild to Severe Alzheimer's Disease Patients." *Internal Journal of Geriatric Psychopharmacology* 1 (1998): 140–144.

Villa, A., J. Santiago, S. Garcia-Silva, Y. Ruiz-Leon, and A. Pascual. "Serum Is Required for Release of Alzheimer's Amyloid Precursor Protein in Neuroblastoma Cells." *Neurochemistry International* 41, no. 4 (2002): 261–269.

Volicer, L., Y. Rheaume, M. E. Riley, J. Karner, and M. Glennon. "Discontinuation of Tube Feeding in Patients With Dementia of the Alzheimer Type." *American Journal of Alzheimer's Care* 5 (1990): 22–25.

Volicer, L., Y. Rheaume, and D. Cyr. "Treatment of Depression in Advanced Alzheimer's Disease Using Sertraline." *Journal of Geriatric Psychiatric Neurology* 7 (1994): 227–229.

Volicer, L., M. Stelly, J. Morris, J. McLaughlin, and B. J. Volicer. "Effects of Dronabinol on Anorexia and Disturbed Behavior in Patients With Alzheimer's Disease." *International Journal of Geriatric Psychiatry* 12 (1997): 913–919.

Walker, L. C., and H. LeVine, III. "Proteopathy: The Next Therapeutic Frontier?" *Current Opinions in Investigational Drugs* 3, no. 5 (May 2002): 782–7.

Wang, J., S. Ikonen, K. Gurevicius, T. van Groen, and H. Tanila. "Alteration of Cortical EEG in Mice Carrying Mutated Human APP Transgene." *Brain Research* 12, no. 943 (2 July 2002): 181–190.

Wavrant-DeVrieze, V. F., R. Crook, P. Holmans, P. Kehoe, M. J. Owen, J. Williams, K. Roehl, D. K. Laliiri, S. Shears, J. Booth, W. Wu, A. Goate, M. C. Chartier-Harlin, J. Hardy, and J. Perez-Tur. "Genetic Variability at the Amyloid-Beta Precursor Protein Locus May Contribute to the Risk of Late-onset Alzheimer's Disease." *Neuroscience Letters* 269 (1999): 67–70.

Wavrant-DeVrieze, F., J. C. Lambert, L. Stas, R. Crook, D. Cottel, F. Pasquier, B. Frigard, M. Lambrechts, E. Thiry, P. Amouyel, J. P. Tur, M. C. Chartier-Harlin, J. Hardy, and F. Van Leuven. "Association Between Coding Variability in the LRP Gene and the Risk of Late-onset Alzheimer's Disease." *Human Genetics* 104 (1999): 432–434.

Wavrant-DeVrieze, F., V. Rudrasingham, J. C. Lambert, S. Chakraverty, P. Kehoe, R. Crook, P. Amouyel, W. Wu, P. Holmans, F. Rice, J. Perez-Tur, B. Frigard, J. C. Morris, S. Carty, D. Cottel, N. Tunstall, S. Lovestone, R. C. Petersen, M. C. Chartier-Harlin, A. Goate, M. J. Owen, J. Williams, and J. Hardy. "No Association Between the Alpha-2 Macroglobulin I1000V Polymorphism and Alzheimer's Disease." *Neuroscience Letters* 262 (1999): 137–139.

Weiner, M. F., R. E. Tractenberg, M. Sano, R. Logsdon, L. Teri, D. Galasko, A. Gamst, R. Thomas, and L. J. Thal. "No Long-Term Effect of Behavioral Treatment on Psychotropic Drug Use for Agitation in Alzheimer's Disease Patients." *Journal of Geriatric Psychiatry and Neurology* 15 no. 2 (Summer 2002): 95–98.

Weinstock, M. "Selectivity of Cholinesterase Inhibition: Clinical Implications for the Treatment of Alzheimer's Disease." *CNS Drugs* 12 (1999): 307–323.

Weintraub, S., M. M. Mesulan, R. Auty, et al. "Lecithin in the Treatment of Alzheimer's Disease." *Archives of Neurology* 40 (1983): 527–528.

Weksler, M. E., N. Relkin, R. Turkenich, S. LaRusse, L. Zhou, and P. Szabo. "Patients with Alzheimer Disease Have Lower Levels of Serum Anti-Amyloid Peptide Antibodies than Healthy Elderly Individuals." *Experimental Gerontology* 37 (7 July 2002): 943–948.

Wisniewski, H. M., W. Silverman, and J. Wegiel. "Ageing, Alzheimer Disease and Mental Retardation." *Journal of Intellectual Disability Research* 38, Pt. 3 (June 1994): 233–239.

Wolfe, M. S., Weiming Xia, B. L. Ostaszewski, T. S. Diehl, W. T. Kimberly, and D. J. Selkoe. "Two Transmembrane Aspartates in Presenilin-1 Required for Presenilin Endoproteolysis and Gamma-Secretase Activity." *Nature* 398 (8 April 1999): 513–517.

Wolstenholme, J. L., P. Fenn, A. M. Gray, J. Keene, R. Jacoby, and T. Hope. "Estimating the relationship between disease progression and cost of care in dementia." *British Journal of Psychiatry* 181 (1 July 2002): 36–42.

Wong, P. C., H. Cai, D. R. Borchelt, and D. L. Price. "Genetically Engineered Mouse Models of Neurodegenerative Diseases." *Nature Neuroscience* 5, no. 7 (July 2002): 633–639.

Wright, C. I., C. Geula, and M. M. Mesulam. "Neurological cholinesterases in the Normal Brain and in Alzheimer's Disease: Relationship to Plaques, Tangles, and Patterns of Selective Vulnerability." *Annals of Neurology* 34 (1993): 373–384.

Wu, Z., C. Kinslow, K. D. Pettigrew, S. I. Rapoport, and M. B. Schapiro. "Role of Familial Factors in Late-onset Alzheimer Disease as a Function of Age." *Alzheimer Disease and Associated Disorders* 12 (1998): 190–197.

Wu, W. S., P. Holmans, F. Wavrant-DeVrieze, S. Shears, P. Kehoe, R. Crook, J. Booth, N. Williams, J. Perez-Tur, K. Roehl, I. Fenton, M. C. Chartier-Harlin, S. Lovestone, J. Williams, M. Hutton, J. Hardy, M. J. Owen, and A. Goate. "Genetic Studies on Chromosome 12 in Late-Onset Alzheimer Disease." *Journal of the American Medical Association* 280 (1998): 619–622.

Yang, D. S., D. H. Small, U. Seydel, et al. "Apolipoprotein E Promotes the Binding and Uptake of Amyloid-B into Chinese Hamster Ovary Cells in an Isoform-Specific Manner." *Neuroscience* 90, no. 4 (1999): 1,217–1,226.

Yasuda, M., N. Hirono, K. Maeda, T. Imamura, E. Mori, and C. Tanaka. "Case-Control Study of Presenilin-1 Intronic Polymorphism in Sporadic Early and Late Onset Alzheimer's Disease." *Journal of Neurology, Neurosurgery, and Psychiatry* 66 (1999): 722–726.

Zhao, L., Q. Chen, and R. D. Brinton. "Neuroprotective and Neurotrophic Efficacy of Phytoestrogens in Cultured Hippocampal Neurons." *Experimental Biology and Medicine* (*Maywood*) 227, no. 7 (July 2002): 509–519.

Zhu, X. D., and E. Giacobini. "Second Generation Cholinesterase Inhibitors: Effect of (L)-huperzine-A on Cortical Biogenic Amines." *Journal of Neuroscience Research* 41 (1995): 828–835.

INDEX